Diet for Natural Beauty

Linda Gaeddes Klau

D1361652

Diet for Natural Beauty

A Natural Anti-aging Formula for Skin and Hair Care

By Aveline Kushi with Wendy Esko and Maya Tiwari

Foreword by Michio Kushi

Japan Publications, Inc.

PART I: The Source of Beauty
PART II: Diet for a Beautiful You

PART III: Natural Beauty Care

Note to the reader: Those with health problems are advised to seek the guidance of a qualified medical or psychological professional in addition to qualified macrobiotic teacher before implementing any of the dietary or other approaches presented in this book. It is essential that any reader who has any reason to suspect serious illness seek appropriate medical, nutritional or psychological advice promptly. Neither this nor any other related book should be used as a substitute for qualified care or treatment.

Published by JAPAN PUBLICATIONS, INC., Tokyo and New York

Distributors:
UNITED STATES: *Kodansha America, Inc., through Farrar, Straus & Giroux, 19 Union Square West, New York, 10003.* CANADA: *Fitzhenry & Whiteside Ltd., 195 Allstate Parkway, Markham, Ontario, L3R 4T8.* BRITISH ISLES AND EUROPEAN CONTINENT: *Premier Book Marketing Ltd., 1 Gower Street, London WC1E 6HA.* AUSTRALIA AND NEW ZEALAND: *Bookwise International, 54 Crittenden Road, Findon, South Australia 5023.* THE FAR EAST AND JAPAN: *Japan Publications Trading Co., Ltd., 1-2-1, Sarugaku-cho, Chiyoda-ku, Tokyo 101.*

First edition: April 1991

LCCC No. 89-63237
ISBN 0-87040-789-9

Printed in U.S.A.

Foreword

Every day we are inundated with the modern image of beauty from the news media. They present an image of artificial beauty adorned with chemically-based cosmetics, jewelry, and expensive clothes. Such attractiveness is bought at the expense of enormous time, effort, and money. As the aging process sets in, those who contribute to these means must employ increasingly artificial methods to maintain their appearance.

Whereas artificial beautification is a superficial and external masking of the internal condition, natural beauty grows from within, and is an expression of simple day to day life. I have met many who personified this ideal. Amongst them is Gloria Swanson who was a close family friend for many years. Gloria maintained a strikingly attractive appearance with the use of minimal natural makeup. She understood from a very early age the importance of maintaining a consistent regimen of diet and natural living. Along with her husband William Dufty she practiced macrobiotics for over twenty years. Due to her respect for nature, her physical, emotional, and spiritual qualities, she matured and grew increasingly beautiful through the years.

Lima Ohsawa is another example of natural beauty. She began macrobiotics in her thirties, and later married George Ohsawa, the founder of the modern macrobiotic movement. Through her study and practice of macrobiotic cooking, she gained an extraordinary degree of natural health and beauty that inspired people all over the world. She accompanied her husband on his many world travels, to India, Africa, Europe, and the United States, amongst other countries and taught macrobiotic cooking to thousands of people. Now in her nineties, she gives regular cooking classes in Japan, and continues to serve as a remarkable example of vitality and radiant natural beauty on both the physical and spiritual levels.

There are many women throughout the world who, like Gloria and Lima perform the same miracle. These women shine as examples, not only for other women, but for all of humanity. As they reach the prime years of their lives, they become guiding lights to millions of people. I hope women everywhere learn to develop such becoming qualities.

Humanity is approaching a difficult stage in its history, as modern materialistic civilization gives way to a more unified and spiritual planetary culture. This is reflected in the widespread increase of illness of every description, as well as personal unhappiness and social unrest. Individuals, families, communities, and the world as a whole are beginning to show the signs of strain. We can no longer depend on such traditional authority as the church, the academic community, the government, or medical profession to guide us, for the individuals who make up these institutions are themselves experiencing decline.

In such a world, women's health—including the elegance, grace, and beauty that arise naturally from good health—is of the utmost importance. Without the participation of women at the core of human affairs, there can be no solution to the world's most serious problems. In this context, I am happy that my wife Aveline, who is a leading voice in macrobiotic education and a pioneer of the natural foods movement in America, has coauthored this book. Aveline has given numerous seminars for women over the years, and with the help of Wendy Esko, a well-known author and teacher of macrobiotic cooking, and Maya Tiwari, a former New York fashion designer, explains in this book how to achieve health and beauty through a diet of whole natural foods, moderate exercise, positive mental attitude, and other natural lifestyle practices.

Diet for Natural Beauty is divided into three parts. Part I begins with a definition of natural beauty, and describes the way daily food contributes to the health of the skin, hair, nails, and condition as a whole. It also includes a discussion of Oriental facial diagnosis, which can be used to understand the relationship between external features and internal condition. Part II includes a description of the standard macrobiotic diet, along with a variety of healthful and delicious recipes. In Part III, Maya Tiwari presents a variety of yoga exercises and natural beauty formulas derived from her study and practice of macrobiotics, yoga, and the traditional Ayurvedic medicine of her native India. Part III complements the first two parts. Together they represent the yin and yang of Eastern thinking about natural health and beauty.

It is my hope that *Diet for Natural Beauty* will become a classic in its field and inspire both men and women to enjoy happier, healthier, and more naturally beautiful lives based on harmony with the universe.

Michio Kushi
Brookline, Massachusettes
August, 1990

Preface

It has been twelve years since I walked into the clear light of wellness, free of cancer. Through these years I have discovered that all diseases permeate the entire being of body and spirit. In my own experience with cancer, I attributed its cause to a long and abiding grief. The degree of pain invariably equals the degree of inquiry and so my pursuit and studies of the holistic sciences of body, mind, and spirit began. Block by block I rebuilt my life through daily practices of learnt disciplines. Through consistency and continued inquiry the old habits subsided. Once the seeking began, the universal grace became abundant. The awareness of the self as an observer to my actions became evident. The confusion of mistaking this limited body, mind, and senses for the limitless "I" dissolved. The self which is *sat*, *chit*, *ananda* (the timeless source of all sources, the spatially limitless and complete self) became the inevitable focus of my renewed life.

In the reflective inertia of my immediate post-cancer years, I journeyed to Boston to meet Aveline and Michio Kushi, the pillars of the macrobiotic movement, whose heroic work in the education of absolute health through the fundamentals is unsurpassed. Macrobiotics provided a firm handle to recondition my living habits. I practiced the synergistic sciences of yoga (*Pranayama*, *Asanas*), shiatsu, and Dō-In (meridian bodywork), and continued my studies in the healing properties of plants. Finally I arrived at the mother of all healing sciences, *Ayurveda*.

Three years ago, Aveline and I were working to formulate a natural cosmetic line. We decided to join efforts in a book revealing the secrets of beauty through macrobiotics and Ayurveda. This effort was further enjoined by the dynamic author of macrobiotics, Wendy Esko. The result of this collaboration is *Diet for Natural Beauty*. Parts I and II of the book are rooted in the macrobiotic diet for internal cleansing. The external beauty program in Part III which I have authored has its basis in Ayurveda. Macrobiotics and Ayurveda, like all valid means of holistic health, necessarily consider the life-force, body, mind, and senses as one unit.

Ayurveda is part of the ancient Vedic sciences of India which existed from the beginning of time. Its practices can be traced to 5000 B.C. It is a dynamic, global system of medicine which incorporates the individual non-separate existence with nature. It has endured great prestige, as well as near demise through the centuries, and it is a miracle that the extensive information preserved by sages and scholars such as Caraka and Agnivesha survived the ravishes of time.

Ayurveda (*Ayu* is life; *Veda* is knowledge) is an eight fold science of internal medicine; eye, ear, nose, throat; general surgery; toxiology; psychology and psychiatry; pediatrics; rejuvenation; and sexology.

Much of the classical treatise on Ayurveda was destroyed amidst a vast body of Vedic sciences during the medieval period of great dissent and chaos in India.

In the sixteenth century B.C., the Buddha paved the way for the various sciences of yoga, Ayurveda, and astrology to spread through the Far East. There is documentation of Ayurvedic use in Persia, and much later in Greece and in Europe, Galen, the Greco-Roman (A.D. 129–199) systematized a form of medicine superior to the empirical knowledge of Western medicine. His system of elemental pathology, based on the body humors, indicate definite roots in Ayurveda. Grecian terminology such as *phyton-therapeia*, which literally means "service through plants," further indicates its basis in the mother science of Ayurveda. Although a clear global history of the influence of Ayurveda is yet to be documented, what is established is that the Vedic sciences are the oldest known knowledge universally.

According to Ayurveda, the human constitution is composed of the five great elements of nature. At the time of birth the maternal humor, maternal foods and activities, paternal humor and the seasonal influence all contribute to determine the child's constitution. The body is comprised of three humors: *Vata* (air/space), *Pitta* (fire/water), *Kapha* (water/earth). These three humors coexist harmoniously to maintain good health. When the humors are out of balance with each other, ill health occurs. The excess of one humor over the others which is known as a dual type, is the most common of the types. For example, the three common body types are Vata-Pitta, Vata-Kapha, and Kapha-Pitta. The four rare body types are *Soma* (the perfect balance of Vata-Pitta-Kapha); solely Vata, solely Pitta, or solely Kapha.

I have introduced this intricate system of health in *Diet for Natural Beauty* to provide a general understanding of the different body types. The formulas are designed for your specific body type with the subtle and potent art of our relationship with plants and minerals. *Diet for Natural Beauty* is a revolutionary and wholesome approach to your total care. All of life is woven in nature, and good health is the result of our harmonious existence with nature. We envision ultimate beauty as synchronous with health. Holistic beauty considers the complete being. The Vedic definition for beauty is a balance between the internal factors and the external factors. Like a scale one side holds the *Alankaras* or external ingredients, the other side holds the *gunas* or internal ingredients, and the act of balancing itself is the third aspect known as *Rasa*. *Rasa* is the cumulative experience or the aesthetic emotions of the individual. *Rasa* deals with time as its essential factor, for only through time can experiences be gathered, and only through the knowledge gained by experience can the individual refine the base or immature emotions. In essence, when the emotion has passed through all five stages of growth, the seed, the sprout, the plant, the flower, and the fruit it becomes *Rasa*. This *Rasa* is the spirit of being fully lived. This is magic. This is maturity. And this is beauty in its fullness.

Diet for Natural Beauty was compiled by Aveline Kushi, Wendy Esko, and myself for the effective prevention of illness and deterioration, and the recuperation of good health.

My deep and abiding gratitude to the many great teachers in my life. A special remembrance for my friend, the late Sally Kirkland. Special thanks to my beloved teacher and friend of twenty-two years, Stella Adler.

I thank Dr. Narasimha Rao, my yoga teacher for his encouragement. And I dedicate my continued efforts to the source of my well-being, Brahman whose grace has brought me the greatest gift of all, my beloved *acarya*, Swami Dayananda Sarawati. I met this great sage and scholar of Vedanta shortly after my father died. His death taught me that nothing in life is ever taken away from us. It is that we hold on too tightly and too long. I recognize Swamiji to be the parting grace of my oldest and dearest teacher, my father Pt. Bhagwan Rampersaud Tiwari. I spent the last three years under the tutelage of Swami Dayananda with the studies of Vedanta and Sanscrit (the language of the Vedas). Vedanta is the end portion of the Vedas which deals with *jnanam* (knowledge of self). It is not a philosophy, but the science of life. This knowledge does not belong to the Hindus, but to every person whose journey is so inclined.

> In the inmost core, the Heart
> Shines as Brahman alone.
> As "I," the Self aware
> Enter deep into the Heart
> By search for Self, or diving deep
> With breath in check.
> Thus abide ever in Atman.
> (*Ramana Gita*, chapter 11, verse 2)

Maya Tiwari

Acknowledgments

I would like to thank everyone who contributed to this book. I extend appreciation to Wendy Esko, who, with the help of her husband Edward Esko, researched and compiled the information in Parts I and II and put it down in written form. Wendy is a well-known author, macrobiotic cooking teacher, and mother of seven. We have worked together on a number of books before and *Diet for Natural Beauty* represents our latest collaboration.

I would like to thank Maya Tiwari, a student and teacher of yoga, Ayurveda, and Vedanta for writing Part III on external beauty care and exercises. The teachings of yoga and Ayurveda represent another way of expressing the macrobiotic principles of balance and harmony with nature, and her part adds a wonderful dimension to our representation.

I also thank my husband, Michio, for contributing the foreword, and for developing the principles and applications of macrobiotic philosophy, upon which much of this book is based.

I thank the staff of the Japan Publications, Inc. in Tokyo for their editorial and production work, including the many illustrations in the book. I would like to express appreciation to Mr. Iwao Yoshizaki and Mr. Yoshiro Fujiwara, respectively president and New York representative of Japan Publications, Inc., for their continuing dedication to publishing books that contribute to health and peace throughout the world. Finally, I thank the millions of men and women in all corners of the globe, who, through their practice of the macrobiotic way of life, are shining examples of health and beauty.

Aveline Kushi

Contents

Chapter 3:   *Sadhanas*—Daily Self-discipline Practices, *185*

Chapter 4:   Natural Beauty Formulas, *210*

PART I

The Source of Beauty

Pure natural beauty
Arises from harmony
Between yin and yang

In ancient Greece, the word *cosmos*, from which the word *cosmetic* derives, was used to describe the order of nature and the universe. According to the classical definition, to be physically beautiful was to be in harmony with nature. Traditional cultures in East and West shared the idea that beauty is the reflection of natural harmony.

Throughout history, another Greek word, *macrobiotics* (from *macro*, or "large," and *bios*, or "life"), was used to describe a way of eating and living in harmony with the cosmos, or order of nature.

The approach to health and beauty that we present in this book is based on macrobiotic understanding. It is holistic and comprehensive, and considers the many factors that combine to create natural beauty. This is in contrast to modern approaches that deal with surface appearances without considering underlying influences on appearance and well-being. In the macrobiotic view, the body is an interconnected whole, not a collection of unrelated parts. Problems with the skin or hair are reflections of problems in the internal condition. Applying moisturizing creams to dry skin, using dandruff shampoos, or taking antibiotics for acne will not change the underlying disorders that produce such complaints. More fundamental changes in diet and lifestyle are necessary if we wish to address the internal imbalances that affect our surface condition.

Dark "circles" under the eyes, for instance, are related to trouble in the internal organs, especially the kidneys and adrenal glands. Problems in these organs are often the result of drinking in excess—including such beverages as coffee, diet soda, and alcohol—as well as eating too many fats or processed foods high in sodium. Rather than recognizing these surface markings as an indication of problems in the internal organs, and then taking positive steps to correct the organ imbalance, we often try to hide the symptoms with cosmetics. As a result, the underlying condition is not dealt with, and new problems are frequently created. The overuse of artificial makeup can degrade the condition of the skin. The result is often a cycle of "chemical dependency" in which increasing amounts of makeup are applied to cover up the cumulative damage from previous applications.

Beauty is not limited to surface appearances, but is a total quality of being. Moreover, there are no absolute standards with which to judge beauty. Beauty is always relative and very much in the eyes of the beholder. There is no such thing as perfection in the relative world. What people consider beautiful varies from person to person, culture to culture, and one time period to the next. One need only look at old films or magazines to see how rapidly styles change. What is "in" one season is often "out" the next. Although this parade of styles can be enjoyable, we also need a more universal definition of beauty based on an awareness of the universe and our place within it. Beauty is dynamic and whole. Often, however, we mistake the static and partial image of beauty for the real thing.

Perhaps the first step in gaining a better awareness of ourselves is to understand the connection between our external appearance and internal condition. It is important to know, for example, what a condition such as acne or dry skin is telling us about the condition of our internal organs and body as a whole. Once we make the connection between the outside of the body and the inside, we can begin to understand the cause of our condition, and take steps to correct it. In this way, we become sensitive to the messages of the body.

Also, as we begin to understand the relationship between our internal condition and appearance, modern fashions may start to appear comic or absurd. The eyebrows, for example, show a person's constitutional vitality. Full eyebrows are a sign of a strong constitution and vitality, while long eyebrows show the potential for long life. However, some people pluck hairs from the eyebrows in order to make them pencil thin. If this were to occur naturally, it would be a sign of sickness. To the eye skilled in Oriental diagnosis, or health evaluation, this "fashion" makes people look like they have some type of illness.

Similarly, to the trained eye, cosmetic surgery to make the lower lip fuller makes people look as though they have chronic constipation. The lower lip reflects the condition of the intestines and when it becomes swollen, it is often a sign of constipation and other digestive disorders.

Increasingly, people are becoming aware that health is something that we create in daily life through our choice of food, activity, and environment, as well as through our attitude and self-image. Like health, natural beauty is something that each of us can create in our day-to-day lives. The tools to produce natural beauty include a balanced natural diet, proper exercise and activity, daily grooming and natural body care, and positive thoughts and emotions.

Achieving natural beauty is actually quite simple. It does not require an advanced degree in organic chemistry or the investment of large sums of money. Wild animals, for example, do not go to beauty salons, yet they know how to eat, exercise, and groom themselves to look their natural best. When we orient daily life in harmony with nature, a beautiful, healthy appearance is the outcome of the foods we eat, the activities we pursue, daily hygiene and grooming, and our view of ourselves and the world that surrounds us.

The Origin of Beauty

Health and beauty come from the same source. Each of us exists at the center of a huge spiral that originates within the infinite universe or God. The dimensions of our environmental spiral include the vegetable kingdom, planetary environment (earth, water, and air), solar environment (light, heat, and radiation), and the universe at large (energy and waves). Over time, these dimensions change into each

Fig. 1 The Spiral of Beauty

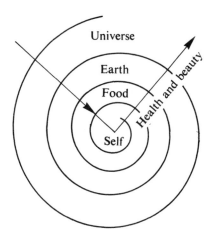

other and ultimately transform themselves into human life. When we see this process of cosmic transformation from our point of view, we can say that we attract or take in the various components of our environment. When we see it from the perspective of the universe, however, it can be said that these factors are condensing and ultimately transforming themselves into human life.

As everyone knows, a clean natural environment, including fresh air, natural sunlight, fresh vegetation, and clean water make it easier to be naturally healthy and beautiful. We are able to control or be selective in the quality of these factors by choosing a certain living place, occupation, leisure activity, and in other ways. On the other hand, the more obscure, invisible components of our environment, including various forms of energy and natural radiation, are continually streaming in toward the planet, and are more or less beyond our control. However, through our choice of food and through activities such as meditation and visualization, we are able to emphasize certain vibrational qualities while de-emphasizing others.

The environmental factor over which we have the most control is our daily food. Daily food and drink are the condensed essence of our larger environment, the material out of which our body and mind are constructed. Moment to moment, new cells, body fluids, and tissues are formed out of what we eat and drink. We are in a sense, the result or creation of what we put into our mouths every day. Our health and appearance are the end products of what we eat. Therefore, understanding how to balance daily food is essential if we wish to be naturally healthy and beautiful.

The key to this understanding is the order of the universe, or the order of change or movement. Our environment is constantly changing. Change is everlasting and occurs at every level of life. New spiral galaxies are constantly forming out of the primordial energy of the universe, while old ones are continually dissolving back into the ocean of energy. In our body, tiny spirals known as cells are constantly forming out of the nutrients and energy supplied by our foods, while old ones are constantly being discharged from the body.

In essence, life is the unfolding of a process of change. Everyone passes through the stages of birth, growth, maturity, and old age. The cycle of life is universal and everlasting. Within the universal process of change, two complementary tendencies appear. One is a movement toward contraction or consolidation that causes energy to become dense and physical. The other is a movement toward expansion or diffusion that ultimately makes things dissolve and return to energy. All things in the universe constantly cycle back and forth between these two tendencies, and move in the form of contracting and expanding spirals.

We perceive this constant movement as the alternation between opposite states. For example, the earth is constantly spinning on its axis, and we experience this as the alternating cycle of day and night. The revolution of the earth around the sun creates the alternation between summer and winter and the cycle of the seasons. All life on earth is governed by alternating cycles such as these. Plants become lush and full in summer and sparse and contracted in winter. Animals become active in warm weather and hibernate in the cold. Our moods and activity also change with these cycles, including the cycle of the tides and waxing and waning of the moon. So, for example, we often feel active and outgoing during the spring and summer or during the full moon, and inward and quiet during the autumn and winter, or during the new moon. Similarly, we feel positive and energetic in the morning, and calm and reflective in the evening.

In ancient India, these universal tendencies were named *Shiva* and *Shakti*. The ancient sages believed that the universe is created by the interaction of these primary energies. In other words, like man and woman, these energies combine and produce "offspring," or all phenomena in the universe. All objects and processes contain elements of both energies in the way that children embody the characteristics of both parents. Ancient cultures throughout the world had a similar view of the cosmos. In China, for example, the names *yin* and *yang* are used to describe these primary energies. The term *yin* describes the primary force of expansion, and *yang*, the primary force of contraction. In all traditional cosmologies, these primary energies were seen as emanating from one infinite universe, or God, which exists beyond the relative world.

Interpreting these cosmologies in modern language, we can say that yin and yang interact to produce energy, movement, or vibration which is the essence of the universe itself. All vibrations carry the basic imprint of yin and yang: they have beginning and end, up-and-down movement, and speeds that accelerate and decelerate. Moreover, they are more yin or more yang in comparison to one another: some are higher in frequency, others lower, some move quickly, others more slowly, and some last for a long time, while others have a short duration. On the whole, however, all vibrations can be categorized into two types: those that are becoming more dense and contracted, and eventually take physical form, and those becoming more diffused and expanded. The movement toward density and contraction is yang, while the movement toward expansion and diffusion is yin.

The basic polarity between yin and yang creates the endless variety of things and distinctions found throughout the universe, such as that between higher and lower speed, downward and upward movement, more compact physical structures and more expanded ones, higher and lower temperatures, and bright, warm colors such as red and orange, and dark, cool ones like green or purple. On the whole, certain

Table 1   Classification of Yin and Yang

Attribute	Yin/Centrifugal ▽	Yang/Centripetal △
Tendency	Expansion	Contraction
Function	Dispersion, decomposition	Assimilation, organization
Movement	More inactive, slower	More active, faster
Vibration	Shorter waves, high frequency	Longer waves, low frequency
Direction	Vertical, ascending	Horizontal, descending
Position	More outward and peripheral	More inward and central
Weight	Lighter	Heavier
Temperature	Colder	Hotter
Light	Darker	Lighter
Humidity	More wet	More dry
Density	Thinner	Thicker
Size	Larger	Smaller
Shape	More expanded, fragile	More contracted, harder
Length	Longer	Shorter
Texture	Softer	Harder
Atomic particle	Electron	Proton
Elements	N, O, K, P, Ca	H, C, Na, As, Mg
Environment	Vibration—air—water—earth	
Climate	Tropical	Arctic
Biology	Vegetable	Animal
Sex	Female	Male
Organ structure	Hollow, expansive	Compact, condensed
Nerves	Orthosympathetic	Parasympathetic
Attitude	Gentle, negative	Active, positive
Work	Psychological and mental	Physical and social
Consciousness	More universal	More specific
Mental function	Dealing with the future	Dealing with the past
Culture	Spiritually oriented	Materially oriented
Color	Purple—blue—green—yellow—brown—orange—red	
Season	Winter	Summer
Dimension	Space	Time
Taste	Hot—sour—sweet—salty—bitter	
Vitamins	Vitamin C	Vitamins K, D
Catalyst	Water	Fire

* For convenience, the symbols ▽ for yin and △ for yang are used.

things are the product of greater yang or contracting energy, while others result from greater yin or expanding force. In Table 1, we classify different things into yin and yang categories depending upon which force is predominant.

The Harmony of Yin and Yang

Beauty arises from the harmonious blending of yin and yang in the human form. We perceive harmony in terms of things such as shape, size, thickness, color, texture, and other attributes, and when these qualities are well balanced, we consider that person to have a beautiful or aesthetically pleasing form or appearance.

The harmony between expansion and contraction is very important in creating a naturally beautiful form. If someone gains weight to the point of obesity, for example, such an overexpanded form strikes us as unbalanced. A swollen, over-expanded form contains too much yin and not enough yang. Conversely, an overly thin or contracted form is also out of balance, this time, because of too much yang and not enough yin. A beautiful or aesthetically pleasing form is in-between these extremes of yin and yang, or expansion and contraction.

Similarly, the balance between wet and dry is important in the harmony of our appearance. If the skin is too dry, for example, we look tight and drawn. If it becomes too wet, the result is a loose, saggy appearance. Beautiful, healthy skin and a uniform, attractive complexion result from the smooth blending of yin and yang in the skin's tone, texture, and moisture content. If we have dark skin, for instance, the appearance of white patches that result from the loss of pigmentation creates disharmony in our appearance. If we have lighter skin, the appearance of dark brown patches, or aging spots, also creates disharmony. As you can see, the even-ness of our complexion is the result of harmony between yin and yang.

The dynamic balance between fast and slow also influences the way we look. Skin cells are formed in the lowest layer of the epidermis, move outward, and are discharged from the body. If this process becomes too slow, old cells accumulate on the surface, creating a thin, flaky film. If it becomes too rapid, crusty patches of skin may start to build up, as they do in psoriasis. Similarly, if the oil-producing glands in the skin manufacture oil too rapidly, the result can be oily skin or acne. If production becomes too slow, the result is dry skin.

From these examples, you can begin to see that harmony in our appearance depends on avoiding extremes of yin and yang, and not becoming one-sided in either tendency. What then are the ideal proportions of expansion and contraction or yin and yang, in the human form? To understand this, we need to see how these primary energies appear on planet earth.

The earth is constantly receiving energy from a countless number of celestial influences, most immediately, from the sun and planets, but beyond these, from stars, constellations, and galaxies. These influences spiral in toward the earth from the far reaches of space. This spiral begins with the most distant celestial bodies, assimilates more immediate influences, and gathers force as it spirals in toward the planet. Since this spiral begins in the universe, we refer to it with the poetic-sounding name "heaven's force," and classify it as a more yang or contracting energy or influence.

Meanwhile, the earth is constantly rotating, and because of this powerful motion, gives off a stream of energy that moves in the opposite direction: from the core of the earth it spirals out toward the infinite reaches of space. Since this more yin spiral begins with the earth, we refer to it as "earth's force."

The interaction of both forces creates the earth, including features such as plains, valleys, moutains, rivers, lakes, ponds, fields, oceans, and continents. It also creates plant and animal life. Heaven's and earth's forces are not equal in strength. The force of the universe is more vast and powerful than that of the earth. This appears as the tendency that things have to fall downward or be "held" on the surface of the planet. The ratio between heaven's downward and earth's rising energy is about

7 to 1. This ratio is an average, and varies slightly according to the time of day, season of the year, and location on the planet.

This ratio is reflected in the overall structure of the human body. The general ratio between the length of the head and the height of the body as a whole averages 1 to 7, as does the width across the narrowest part of the waist to the overall height of the body. If the head is much larger or smaller than this, that form strikes us as being somewhat out of balance with the surrounding environment, while if someone expands around the waist as the result of gaining excess weight, we feel that their form is not the most ideal or beautiful. So, if our waistline begins expanding beyond this proportion, we sense that we are getting "out of shape" and go on a diet or begin exercising in order to "shape-up" and return our body to this 1 to 7 ratio.

The Harmony of Food

Food is the primary means through which we maintain harmony between yin and yang and keep our physical condition and appearance in optimal balance with the environment.

Like everything else in the universe, foods can be classified into yin and yang. In general, eggs, meat, cheese, chicken, fish, seafood, and other animal foods produce constrictive or tightening effects in the body. They are rich in hemoglobin, sodium (a contractive element), and other mineral salts, and the fat they contain is more heavy, dense, and saturated. On the other hand, vegetable foods produce cooling and relaxing effects. They are rich in chlorophyll and potassium (an expansive element), and the oil they contain is usually lighter, less dense, and unsaturated. In general, animal foods are more yang or contractive, while vegetable foods, including grains, beans, seeds, and fruits, are more yin or expansive.

A wide range of variation exists within each of these broad categories. Some animal foods are more contractive than others, while certain vegetables are more expansive than others. Within the realm of animal foods, including fish, shellfish, birds, reptiles, and mammals, inactive or slow-moving species are more yin than fast-moving, active species. So, slow-moving carp are generally more yin than fast-moving bluefish or tuna, while an octopus, which moves slowly through the water, is more yin than rapidly darting shrimp. At the same time, cold-blooded species such as fish and shellfish, which are less biologically developed, are more yin than highly evolved warm-blooded species such as birds and mammals. Also, species that live in cold climates are yang in comparison to those in warm regions, as are species that live on dry land in comparison to aquatic species.

Among the factors used in judging the yin and yang quality of vegetables, climate of origin is one of the most important. As the climate becomes colder, or more yin, vegetables make balance by becoming smaller and more compact, or more yang. Conversely, as the climate becomes warmer, plants make balance by becoming more yin or expanded. So, tropical fruits, such as pineapples and grapefruit, are expanded, juicy, and acidic, and are more yin than temperate varieties such as apples or pears which are less juicy and acidic. Avocados, which grow in southern regions, are more yin than turnips or cabbage grown in the north, while vegetables that originated in the tropics and were imported into the north, such as tomatoes, potatoes, and eggplant, are also more yin or expansive. Vegetables that are higher in potassium (more yin) and lower in sodium (more yang) are also more yin, while those with more sodium and less potassium are generally more yang.

The seasonal cycle also plays a role in determining the yin and yang quality of vegetable foods. Foods that grow in spring or summer, such as summer wheat, barley, and vegetables like lettuce or Chinese cabbage, are generally more yin, while winter varieties such as winter wheat or barley, and hearty, cold-weather vegetables like kale or watercress are generally more yang or contracted.

In Figure 2, foods are classified according to their yin and yang energies. As we saw earlier, yin and yang appear on the planet as the forces of heaven and earth. Foods that are more yin have a stronger charge of earth's force and a weaker charge of heaven's force; while more yang foods have a stronger charge of heaven's

Fig. 2　General Yin (▽) and Yang (△) Categories of Foods

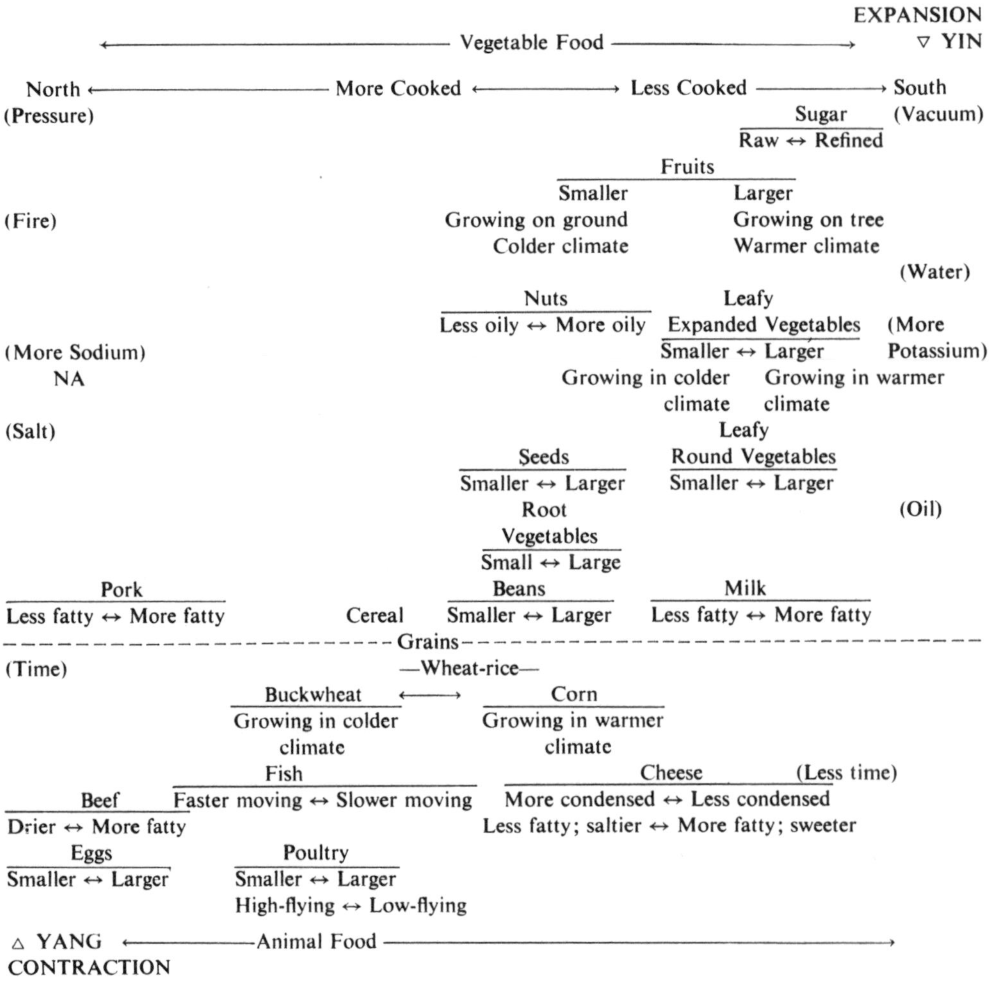

EXPANSION
▽ YIN

←———————————————— Vegetable Food ————————————————→

North ←——————————— More Cooked ←————————→ Less Cooked ———————→ South
(Pressure)

		Sugar	(Vacuum)
		Raw ↔ Refined	

Fruits

(Fire)　　　　　　　Smaller　　　　　Larger
　　　　　　　Growing on ground　　Growing on tree
　　　　　　　Colder climate　　　Warmer climate

(Water)

Nuts　　　　　Leafy
Less oily ↔ More oily　Expanded Vegetables　(More
(More Sodium)　　　　　Smaller ↔ Larger　Potassium)
NA　　　　　　Growing in colder　Growing in warmer
　　　　　　　climate　　climate

(Salt)　　　　　　　　　　　Leafy
　　　　　　Seeds　　Round Vegetables
　　Smaller ↔ Larger　Smaller ↔ Larger
　　　　　Root　　　　　　　　(Oil)
　　Vegetables
　　Small ↔ Large

Pork　　　　　Beans　　　　Milk
Less fatty ↔ More fatty　Cereal　Smaller ↔ Larger　Less fatty ↔ More fatty
– – – – – – – – – – – – – – – – – – – Grains –
(Time)　　　　　　—Wheat-rice—
　　　　Buckwheat　←——→　Corn
　　Growing in colder　Growing in warmer
　　climate　　　climate
　　　Fish　　　　Cheese　　(Less time)
Beef　Faster moving ↔ Slower moving　More condensed ↔ Less condensed
Drier ↔ More fatty　　Less fatty; saltier ↔ More fatty; sweeter
Eggs　　　Poultry
Smaller ↔ Larger　Smaller ↔ Larger
　　　　High-flying ↔ Low-flying

△ YANG ←———————Animal Food ————————————————————→
CONTRACTION

force and a weaker charge of earth's force. However, all foods have both yin and yang energies: this classification is based on which of the two forces is predominant.

Eggs, which are the compact form of a new life, are generally the most yang among animal foods. Smaller eggs, such as those laid by wild birds, are more yang than larger varieties, as are those which are fertilized and non-chemicalized compared to those produced by chickens kept in artificial environments and fed hormones and antibiotics. Various types of meat are also more yang; those which are drier and less fatty more so than those which are higher in fat. Poultry and fish are generally less yang than meat, with low-fat, white-meat fish generally the least yang among them. Among dairy products, dry, salty cheeses are yang, while milk or cottage cheese, which are watery, higher in fat, and have a sweeter taste, are more yin. Modern commercial yogurts, which are often processed with fruit and sugar, are very yin or expansive, as is ice cream.

Among vegetable foods, whole grains, which represent the fusion of fruit and seed into one compact unit, occupy the center of the food spectrum. Whole grains come closest to counterbalancing the 7 to 1 ratio between heaven's and earth's forces on the planet, and this is generally reflected in the ratio of minerals to proteins to carbohydrates they contain. The relatively compact structure of grains (when compared to other vegetable foods) is reflected in the quality of carbohydrate they contain. The complex carbohydrates in grains are made up of many small molecules of glucose that are tightly bound together. This structure results from the predominance of strong centripetal or contracting force. In contrast, simple sugars, such as those in fruit or concentrated sweeteners, are made up of many loose molecules of glucose and lack the cohesiveness of complex carbohydrates. Because they are more contracted, complex carbohydrates, which are also found in beans, vegetables, and sea vegetables, require thorough chewing to be digested properly. They are gradually broken down and not absorbed until they reach the small intestine. More yin, simple sugars bypass the normal digestive process and are rapidly absorbed into the bloodstream, producing chaotic fluctuations in the body's metabolism.

Although whole grains in general are centrally balanced, certain varieties are more yin and others are more yang. Buckwheat grows in cold, northern climates and is more yang, while corn, which grows in warm, sunny climates, is more yin. Brown rice and whole wheat are generally in the middle, with wheat, a hardier, colder-climate grain, being somewhat more yang than rice. We can see this difference reflected in their structure. Whole wheat berries have a hard outer shell and remain somewhat tough even after being cooked. In order to balance this more yang quality, wheat is usually made more yin by crushing or fragmenting the grains into flour or partially milling them into a food such as couscous or bulgur. In comparison, brown rice becomes soft and easily digestible when cooked in water.

Beans are generally larger and more expanded than grains and are higher in fat and protein. They are generally more yin. However, smaller, low-fat varieties such as *azuki* beans are more yang than beans such as lima or pinto that are larger and higher in fat. On the whole, vegetables are more yin than grains and beans, but again, a wide range of variation is found among them. Root vegetables, such as carrots, burdock, and turnips, are generally more yang; round-shaped vegetables, such as cabbage, squash, and onions are in-between; while expanded leafy vegetables, such as mustard greens and Chinese cabbage, are more yin. Sea vegetables also have a different quality. Because of their high mineral content, sea vegetables are generally more yang or contracted than land varieties.

Seeds and nuts, which are higher in fat and oil than grains or beans, are generally more yin or expansive. Between the two, nuts—which are oilier—are more yin than most varieties of seeds. Low-fat seeds such as pumpkin are more yang, while sunflower seeds contain more oil and are more yin. Tropical nuts, such as cashews and Brazil nuts, are more oily, yin, and expansive than temperate varieties such as walnuts or chestnuts.

On the whole, fruits are more expansive than the types of vegetables we have discussed so far. They are juicier, grow mostly in warmer seasons, decompose fairly rapidly, contain a form of simple sugar known as *fructose*, and are acidic. Among fruits, those grown in northern latitudes are more yang than those grown in warm, tropical zones. Strawberries, berries, and other small fruits, are generally more yang than melons or larger fruits, while varieties that grow above the ground in trees are often more yin than those growing closer to the ground.

On the whole, concentrated sweeteners such as refined sugar, honey, and maple syrup are highly expansive. Refined sugar is the most yin among these substances, as are chemicalized sugar substitutes. However, among concentrated sweeteners, those derived from the complex carbohydrates in whole grains—such as brown rice syrup or barley malt—are less extreme than those that come from the simpler sugars in sugar cane or maple sap.

Although not listed in Figure 2, tropical products such as spices, chocolate, and coffee are strongly yin, as is alcohol and most drugs and medications, including antibiotics, aspirin, and cortisone. The artificial fertilizers and insecticides used in modern agriculture are also strongly yin, as are illicit drugs such as cocaine and marijuana.

A variety of other factors influence the energy of food. The factors used in cooking and food processing are especially important, as they change the yin and yang quality of foods and beverages. In general, fire, pressure, salt, and time (aging) are yangizing. They cause foods to become more contracted. On the other hand, using little or no pressure, adding water or oil, or using fresh foods makes the quality of our meals more yin. Cooking and food processing employ these complementary influences in varying degrees, in order to rebalance the energy of food, and if they are well managed, to help us create harmony with the environment and our needs and preferences.

Another way to understand the energies in foods is to classify them in three categories: (1) foods that are excessively yang, (2) those that are excessively yin (both categories are best avoided for optimal health) and, (3) foods that are more centrally balanced and suitable for regular consumption in a temperate zone. These categories are summarized in Table 2. The foods in the strong yang column are primarily animal foods and are naturally eaten in higher proportions in colder regions of the world. The foods in the strong yin column are mostly vegetable-

Table 2   Three Categories of Food

Strong Yang Foods	More Balanced Foods	Strong Yin Foods
Refined salt	Whole cereal grains	White rice, white flour
Eggs	Beans and bean products	Frozen and canned foods
Meat	Root, round, and leafy	Tropical fruits and vegetables
Cheese	green vegetables	Milk, cream, yogurt, and ice cream
Poutry	Sea vegetables	Refined oils
Fish	Unrefined sea salt, vegetable oil,	Spices (pepper, curry, nutmeg, etc.)
Seafood	and other seasonings (if moderately used)	Aromatic and stimulant beverages (coffee, black tea, mint tea, etc.)
	Spring water and well water	Honey, sugar, and refined sweeteners
	Nonaromatic, nonstimulant teas and beverages	Alcohol
	Seeds and nuts	Foods containing chemicals, preservatives, dyes, pesticides
	Temperate-climate fruit	Drugs (marijuana, cocaine, etc., with some exceptions)
	Rice syrup, barley malt, and other grain-based natural sweeteners (if moderately used)	Medications (tranquilizers, antibiotics, etc., with some exceptions)

quality foods and are primarily native to the tropics. Those in the middle column are common to the temperate zones.

From this list we can see that most diets today combine foods mostly from the strong yang category and the strong yin category. Historically, most of these foods originated in either colder northern climates or in hotter southern climates, even though they are now produced in temperate zones owing to the development of modern technology. In their original habitats, some of these foods are part of a balanced natural diet, for example, curry and spices in India, coconuts in the Pacific Islands, and meat and dairy food in Siberia and Alaska. However, when consumed on a regular basis in a four-season climate, strong yin and strong yang foods are unnatural and create imbalance in the body.

It is important when eating for health and beauty to base your diet on foods from your own climate or one that is similar to yours. Therefore if you live in the temperate zones, eating avocados, pineapples, mangoes, and other tropical fruits results in imbalance, as does including vegetables such as tomatoes, potatoes, eggplant, and other members of the nightshade family that originated in the equatorial zones before being imported to Europe and North America.

Yin and yang attract one another like man and woman or the oppositely charged poles of a magnet. When we eat plenty of foods with extreme yang energy we are inevitably attracted to yin extremes, and vice versa. This extreme pattern prevails today, and is a major factor in the widespread incidence of degenerative illnesses. Below are examples of extreme combinations common in diets today.

When the diet is based on extremes, the body is forced to cope with unnecessary or excessive factors, including plenty of saturated fat, cholesterol, and simple sugars. Moreover, foods high in fat, cholesterol, and refined sugar tend to displace nutritious, centrally balanced grains, beans, and fresh local vegetables. Overall balance

Table 3 Opposites Attract

YANG EXTREMES When you eat:	YIN EXTREMES You are attracted to:
Steak	Potatoes, Scotch whiskey, ice cream
Hamburger, pizza	French fries, soft drinks, donuts
Eggs and bacon	Fried potatoes, white bread, frozen orange juice, sugared iam, coffee with cream and sugar
Cheese, chicken	Wine, raw salad, chocolate, raw fruit
Tuna fish	Cottage cheese, yogurt, raw tropical fruits, diet soft drinks
Salty popcorn, chips	Soft drinks, candy
Hot dogs	Mustard, beer, soft drinks, ice cream
Turkey	Mashed potatoes, sugared cranberry sauce, sweet potatoes, yams
Spaghetti with meat balls	Tomatoes, spices, garlic, white bread, alcohol
Sushi (raw fish) dipped in high-sodium commercial soy sauce	Alcohol, mustard, ice cream, and artificial chemicals
Meat-centered diet	Sugar, alcohol, soft drinks, spices, chocolate, drugs

between yin and yang becomes much harder to maintain, and we lose harmony with our environment and in our health and appearance. Imbalance in the body eventually appears on the surface in the form of abnormal conditions of the skin, hair, nails, facial features, and body-build, all of which affect the way we look.

The quality of the yin and yang elements in our diet is the central issue in a naturally balanced way of eating. Foods such as whole grains, beans, fresh local vegetables and sea vegetables contain high-quality yin and yang factors that exist in naturally balanced proportions. Sea vegetables, for example, are very soft and flexible (more yin qualities), yet strong and resilient (more yang qualities) due to the minerals they contain. A similar balance exists in a condiment such as *gomashio*, or seasame salt. (Gomashio is made by roasting sesame seeds in a dry skillet and crushing them together with sea salt in a small grinding bowl.) Sesame seeds contain natural oils that help keep the skin soft, flexible, and resilient. The sea salt in gomashio contains trace minerals that keep the skin firm and well-toned. When eaten in the proper amounts, along with other natural foods, gomashio adds high-quality yin and yang elements to the diet. Natural health and beauty result from the right combination of foods that produce beautiful yin and beautiful yang qualities in the body.

On the other hand, extremes such as meat and sugar, poultry and ice cream, eggs and tropical fruits contain poor-quality yin and yang factors. Excessive consumption of these foods results in a gradual loss of natural health and beauty. Rather than keeping the body firm and well-toned, poor-quality yang foods cause it to become hard, tight, and rigid. Instead of keeping the body flexible and supple, and the skin smooth and soft, poor-quality yin foods cause looseness, swelling, and lack of definition.

How Food Affects Our Appearance

As you will discover in this book, diet has a direct influence on the way we look, and eating well provides the foundation for natural health and beauty. In the chapters that follow, we show how diet and lifestyle influence our appearance by examining their effect on the skin, hair, nails, and facial features. We will also see how living and eating well can help restore the body to a naturally healthy and beautiful condition.

Increasingly, the connection between diet, health, and appearance is gaining recognition among doctors, nutritionists, and researchers. Of course, the relationship between a diet high in fat, sugar, and processed foods and overweight (which for many is the number one obstacle to looking and feeling good) is a matter of common sense. However, researchers have started to link problems such as acne with a diet high in fat and protein (such as the modern diet), and are recommending dietary change in the direction of macrobiotics as a possible method for preventing and improving the condition. Writing in *Your Skin*, dermatologist Fredric Haberman, M.D. states, "The link between acne and your overall diet is not necessarily farfetched. Scientists have already demonstrated the role of diet in a more serious disease, breast cancer. (This too tends to be far more prevalent in countries with high-fat, high-protein, and refined-food diets.) Of course, until all the evidence is in, the best policy is still moderation. The recently established U.S. Dietary Goals are probably the most sensible and well-justified guidelines to date."

Like the guidelines of macrobiotics, *Dietary Goals for the United States* (released in 1977 by the U.S. Senate Select Committee on Nutrition and Human Needs) recommended increasing the intake of complex carbohydrates, including whole grains, beans, and fresh, local vegetables, and decreasing the intake of saturated and unsaturated fat, cholesterol, sodium, and refined sugar.

Diet influences appearance in two important ways. It creates our basic constitution, including the facial features, body type, skin pigmentation, and hair color that we are born with, and influences our day-to-day health and condition. Your constitution is like the foundation of a house, and is determined largely by your mother's diet and daily life during the time she was pregnant with you. The way you ate while growing up also plays a role in forming your basic constitution. Your condition is like the decoration and furnishings of a house and is created largely by the influence of your recent diet and lifestyle.

Because it is so basic, our constitution changes very slowly, if at all, while our condition changes day to day depending on what we eat, how active we are, and the thoughts and emotions we experience. Congenital conditions, for example, are constitutional. A problem such as cleft palate arises during the embryonic period when the left and right sides of the face merge into one. This coming together occurs as the result of the contracting influence provided by nutrients in the mother's diet, especially minerals and complex carbohydrates. However, if the mother's diet is especially high in yin extremes, such as sugar, tropical fruits, alcohol, chocolate, or drugs or medications, and deficient in minerals and complex carbohydrates, the embryo may not develop enough contracting power for both sides of the palate or upper lip to completely fuse. Although this more extreme example is not common, it illustrates the importance of proper diet during pregnancy. By eating well, a mother is helping her child create a strong and well-balanced constitution that can serve as the foundation of natural health and beauty throughout life.

In contrast to our constitutional appearance, a condition such as dry skin is caused by our more immediate diet, especially the overintake of cholesterol and saturated fat that block the flow of moisture in the skin. Dry skin can be remedied fairly easily by avoiding foods that are high in fat and cholesterol, and changing to a more natural diet and way of life. Other conditions, such as split ends, eyebags, and falling hair can also be changed through diet and lifestyle.

As you can see from the above, creating natural beauty involves three important aspects. The first is prenatal education and care to provide children with the foundation of health and beauty. In Oriental countries, prenatal care along these lines was known as *Tai-Kyo*, or "embryonic education," and was based on the avoidance of extremes in diet and lifestyle. The second aspect is the daily management of our own diet, activity, and thinking, and for this, yin and yang are indispensable tools. They help us navigate through extremes and find the most appropriate balance for our health and condition. The third consists of natural hygiene and daily care, and, as with food, we recommend using natural beauty-care products rather than artificial, chemicalized ones.

The Harmony of Daily Life

Balancing yin and yang in other aspects of daily life such as between activity and rest, stress and relaxation, time spent indoors and time spent outdoors, and mental and physical activity is also important for natural health and beauty. If you work in an artificially lit office and spend a great deal of time in front of a computer, it is important to make balance by exercising, preferably outdoors. Also, if you live or work in the city surrounded by car exhaust, concrete, and crowds, it is important to spend time in nature surrounded by trees, fresh air, and quiet.

As you can see, yin and yang are invaluable in helping us to avoid becoming one-sided or extreme in our daily life pattern. No matter how busy you become in daily life, it is important to take time each day to reflect on what you are doing and when necessary, make the appropriate adjustments in your routine.

Yin and yang also clarify the relationship between body and mind, thinking and physical condition. How we view ourselves is of the utmost importance in how we look and what we become. Beauty begins with our self-image. Try to cultivate a happy, peaceful mind and a positive self-image, in which you see yourself as healthy and beautiful, and then seek to realize that image day to day by eating and living in harmony with nature. This type of creative visualization is more constructive than the type in which we dwell on various flaws or imperfections. Keep in mind that there is no such thing as perfection when it comes to health or beauty. Accentuate the positive in your appearance and visualize yourself as healthy and attractive. Remember, as you imagine, so you become.

As your daily life becomes more natural and harmonious, your desire for natural harmony will extend to your environment and relationships with others. Keep your home and surroundings clean, orderly and aesthetically pleasing, and your relationships with others courteous, considerate, and respectful. Begin to radiate an invisible, spriritual beauty that illuminates every aspect of life. Intangible spiritual beauty never fades with age but grows brighter as time goes by.

Chapter 2 *Healthy and Beautiful Skin*

Smooth radiant skin
Is as fresh as the morning
After a spring rain

When we see someone with beautiful, healthy skin, we are perceiving this on two levels. One is the obvious physical appearance of the skin—whether it is smooth, clear, and free of markings or discolorations. The other, more intangible aspect is the quality of radiance, freshness, or aliveness that transcends the person's physical characteristics. These qualities arise from the nature of a person's energy, which we perceive intuitively as a part of the total impression we have of them.

In this chapter, we look at the skin from both points of view. We will see how the foods we eat and the way we live influence the physical characteristics of the skin as well as the invisible flow of energy that gives it life.

Radiant Health and Beauty

What is the source of radiant natural beauty? As we saw in chapter 1, there are two huge streams of energy in our environment. One is comprised of vast currents that stream in toward the earth from space. We call this stream *heaven's force*. Because it moves in a downward or inward direction, we classify it as more yang. The other is made up of powerful currents that move outward from the earth toward space. We call it *earth's force* and classify it as more yin due to its expanding nature. These forces make up the invisible energy blueprint within which the human body takes shape, and constantly charge it with life energy. Ultimately, then, heaven and earth are the source of radiant health and beauty.

Heaven's force enters at the hair spiral on the top of the head. It passes down through the center of the body and exits in the region of the sexual organs. Meanwhile, earth's force is continuously flowing into the region of the sexual organs. It moves upward and exits through the hair spiral. These upward and downward currents run along a central line of energy. This central channel carries the primary charge that creates "aliveness" and supplies every cell with the energy needed for life.

At certain places along this central line, heaven's and earth's forces intersect and create highly charged spirals. Five spirals arise within the body, and when counted along with the two areas where heaven's and earth's forces enter and leave the body, produce a total of seven highly charged regions. In ancient India, these highly charged centers were named *chakras*, or "spiral wheels" of energy. The chakras feed energy to the entire body. They supply it to organs, glands, and systems deep within the body, as well as to the skin, hair, and nails at the periphery.

The seventh chakra, located at the top of the head, charges the left and right hemispheres of the brain, as does the sixth chakra, located in the region of the midbrain. Our thinking and consciousness arise from the energy produced here. The fifth, or throat chakra energizes the thyroid and parathyroid glands as well as the vocal cords, while the heart and lungs are activated primarily by the fourth, or heart chakra, located deep in the chest. The organs in the central part of the body—the stomach, spleen, pancreas, liver, and gallbladder—are especially charged by the third, or stomach chakra, in the solar plexus. The second, or *hara* chakra, located deep within the small intestine, activates the small and large intestines and kidneys; while the first, or sexual chakra, charges the bladder and reproductive organs. All of the functions of the body are animated by the energy supplied by the chakras.

Fig. 3 The Seven Chakras

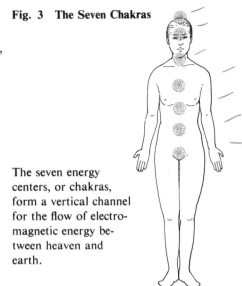

The seven energy centers, or chakras, form a vertical channel for the flow of electromagnetic energy between heaven and earth.

If we visualize the central line of energy as a river, then the chakras are like powerful whirlpools that arise within the ongoing current. Meanwhile, the main river branches off into smaller streams, and these are known as *meridians*. The meridians (there are twelve major ones that correspond to internal organs and body functions) run just below the skin. The meridians branch out from the central channel in the way that the ridges of a pumpkin radiate out from its central core.

The twelve meridians are as follows:

Less-active meridians — balanced by — Active meridians*

Less-active meridians	Active meridians*
Liver	Gallbladder
Heart	Small intestine
Spleen (pancreas)	Stomach
Lung	Large intestine
Kidney	Bladder
Heart governor (blood and body-fluid circulation)	Triple heater (generation of heat and caloric energy)

Each meridian then subdivides into smaller and smaller branches that ultimately lead to the smallest biological units of the body: the cells. Each cell, including those of the skin, is constantly supplied with energy by the meridians, which in turn receive energy from the central channel and chakras. Energy continually flows from

---

* Compact organs, such as the kidney and liver, generally have a less-active meridian flow, while hollow or expanded organs, such as the small intestine and stomach, generally have a more active flow. The heart governor does not refer to a specific organ but to the body-wide circulation of blood, lymph, and other body fluids. The triple heater refers to the overall function of body metabolism.

the center of the body toward the periphery, and is ultimately discharged through the skin, hair, and nails.

The skin, hair, and nails also act as receptors for heaven's and earth's forces. Energy is attracted to numerous points just below the surface of the skin and they in turn feed it to the meridians. From here it flows into the central channel and chakras. Natural health and beauty depend on the proper balance of yin and yang, or complementary streams of incoming and outgoing energy in the body.

Radiant health and beauty are more than skin deep. They are the product of the quality of energy that charges the body as a whole. When energy is unblocked and vibrant, the body as a whole is healthy and alive, and we perceive this as natural radiance.

Diet and Energy Flow

In order to maintain naturally radiant beauty throughout life, we need to understand the factors that cause the body's energy flow to remain healthy and active, as well as those that cause it to stagnate. Perhaps the most important factor in determining the quality of energy in the body is the food we eat each day. Food creates blood and body fluids which in turn nourish and create cells. If our food is well-balanced, then the quality of our cells, including those of the skin, will be healthy, which means that they actively conduct energy.

The skin is the most peripheral part of the body's energy system, and is a mirror of our total health. How we eat and drink, the type of exercise and activity we pursue, and our mental outlook are the primary factors that combine to create smooth and active energy flow, good overall health, and radiantly beautiful skin.

Among nutrients, complex carbohydrates, such as those in whole grains, beans, bean products, vegetables, and sea vegetables, provide the most steady, even release of energy. They supply the chakras, meridians, meridian branches, and cells with constant energy for metabolism and life functions. Eating them creates a fresh, healthy looking appearance. Moreover, these foods are good sources of fiber, vitamins, minerals, and trace elements that promote healthy skin and smooth functioning in the intestines and digestive tract. Constipation and other intestinal disorders are far less common among people who eat adequate fiber in their diets. When the intestines and digestive tract function smoothly, waste products are eliminated regularly. This helps to ensure a smooth flow of energy and nutrients through the body and keeps the skin clear and healthy looking.

High-quality minerals, such as those found naturally in whole grains, vegetables, sea vegetables, and natural sea salt are also important in maintaining radiant health. Minerals conduct electromagnetic energy from the environment, and when eaten as a part of the whole foods they are found in, activate the charge of energy in the meridians, chakras, and central channel. They also promote smooth digestion and elimination, and thus help keep the body free of toxic accumulations.

The cleanest protein for natural beauty comes from whole grains, beans (including soybean products), seeds, and other vegetable sources. Unlike the proteins found in animal foods, vegetable-quality protein does not come with plenty of saturated fat and cholesterol. The accumulation of cholesterol and fat throughout the body blocks the flow of energy through the chakras and meridians, so that less energy reaches the skin and other organs. On the other hand, unsaturated vegetable oils, such as those found in grains, beans, and seeds, help lubricate the tissues and keep the skin smooth and supple. This enhances the flow of energy in the body.

Today, however, modern diets often lack the proper balance of energy and nutrients. They are excessive in some, and deficient in others. The dietary extremes so common today have negative effects on the quality of energy in the body and as a result, on the condition and appearance of the skin. Several examples are described below.

Saturated Fat and Cholesterol

In the United States today, fat accounts for about 42 percent of the average diet, mostly in the form of hard, saturated fat such as that in meat, eggs, dairy products, poultry, and other animal foods. Foods such as hamburgers, pizza, fried chicken, yogurt, French fries fried in animal fats, and processed snack foods are among the leading sources of saturated fat in the modern diet. *Saturated fats*, which are solid at room temperature, are more dense and compact (more yang) than *unsaturated vegetable oils* which are liquid at room temperature (more yin).

Overintake of the foods mentioned above causes saturated fat to eventually accumulate in the blood vessels, tissues, and cells, making the body hard and inflexible. When fats accumulate in and around the organs, the flow of energy through the chakras and central channel becomes blocked, and as they accumulate in the

Fig. 4   Relationship between Breast Cancer and Dietary Fat Intake*
(Carroll, 1975)

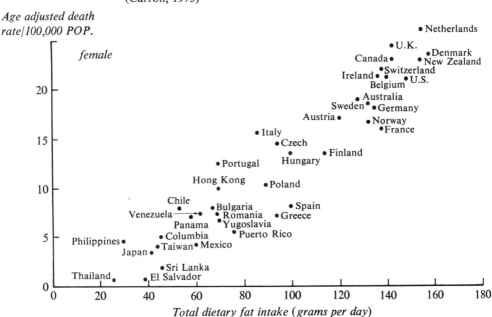

*From *Cancer and Heart Disease: The Macrobiotic Appproach to Degenerative Disorders* by Michio Kushi, Japan Publications, Inc., 1986.

blood vessels, muscles, and under the skin, they block the smooth flow of energy along the meridians. Animal foods are also the source of cholesterol, a substance that accumulates in the arteries and blood vessels, leading often to heart disease.

The accumulation of fat from animal foods is also linked with breast cancer. In a study conducted on women in northwestern Italy's province of Vercelli, and reported in *Science News*, February 18, 1989, saturated fat and animal proteins were found to be the most potent dietary risk factors for breast cancer. Researcher Paolo Toniolo compared the diets of 250 breast cancer patients against those of 499 healthy women of about the same age and found that the biggest difference between the groups was that women with breast cancer tended to consume considerably more milk, butter, and high-fat cheese. According to a report on the study in the February 15, 1989 *Journal of the National Cancer Institute*, breast cancer risk was highest—three times normal for this population—among women who consumed about half their calories as fat, 13 to 23 percent as saturated fat, and 8 to 20 percent as animal protein. Lowering the intake of fat, saturated fat, and animal protein was found to reduce the risk of breast cancer.

Eating too many foods high in cholesterol and saturated fat contributes to hardening of the skin and can give it a tight, dry, and weather-beaten look. Wrinkles on the face, including deep vertical lines between the eyebrows, become more permanently etched when skin is hard and inflexible. Overconsumption of saturated fat creates unnecessary and unnatural aging of the skin.

Simple Sugars

Today, people eat a large volume of simple sugar (such as that in refined white sugar) and not enough complex carbohydrate, such as that in whole grains, beans, and fresh vegetables. Simple sugars are made up of loose or fragmented molecules of glucose and are more yin or expansive than complex casrbohydrates. The glucose molecules in complex carbohydrates are tightly bound into long chains. Simple sugars are found in foods such as candy, chocolate, cookies, honey, maple syrup, orange juice, soda, and sweetened snack foods. They are also added to breads, cereals, salad dressings, and many other common foods so that it is possible to eat a large volume of simple sugar even when white sugar is eliminated from the diet.

Because of their molecular structure, simple sugars are rapidly absorbed by the body, causing the level of glucose in the blood to quickly rise. In response, the pancreas—the organ that regulates blood sugar—secretes insulin that allows excess sugar in the blood to be removed and enter the cells. This causes the blood sugar to drop, resulting in rapid fluctuations in metabolism—a sugar "high" followed rapidly by a drop in blood sugar and an inevitable "low." This extreme pattern eventually depletes the chakras, meridians, and cells, and can result in a "burnt-out" or fatigued appearance. Moreover, refined sugar is an extremely alkaloid substance. It causes acid reactions in the body that deplete minerals from the blood, bones, and teeth.

Simple sugars contribute to uneven coloring of the skin, and are a leading cause of red blotches caused by overexpansion of blood capillaries near the surface, as well as freckles and large brown "age spots." These markings are caused by the extremely expanding effects of simple sugars and the discharge of excess energy they contain. The depletion of calcuim and other minerals caused by simple sugars contributes to a loosening of the body's tissues and to an overall puffiness and sagging of the skin.

Poor-quality Salt

The modern diet is very high in sodium. Processed snack foods such as potato chips, popcorn, salted nuts, and others are very high in sodium, as are canned and fast foods, and many animal foods. Salt, and especially refined table salt, is a more yang or contractive substance. It causes the tissues to constrict or tighten, and when taken excessively, inhibits the flow of energy through the chakras and meridians. It also hardens deposits of saturated fat and cholesterol in the body, and when taken excessively, contributes to drying, tightening, and shriveling of the skin and hair. Naturally processed sea salt contains many trace minerals in addition to sodium chloride. It has a much milder effect on the body when used properly in cooking.

Poor-quality Liquid

Today, it is not unusual for people to drink ten cups of coffee, four or five cans of diet soda, as well as beer, wine, frozen orange juice, and milk on a daily basis. Their consumption of fluid goes beyond what the body actually needs. Part of the reason why people are so attracted to so many liquids is because they consume too much animal food and salt. This is an example of opposites attracting. Salt, which is yang, causes attraction to liquids which are yin. Moreover, animal foods contain plenty of fat which causes the body to retain heat. This fuels the craving for ice-cold foods and beverages. However, overconsumption of liquid expands and loosens cells and tissues and diminishes their ability to conduct energy. It also increases the volume of fluid in the circulatory system, and causes the heart, kidneys, bladder, and sweat glands to overwork, leading to chronic fatigue, frequent urination, and excessive perspiration. Too many liquids can make the skin flabbly and loose, and give it a "washed out" appearance. The habit of overconsuming liquids promotes a general lack of firmness in the body and its features. Many wrinkles in the face, including deep horizontal lines in the forehead and eyebags, are the result of the excessive consumption of fluid.

Processed Foods

At one time, fresh, farm and garden grains, beans, vegetables, seasonal fruits, and other foods made up the mainstay of people's diets. For most people today, however, these fresh, natural foods have been replaced by canned, frozen, refined, and processed versions. Modern processed foods lack freshness, vitality, and life energy. Eating them depletes the flow of energy in the body, contributes to a stale or wilted look, and makes it more difficult for some to appear fresh and vibrant.

Too Much Protein ——————————————————————————————

The effects of protein deficiency on the way we look are well-known. Lack of protein contributes to a sunken, hollowed outlook in the face and other parts of the body. However, for most people in the modern industrialized world, problems with protein are not caused by too little but by too much.

For adults, the body's primary requirement from food is for energy to carry on regular activities, and only secondarily for the formation and maintenance of cells and tissues. The ratio of nutrients used for body construction to those used for daily activity is, on average, about 1 to 7. This fluctuates between 1 to 5 and 1 to 10 depending on age, activity, and climate. Generally, protein is used for body construction and maintenance and carbohydrates for daily activity, though these nutrients are somewhat interchangeable. Under normal circumstances, adults require a much greater volume of carbohydrates in the diet than protein. However, the modern diet is based largely on such high-protein foods as meat, eggs, chicken, and cheese which means that most people consume more protein than the body needs.

Compared to the proteins found in plant foods, animal proteins are highly unstable. They decompose rapidly into toxic compounds including ammonia and uric acids as well as toxic bacteria. Uric acids, sulfates, and other by-products of a diet high in animal protein weaken two of the body's key organs of discharge: the kidneys and intestines, causing toxins to build up in the bloodstream and throughout the body. Skin cells, which are like the leaves of a plant that are nourished by the bloodstream, become unhealthy and wither as a result of this toxic buildup. Consumption of too much animal protein also leaches calcium and other minerals from the bones. This may be a leading cause of the current epidemic of *osteoporosis* (thinning of the bones) and fractures that occur in later life. The body becomes more frail and brittle as a result of this imbalance.

Excess protein is discharged outward through the meridians and accumulates on the surface of the body in the form of unnecessary and excessive growths on the skin, including warts, moles, callouses, and excess body hair. Overintake of animal protein contributes to an uneven-textured skin and to unsightly growths and markings.

Vitamin Imbalances ——————————————————————————————

Vitamins exist naturally in whole foods and are best eaten in their whole form as a part of the food itself rather than as artificial supplements. Vitamin pills and other nutritional supplements became popular in recent decades to offset the deficiencies, and in extreme cases, deficiency diseases, caused by modern food processing. In essence, the vitamins and minerals that are taken out of whole foods are sold back to the consumer in capsule form. When taken in this unnatural way, vitamin pills produce a chaotic effect on the body's metabolism and energy flow and contribute to an uneven complexion and artificial looking skin.

Chemicals and Additives

The chemicals used in modern agriculture deplete the soil, and produce a weaker quality of food. Chemicalized soil often has a dry, parched, and depleted look, while natural organic soil is rich in nutrients and has a deep, rich, and vibrantly alive appearance. Chemicals affect the health and appearance of the skin in a similar way.

Over the past twenty years, many people have become aware of the harmful effects on the skin and hair that can result from continual use of chemicalized beauty-care products, including makeup, shampoo, facial creams, and soaps. As a result, a growing natural cosmetic and body-care industry has arisen to provide consumers with safer and more natural alternatives. However, although helpful, using natural beauty products while continuing to eat a highly refined and chemicalized diet only deals with the surface problem. According to some estimates, more than 3,000 chemicals have found their way into the food supply since World War II. These artificial substances affect not only the internal condition, including the health of the organs, glands, and cells, but also the health and appearance of the skin. Most of these chemicals have an extreme yin, or expansive quality that weakens and depletes the flow of energy in the body, including the chakras, meridians, and cells. A diet that is high in chemicalized, artificial foods causes the quality of skin cells to deteriorate, and can produce synthetic, plastic-looking skin. The chemicals ingested through food affect the skin just as much as those applied to it from the outside.

So far we have looked at the skin as a part of the body's energy system. Now we turn to the physical qualities of the skin, in order to better understand how our diet and way of life influence its health and appearance.

Beauty Is More Than Skin Deep

Skin, nails, and hair occupy the most yin or peripheral position in the body. They correspond to and counterbalance the bones, blood vessels, organs, and glands located deep within the body. The skin reflects the condition of these internal features and that of the body as a whole.

The largest and one of the most complex systems in the body, skin comprises about 15 percent of body weight and receives about a third of its circulating blood. Skin varies from one-thirty-second to one-eighth of an inch in thickness.

The body's outer coat is constantly renewing itself. Skin is a dramatic example of the changing nature of human life itself. To study the skin is to become aware of a process of dynamic change or movement. The direction of movement is yin— from the center of the body toward the surface, and this process of constant change represents the life of skin cells themselves. The skin and layer of tissues below it can be divided into seven layers.

Energy from the environment constantly enters the body through numerous invisible holes or "points" in the skin, and flows into the meridians that run just

Surface

	7.	Stratum corneum
Epidermis............	6.	Stratum lucidum
	5.	Stratum granulosum
	4.	Stratum germinativum
Dermis..............	3.	Papillary layer
	2.	Reticular layer
Subcutaneous		
Layer...............	1.	Made up of soft fatty tissue underlying the skin

Inside

below the surface. When this incoming stream reaches the stratum germinativum (in the middle of the seven layers), it encounters the stream of energy and nutrients coming out from the chakras, meridians, and bloodstream. The collision of these opposite streams produces a strong charge of energy that stimulates the division of cells. It is here that amino acids, fatty acids, and other substances provided by the blood are constantly transformed into new skin cells. Newborn skin cells gradually migrate toward the surface of the body, and become more yang as they move upward through the layers of the epidermis: they flatten out, lose moisture, and eventually become so yang that they shed their more yang nuclei (a wonderful example of like repelling like).

Before they reach the uppermost layer of the epidermis, cells contain granules of a protein known as *eleidin*. As they approach the surface, eleidin condenses into *keratin*, a more yang or tough protein substance (the word *keratin* is from the Latin word "horn"). By the time cells reach the outermost layer, they die. Dead cells are shed after a week or two and are constantly replaced by new ones (a process known as *keratinization*) in a cycle that continues as long as we live.

Dermatologists refer to the time it takes for skin cells to develop, migrate to the outermost layer of the epidermis, and be sloughed off as the *cell transit time*. Skin cell transit time differs from person to person according to a number of factors. In one study, people age 19 to 30 were found to have average transit times of about 20 days, while in people 70 to 80 years old, transit time was found to average 37 days. The average transit time is about 28 days. Although age is obviously a factor in the transit time of skin cells, other factors, especially diet, also play a role in the life cycle of skin cells.

The underlying dermis supports the outer layers of skin in the way that the foundation of a building supports the structure. Within the dermis are two types of connective tissue known as *collagen* and *elastin*. Collagen, which is more yang, gives skin its strength and toughness, while elastin, which is more yin, makes the skin elastic and flexible. Collagen is a form of protein found throughout the body (it makes up about a third of the body's total amount of protein), including the blood vessels. In the dermis, collagen takes the form of fibrous bundles that interlace, forming a felt-like network. Fibers of elastin are interspersed among the

Fig. 5   Cross Section of Skin

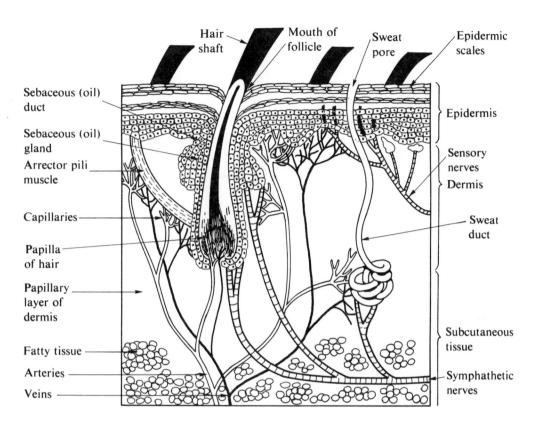

Hair shaft · Mouth of follicle · Sweat pore · Epidermic scales

Sebaceous (oil) duct · Sebaceous (oil) gland · Arrector pili muscle · Capillaries · Papilla of hair · Papillary layer of dermis · Fatty tissue · Arteries · Veins

Epidermis · Sensory nerves · Dermis · Sweat duct · Subcutaneous tissue · Symphathetic nerves

collagen fibers. Smooth, healthy skin depends on the health of these complementary connective tissues. And, as we shall see, this depends largely on the proper balance of yin and yang in the diet.

A rich supply of blood capillaries, lymphatic vessels, and nerves are found in the dermis. The upper, papillary layer receives a rich supply of blood and provides nutrients to the epidermis. Pain and touch receptors are also located here. In the deep reticular layer are found blood vessels, oil and sweat glands, hair follicles, and nerves that are sensitive to pressure.

About two million sweat glands are located in the dermis. (There are about 650 in a square inch of skin.) They take the form of coiled tubes that spiral upward through the epidermis, creating tiny openings known as *pores* (from the Greek word *poros*, or "passage"). Every day they discharge about a pint-and-a-half of clear alkaline fluid containing mostly water, with a small percentage of salt and urea. Sweat glands are most numerous in the palms and soles of the feet.

Aside from their function in discharging excess, sweat glands work along with the capillaries in the dermis to regulate body temperature. When the temperature outside or inside the body rises (heat is a more yang influence), the blood capillaries dilate to make balance (expansion is more yin). This allows blood to flow toward the surface and the heat it contains to leave the body. Conversely, when the temperature outside or inside the body becomes lower (cold is a more yin influence),

Table 4   Balancing Reactions of Skin to Changes in Temperature

Higher Temperatures (more yang)	Lower Temperatures (more yin)
Expansion of dermal capillaries	Contraction of dermal capillaries
Increase in sweat production (more yin)	Decrease in sweat production (more yang)

the blood vessels make balance by constricting (contraction is a more yang movement). This keeps blood in the center of the body and helps retain heat.

High temperatures also stimulate activity in the sweat glands, causing them to increase production of perspiration. As perspiration reaches the surface it evaporates and cools the body. In cold temperatures, the production of sweat decreases, so that evaporation and heat loss are thus reduced.

Sebaceous glands, which secrete an oily substance known as *sebum,* are also located in the dermal layer. About a hundred of these glands are found in a square inch of skin. Most empty into hair follicles, but some open directly to the outside. The sebum they secrete serves to keep the skin naturally moist and softens the outer layers. Sebum is slightly acid (counterbalancing the slightly alkaline bloodstream), and provides a natural immune function by discouraging bacteria from growing on the skin. Sebum also keeps the hair shiny and moist.

Just below the dermis lies the *subcutaneous layer* made up of stored fat cells and strands of connective tissue. Fats stored in the cells of the subcutaneous layer are normally soft and resilient. This layer acts as a cushion and provides contour and evenness to the skin. It also holds heat in the body, insulating it from outside changes in temperature.

Diet and Skin Condition

As we saw above, food influences the skin by changing the quality of energy that flows through the body. Food affects the skin in another way: by changing the quality of blood that nourishes new skin cells and produces the secretions of the sweat and oil glands. Skin receives about a third of the body's blood supply. Nutrients provided by food are absorbed into the bloodstream and supplied to the cells of the skin. The health of the epidermis, dermis, sebum, fatty layer, and connective tissues depends on the quality of nutrients they receive from the bloodstream.

Yin and yang are wonderful tools for understanding the way that food affects the condition and appearance of the skin. As we saw in chapter 1, animal foods are generally more yang or contracting than vegetable foods. Among vegetable foods, whole grains, beans, temperate vegetables, and fruits are more centrally balanced in terms of yin and yang energies. Tropical fruits, spices, chocolate, sugar, and concentrated sweeteners are extremely yin. For the most part, food additives, dyes, and preservatives are even more extreme, as are most drugs and medications. Radiantly healthy skin comes from keeping the proper balance of yin and yang in the diet, as well as in activity and rest, exposure to wind and sunlight, and time spent indoors, and other aspects of daily living. Basing the diet on foods that are centrally balanced is an important part of maintaining balance in life as a whole, and is essential in keeping the skin naturally healthy and beautiful.

Dermatologists classify skin into four general types: (1) *normal skin*, or skin that has a smooth, firm, flexible surface with a good balance between oil and moisture, and a clear, fresh, well-scrubbed look; (2) *dry skin*, or skin that feels tight, spiny, and rough after washing; (3) *oily skin*, or skin that feels sticky or clammy (often with large visible pores) because of excess oil on the surface; and (4) *combination skin*, or skin that is oily around the foreshead, nose, and chin, but dry and flaky near the eyes, cheeks, and mouth. These differences are due to differences in dietary practice. For example, oily skin is caused by too many fats and oils in the diet, and is an indication that the body is trying to discharge this excess through the surface. However, when hard fats begin to accumulate in the pores and sweat glands, they may start to block the flow of moisture to the surface and certain areas may become dry, such as in combination skin. If this condition spreads to the entire body, the result is often dry skin. Below we study the problem of dryness and unnatural aging in detail in order to illustrate the vital role played by diet in the health and appearance of the skin.

Dryness and Unnatural Aging

Medical science is becoming increasingly aware of the way that the modern high-fat diet affects the heart and circulatory system. The potentially harmful effects of over-consuming meat, eggs, dairy products, and other animal products that are high in fat and cholesterol are becoming increasingly well-known. Less well understood is the way in which foods such as these influence the condition and appearance of the skin. However, as we explain below, the way that diet affects the blood vessels is mirrored in the influence it has on the skin.

The blood vessels are made of collagen and elastin, the connective tissues also found in the skin. When the diet is high in animal foods that contain saturated fat and cholesterol, a variety of things happen to the blood vessels, skin, and other tissues in the body. When eaten excessively, these foods cause the ratio of collagen and elastin, which represent contraction and expansion, to shift. A diet high in animal food causes a steady depletion of elastin, so that collagen (which is tougher, or more yang) becomes prevalent. As a result, the skin and circulatory vessels lose their normal flexiblility and resilience and become hard and inelastic. Extreme yin foods, such as sugar, tropical fruits, spices, nightshade vegetables, soft drinks, and chemical additives also affect the body's connective tissues. A high intake of extreme yin foods can cause overall thinning and depletion of the body's connective tissues.

Overconsumption of fat also changes the quality of collagen in the body. It accelerates a process known as *cross-linking*, in which collagen changes from its soluble to unsoluble form. In young people, collagen exists in the form of short cables of molecules that are separate from one another. As fats accumulate in the body, however, the collagen bundles gradually become knotted with tough elastic fibers that bind the molecules together. The result is a stiffening, hardening, and loss of elasticity in the skin. The skin loses its youthful softness and becomes dry, thin, wrinkled, and inelastic.

Cross-linking of collagen—accelerated by dietary imbalance—is a body-wide phenomenon. It affects the connective tissue throughout the body. When it occurs in the arteries, the result is hardening of the arteries and blood vessels. When it takes place in the eyes, the result is the formation of cataracts. An extreme or unbalanced diet causes the body to become stiff and less flexible in a process we refer to as "unnatural aging." Today this process begins at a very young age due to the modern high-fat diet and the lack of centrally balanced foods.

In extreme cases, overconsumption of chicken, cheese, eggs, meat, and other animal foods can cause the body to overproduce collagen. This condition, known as *scleroderma*, or "hard skin," can lead to thickening and hardening of the skin, and in advanced stages, to atrophy of the body and internal organs. Over 500,000 people in the United States suffer from this disease, mostly middle-aged women. More than half of the patients with advanced scleroderma die within several years.

Scleroderma is the result of dietary imbalances. It can be prevented and overcome by avoiding the foods that cause it and by eating a naturally balanced diet. In the book, *Macrobiotic Health Education Series: Arthritis*, by Michio Kushi, Japan Publications, Inc., 1988, is the following description of a woman's experience with and recovery from the disease through macrobiotics:

> In 1983, at age 36, Beverly Lemar began experiencing strange sensations in her body. Her hands began to swell and her fingers stiffened; she was feeling unusually tired and was cold most of the time. She took time off from her job but the symptoms persisted. After visiting doctors and receiving opinions about her condition, she was finally diagnosed as having scleroderma.
>
> Beverly's condition rapidly weakened over the next seven months and she was forced to take a leave of absence from her job. At one point she was hospitalized. A numbness eventually spread over her arms and legs, and she became unable to feed and clothe herself. Her weight dropped to 85 pounds and her skin had toughened like an alligator hide. Her armpits and neck had fused to the rest of her body. "It was the most horrible thing you could imagine," Beverly explained. "My body just slowly hardened and thickened before my eyes and I lost all feeling in it." Eventually she had trouble breathing and digesting her food, and was told by her doctor not to be too optimistic about the future.
>
> After seeing a nutritionist, Beverly decided to adopt a macrobiotic diet. Over the next year she strictly adhered to her diet, had daily massage, wore simple cotton clothing, and did positive affirmations. She also walked every day, even

though she could only go about 800 feet at a time, and was exhausted by the effort.

She began to see improvement after three months. "I can remember the turning point in August, 1984," she recalled. "That day my mouth, which was frozen almost completely shut, began to open a little, and I regained some movement in my lips. I knew that day I was going to beat this terrible disease."

Gradually throughout the next two years, Beverly's face began to unfreeze, her arms and legs lost their roughness, and her skin softened as her body slowly uncurled from its paralyzed state. She now shows few signs of the disease that nearly took her life. The only remnants are seen in her fingers, which are still slightly curled. She can do almost everything she did before getting sick, except completely open her fingers. Beverly's plans include continuing with the macrobiotic diet indefinitely, as well as keeping up with the other positive changes she incorporated in her life over the past five years. (*Source: Beverly Lemar Case History*, by Cynthia Smith)

Saturated fat and cholesterol also change the subcutaneous layer below the skin. Normally, the fat in the subcutaneous layer is soft and elastic, and provides cushion and contour to the skin. This layer of soft fat is usually more ample in women than men. As a result, the female form is generally softer and more well-rounded, and a woman's skin is softer and smoother. These differences become apparent at puberty when estrogen and other female hormones become active. These more yin hormones cause the breasts to enlarge and develop, and produce other feminine characteristics. When eaten in excess, animal foods, which are extremely yang, suppress the body's production of these hormones or weaken their quality. As a result, overconsumption of animal food can cause a gradual thinning and depletion of the soft fat in the subcutaneous layer, giving the skin a saggy, wrinkled, and hollowed outlook. However, these effects are somewhat offset when livestock are fed synthetic estrogens and other growth hormones. The intake of hormone-fed livestock, for example, in combination with the widespread intake of milk, ice cream, yogurt, sugary sweets, and other more extreme yin foods, can cause people to begin producing too much estrogen. Among women, the result has been a steady increase in the incidence of breast cancer, fibroid tumors, and other estrogen-dependent conditions, while among men, a growing number have started developing breasts and other feminine characteristics. The problem of breast cancer has also started among men.

Overintake of animal food also affects the activity of the sweat and sebaceous glands. Hardening and drying of the skin causes these glands to constrict and become less active. Further, hard fat may begin to accumulate in the glands and sweat ducts, similar to the way it accumulates in the blood vessels. These conditions block the secretion of moisture and oil that keep the skin smooth and soft. If the epidermis does not receive enough moisture, it becomes hard and dry, and cracks easily.

The skin is richly supplied with blood vessels, and any changes that occur in their condition directly affect the skin. If saturated fat and cholesterol accumulate in the blood vessels, the skin receives less blood, as well as less oxygen and nutrients. Further, the ability of the blood to remove the waste products of cell metabolism also declines. The result is an overall condition of stagnation and an accumulation of toxic excess that gives the skin a stale appearance.

Cells depend on oxygen and nutrients for life. If the supply of these vital factors diminishes, cells take longer to renew themselves. Moreover, the accumulation of toxins causes new cells to develop abnormally, giving the skin an unhealthy and uneven look. Also, as the skin becomes tighter and more contracted, it becomes harder for skin cells to migrate outward, and cell transit time increases. The slowing of cell transit time makes the complexion lose much of its vitality and tone. Fatty accumulations compound the problem by causing cells to stick to each other. As a result, a dull, flaky film accumulates on the surface of the body as dead, dehydrated cells accumulate.

In this condition, the flow of energy along the meridians becomes less active. A person loses the natural radiance that comes from the active flow of energy and nutrients. As a result, natural beauty and youthfulness fade in the way that the leaves of a plant wither when deprived of adequate nourishment.

Other factors—both dietary and environmental—also influence this process. Too much poor-quality salt can constrict blood vessels, fatty tissue, and collagen, and cause the skin to become dry and tight. Too many baked flour products in the diet, including bread, muffins, cookies, pancakes, and others, also contribute to a hardening and drying of the skin.

Furthermore, a lack of freshness in the diet, including fresh vegetables, accelerates this process, as does a lack of fiber. Fiber strengthens the large intestine, a major discharge organ, and helps keep elimination smooth and regular. The modern high-fat, low-fiber diet leads to stagnation in the intestines and digestive tract. The body becomes less able to discharge excess fat and cholesterol, and these circulate in the bloodstream, eventually to be deposited in the connective tissues, blood vessels, and internal organs.

When the diet is high in fat and cholesterol, overexposure to sunlight—a yangizing environmental influence—contributes to cross-linking of collagen and can accelerate unnatural aging. Modern heating systems that make the air very dry in winter also promote loss of moisture in the skin and contribute to unnatural dryness.

When combined with a naturally balanced diet, exercise and movement stimulate energy flow and blood circulation, and directly benefit the skin. Active circulation keeps the skin well supplied with oxygen and nutrients, and facilitates the speedy removal of waste products. On the other hand, lack of exercise causes circulation to stagnate. Artificial fabrics, such as nylon and polyesters, also block the smooth flow of energy in the body, and interfere with the skin's ability to discharge. Watching television—especially color television—for too long drains energy from the meridians and chakras, as does spending too much time in front of computer display terminals. Also, spending the day in an artificially dry, heated or air-conditioned office drains moisture from the skin and energy from the body, especially when not enough counterbalancing time is spent out of doors.

As we can see, the way we eat creates the underlying condition that determines the health of the skin. By eating a naturally balanced diet, getting the proper exercise and rest, and being aware of the effects of too much strong sun, we can avoid unnatural aging and enjoy beautifully healthy skin throughout life.

Diet for Beautiful Skin

Whole grains, beans, fresh vegetables, sea vegetables, and other whole, natural foods included in the macrobiotic diet contain the proper balance of nutrients that we need to keep the skin healthy and beautiful. Eating foods in their whole form is especially important. Whole grains, for example, include the outside skin, as do beans, many vegetables, sea vegetables, seeds, and other natural foods. The outer layers of whole grains, including the thin, cellophanelike skin, are especially rich in vitamins, minerals, oils, and proteins that keep the skin firm, smooth, and supple. When grains are refined, however, these nutrients are stripped away, and when we eat them, we deprive the skin of many of the essential nutrients it needs. Table 5 shows how the vitamins found in whole, natural foods benefit the health and appearance of the skin.

When whole grains and other natural foods are cooked properly, their outside

Table 5 Vitamins and the Skin

Vitamins are found in abundance in whole, natural foods and are best consumed in whole form as a part of the food itself. Vitamin pills may contribute to chaotic metabolism and other symptoms of imbalance. Some of the major vitamins essential to the health of the skin are listed below, along with their best sources.

Vitamin A	Retinol and beta-carotene, are necessary for smooth and healthy skin. Vitamin A keeps skin elastic and prevents dryness, wrinkling, and unnatural aging. Deficiency may result in flakiness, itching, roughness, pimples, accumulation of dandruff, and splitting and peeling of the nails. Best sources: carrots, winter squash, rutabaga, and other yellow or orange vegetables; broccoli, kale, and other dark green leafy vegetables; and *nori* sea vegetable.
Vitamin B_2	Riboflavin, aids in transport of oxygen and is essential to carbohydrate metabolism. It protects eyes, skin, and mucous membranes. Deficiency produces lining and wrinkling of the lips, oily skin on the nose and chin—with the appearance of tiny fat deposits or "whiteheads"— and fissures at the corners of the mouth and eyelids. Oily hair may also result from deficiency. Best sources: whole grains, beans, leafy green vegetables, nori and *wakame*
Vitamin B_3	Niacin, keeps the circulation smooth and active, thus ensuring an adequate supply of oxygen and nutrients to the skin, hair, and nails. It contributes to the health of the tongue, skin, and other organs and tissues; aids in fat synthesis, carbohydrate utilization, and tissue respiration; and protects against pellagra, a chronic disease characterized by skin eruptions and nervous disorders. Deficiency has been linked with dermatitis, including redness, dryness, and scaling of the skin. Best sources: whole grains and their products, beans, green leafy vegetables, *shiitake* mushrooms, seeds and nuts, and fish and seafood.

Vitamin B_5	Pantothenic acid, is essential in the conversion of carbohydrates into energy. It is also considered an anti-dermatitis factor necessary for healthy skin, and is sometimes referred to as the "anti-stress" vitamin. Best sources: whole grains, broccoli, cabbage, and other green vegetables, cauliflower, corn, sunflower seeds, and unrefined vegetable oils.
Vitamin B_6	Pyridoxine, assists in carbohydrate, protein, and *lipid* (fat) metabolism. It plays a major role in the functioning of skin and nerves and in hormone production. Deficiency results in dry, oily, or scaly skin, dandruff, and skin rashes. Best sources: whole grains including brown rice and buckwheat flour, beans, carrots, cabbage, sunflower seeds, and fresh fish.
Vitamin B_9	Folic acid, aids in red blood cell formation and in the body's utilization of fats. Deficiency can result in anemia and reduced nutrition to the skin and hair cells, and in blemished skin with a grayish-brown pigmentation. Hangnails are an indication of a deficiency of folic acid, together with vitamin C and protein. Best sources: whole grains, green leafy vegetables, *tempeh*, and sea vegetables, especially nori and *hijiki*.
Biotin	Vitamin H, stimulates the growth of body cells and plays a role in the growth of hair. Best sources: whole grains, beans, fish.
Inositol	A part of the B complex, is found in abundance throughout the body. It is associated with hair growth, and has been used to reverse hair loss. Deficiency can result in eczema. Best sources: barley, oats, and other whole grains, beans, and seeds.
Vitamin C	Ascorbic acid, cooperates with protein in the formation of collagen and elastin, both essential for soft, well-toned skin; contributes to healing of wounds and broken bones; aids in red blood cell formation; protects against capillary wall ruptures, bruising, and scurvy. It is essential to the strength and elasticity of blood vessel walls and healthy cell membranes. Deficiency can result in collagen deterioration, with wrinkles, flabbiness, skin discolorations and other signs of unnatural aging. The need for vitamin C, a more yin vitamin, increases as the intake of animal food rises. Many signs associated with aging, such as dry skin, wrinkles, and loss of elasticity, may actually be the result of scurvy, or vitamin C deficiency resulting from overconsumption of animal food, salt, and a lack of fresh vegetables and other foods in the diet. Best sources: broccoli, mustard greens, kale, parsley, watercress, turnip greens, cabbage, dandelion, and other leafy green vegetables, strawberries, cantaloupe, cherries, apricots, and other fresh, seasonal, temperate climate fruits.
Vitamin D	Calciferol, promotes calcium absorption essential in formation of bones and teeth; protects against rickets. Best sources: sunlight, fish liver oils.
Vitamin E	Tocopherol, prevents oxidation of unsaturated fatty acids, vitamins A and C, and other substances in the body; lowers serum cholesterol and facilitates blood circulation. It is believed to keep skin healthy and youthful by slowing the aging of cells resulting from the interaction of oxygen with other chemicals in the body. Best sources: green leafy vegetables, unrefined vegetable oils, whole grains, soybeans and other beans.

layer becomes soft and edible. Yet, each grain still retains its shape and definition. These qualities help keep the skin soft, smooth, yet firm and well-toned.

In contrast, animal foods are less often eaten with the outside skin of the animal. The skin is either unedible, or in the case of chicken or turkey, much higher in cholesterol and saturated fat than the meat inside. These partial foods lack a complete balance of nutrients and energy. The same is true for white sugar, white flour, and other refined and chemically synthesized foods.

The foods we eat create us, and we become like them. The conversion of plant foods into animal cells and tissues, or chlorophyll into hemoglobin, that occurs in the human body is perhaps the most dramatic example of this dynamic process of change. Ultimately, all animals owe their existence to a similar process. When we eat plant foods, the nutrients and energy they provide are converted into blood, cells, and tissues that are unique to human beings, in a dramatic example of yin changing into yang. When we base our diet on animal foods, however, this conversion is not as complete. Some of their components—especially fats and proteins—are broken down and then reassembled in a form not unlike that of the animal tissues from which they came. As a result, we begin to take on characteristics of the foods we are eating.

Eating a large volume of chicken or eggs, for instance, can make the skin take on characteristics of chicken skin. This is often apparent in the arms, hands, fingers, feet, and toes. The joints in the fingers and toes, for example, may become hard and nobby, and these digits may start to curl inward, so that they resemble chicken feet. The skin on the fingers often becomes hard, dried, and shriveled, not unlike the skin of chicken's legs. Similarly, a diet high in beef or cheese often produces dry, tough, and hard skin that resembles the tough hide of a steer. These and other degenerative changes take place over time, and are usually noticeable after age 40. If we do not change our diets, they become more pronounced with age.

A naturally balanced diet based on whole grains, beans, fresh local vegetables, and other whole foods is the best way to avoid degenerative changes such as these and keep the skin soft, flexible, and naturally beautiful throughout life. Moreover, a naturally balanced diet can help melt deposits of cholesterol and fat, and over time, reverse these degenerative changes and restore the skin and body as a whole to its healthy natural state. Of course, exercise and simple daily care, including body scrubbing (see Part III), can help speed the renewing effects of a naturally balanced diet.

Chapter 3 *Problem Skin*

A balanced diet
Clears and beautifies the skin
From the inside out

In the modern world, complaints such as acne, premature wrinkles, aging spots, and skin markings are common, so common, in fact, that they are often thought to be part of the normal process of adolescence or of aging. Of the many theories about why these conditions appear, none really explains what the underlying causes are or offers a simple, natural method to prevent them from occurring. However, acne, wrinkles, and skin markings are primarily the result of our diet and lifestyle. Many of these markings show that something is out of balance in our internal condition. Nothing occurs in isolation in the body, and when something appears on the surface, it is the result of something else that is taking place on the inside.

Deep wrinkles offer a good example of this process. As we saw in the preceding chapter, repeated consumption of cholesterol and saturated fat causes collagen, which is the protein found in the skin, to become hard and inflexible. This makes the skin less resilient, and can cause lines or wrinkles to become deeply etched in the face. Unfortunately, however, instead of suggesting dietary change as a method to prevent or even reverse wrinkling, modern approaches, including cosmetic surgery, isolate the wrinkles and try to hide or cover them up. In one method, liquid silicone or collagen taken from the skin of cows is injected to puff up the skin around the wrinkle, thereby causing it to become less pronounced. These methods are frequently used to cover up deep vertical lines between the eyebrows which are sometimes referred to as *glabella*, or as "scowl lines." As we will see later, these lines appear as the result of trouble in the liver. Injecting bovine collagen or liquid silicone merely hides the wrinkles without dealing with the underlying problem in the liver or seeking to correct the case of the condition. Besides, these artificial substances disturb the flow of energy through the facial meridians and block the natural discharge function of the skin.

In the sections that follow, we see how diet and lifestyle contribute to acne, skin markings, excess facial hair, and other conditions that diminish natural beauty and attractiveness. We also describe a natural, macrobiotic approach to these problems that is based on changing their fundamental causes.

Acne

The numerous oil-producing glands found in skin are most plentiful in the face, back, and chest. As many as five thousand can be found in each square inch of skin in these areas. Acne results when the volume and quality of sebum secreted by these glands becomes abnormal.

A diet too high in saturated animal fat underlies most cases of acne. Foods such as hamburgers, fried chicken, pizza, eggs, bacon, grilled cheese sandwiches are major contributors to problem skin. Other sticky fats, such as those produced by milk, simple sugars, chocolate, nuts and nut butters, and other oily items also contribute when consumed excessively.

Acne is a visible symptom of imbalance in the body. It represents the discharge of unnecessary and potentially toxic substances. Because acne takes time to develop, short-term studies that have attempted to show a connection between certain foods and outbreaks of acne were inconclusive. In these studies, subjects were given a large quantity of a particular food that had been suspected of causing acne (such as chocolate or peanuts) for several days. Since no changes in the subjects' skin condition were apparent in that brief period, the researchers mistakenly concluded that there was no relationship between diet and acne. However, acne does not appear overnight. It takes time to develop. Moreover, acne usually develops as the result of a person's overall dietary pattern rather than as a reaction to one specific food.

The cells in the sebaceous glands act as tiny processing plants for nutrients provided by the bloodstream. They take fatty acids and other substances in the blood, which originally come from the diet, and resynthesize them in the form of the fatty secretion known as sebum. That is why the fatty acids in food do not perfectly match those in sebum, leading some researchers to conclude that there is no relationship between fats in the diet and those secreted by the skin. However, the sebaceous glands alter these fatty acids, and the quality of blood determines both the quality and amount of sebum they produce. Fatty, oily, and sticky foods create a sticky, fat-filled bloodstream. They promote a clumping or sticking together of red blood cells, causing a reduction in their capacity to bind and transport oxygen to the trillions of cells throughout the body, including the cells of the skin. Fats, especially hard saturated fats, have a similar effect on the sebum produced in the glands, as do the fatty acids produced by excessive consumption of refined sugar. They influence the sebaceous glands to secrete a thicker, stickier quality sebum that does not flow smoothly through the hair follicles or sebaceous ducts. Just as they slow the transit time of skin cells, these fats also slow the transit time of sebum. The result is often blockage or stagnation in the follicle or duct.

Normally, the flow of oil carries dead skin cells with it that flake off from the inside of the follicle or duct. When oil does not flow freely, these cells clump or stick together, similar to the way that red blood cells clump, and form a plug that blocks the movement of oil to the surface. When this occurs, bacteria that normally live at the base of the gland begin to feed on the dead, oily cells. They also release an enzyme that breaks the oil down into free fatty acids and other toxic by-products.

Ultimately, the dead cells, oil, and bacteria completely block the opening. The oil pore or follicle then enlarges and this appears as a tiny swollen bump on the skin. In some cases, the blockage stretches the opening of the duct and the pore appears to be filled with dark matter. The black material that develops in the clogged pore—or "blackhead"— is *melanin*, a dark skin pigment that takes on a dark color when exposed to air. It is not trapped dirt as many people believe.

If pressure builds inside the follicle, the debris within it breaks through the oil-gland walls and spills into the dermis below. This causes blood capillaries to dilate and white blood cells to gather in the area in order to neutralize the infection. The result is inflammation, with redness, irritation, swelling, and pus. At this stage, pimples (which are red and tender), *pustules* (white-capped pimples), or large cysts and boils can result. These are symptoms of full-blown acne.

Among the many hormones secreted by the body, androgens, including testosterone, influence the development of acne. *Testosterone*, a more yang male hormone, activates the sebaceous glands. These effects are normally balanced by estrogen and other more yin female hormones. Testosterone exerts a contractive and activating influence: it causes fatty acids and other substances in the bloodstream to gather in and around the sebaceous glands where they are converted into sebum and discharged. *Estrogen* has the opposite effect: it slows the movement of fatty acids and other substances toward the sebaceous glands. Instead they circulate more freely and may eventually accumulate in the lymph glands and fatty tissue in the breasts and other parts of the body. (High estrogen birth control pills are sometimes recommended for women with severe acne. However, as several recent studies have shown, oral contraceptives may increase the risk of breast cancer and are also associated with a range of negative side effects.)

The production of testosterone is accelerated by overintake of extreme yang foods, especially animal foods that contain saturated fat and cholesterol. In some cases, a diet high in animal food causes the body to step up production of testosterone, and in others it causes the body to produce stronger and more potent forms of the hormone.

Testosterone and other sex hormones become active during puberty and adolescence, the age at which acne is most prevalent, although it also occurs in adults. In the past, when diets were based more around grains and vegetables, puberty began at a later age than it does today. It usually started around age 16 for boys and 14 for girls. Now because of the high consumption of animal food, it usually begins around age 12 or 13. The more extreme modern diet causes young people to begin producing sex hormones at a younger age, and increases the likelihood of acne.

Although acne is unsightly and inconvenient, it is actually a natural, self-protective response. It helps the body discharge toxic excess that otherwise would cause trouble in the internal organs. Animal foods, which have extreme yang or contractive effects, create disequilibrium in the body, especially in combination with more yang androgens in the body. The combination of the two triggers a variety of natural discharge mechanisms. One is the action of the oil-producing glands in the skin. Uncontrollable behavior, which is common among teenage boys in modern industrialized countries where animal food forms the basis of the diet, is another form of discharge. By triggering the discharge of fats, the stepped up activity of the sebaceous glands prevents some of this excess from being deposited internally, and to a certain extent, protects the circulatory system and other vital functions from these internal accumulations.

Similar reactions to unbalanced foods occur all the time. For example, when newborns are given cow's milk formulas, which are high in saturated fat and cholesterol, many experience immediate reactions in the form of digestive upsets, diarrhea, skin rashes, and other symptoms. These are simply the body's attempt to discharge the excessive factors contained in cow's milk. Like acne, these reactions slow the accumulation of fats and other substances in the blood vessels, internal organs, and other parts of the body.

No one need suffer from acne. This condition is the result of an unbalanced diet and can be prevented or improved simply by changing the way we eat. Unfortunately, however, modern approaches to acne are symptomatic—they deal only with the surface appearance of pimples—and in many cases carry the risk of side effects, some of which can be serious. One of the more popular methods today is to use powerful antibiotics, often from the tetracycline family, to kill bacteria within the oil-producing follicles. However, well-known side effects of tetracyclines include diarrhea, abdominal cramps, vaginal discharge (triggered by the overgrowth of *monilia*), and increased sensitivity to sunlight. Tetracyclines can also cause birth defects when taken during pregnancy. Moreover, antibiotics, including those recommended for acne, disrupt normal digestion and absorption by depleting the body's stock of beneficial intestinal flora. They also depress natural immunity and overuse could contribute to the widespread incidence of immune deficiencies occurring today, as well as the prevalence of related conditions such as *candida* and *chronic fatigue syndrome* (CFS).

Drugs also suppress acne by inhibiting the body's ability to discharge toxic excess. One compound currently in use, 13-cis-retinoic acid, suppresses the production of sebum in the oil glands by as much as 80 percent. As a result, excess backs up in the bloodstream or internal organs, and if the diet is not changed, can accumulate and contribute to future heart disease or cancer. One of the side effects of this treatment is *hypertriglyceridemia* (elevated levels of blood fats, or *triglycerides*), showing that fats and other toxins are accumulating in the bloodstream rather than being discharged through the skin.

Using powerful drugs to suppress acne is an extreme measure. A well-balanced natural foods diet is a far simpler and less harmful way to prevent and control acne, without the risk of negative side effects.

What Your Pimples Reveal

In general, pimples are more yin or expansive in nature. Even when animal foods are the underlying cause, pimples arise from the discharge of fats and other more yin components rather than from the discharge of the minerals and other more yang components the food contains. Pimples normally have a reddish-white color due to the expansion of blood capillaries and the accumulation and discharge of fats. They appear most frequently on the upper regions of the body, which are more yin, rather than on the lower parts, and are found most commonly on the cheeks, forehead, nose, and area around the mouth, jaws, shoulders, chest, and upper back.

The dietary extremes that create pimples affect not only the skin, but the internal organs as well. Pimples show that fats and mucus are accumulating throughout the body, and as we saw, help the body discharge some of this excess. The location of

Table 6   Correspondences between the Internal Organs and the Location of Pimples

Location of Pimples	Organ or Part of Body
Forehead	Intestinal area
Cheeks	Lung and breast area
Nose	Heart area
Around the mouth	Reproductive area
Jaws	Kidney area
Shoulders	Digestive area
Chest	Lung and heart area
Upper back	Lung area

pimples tells us which of the internal organs are primarily affected by these accumulations. The correspondence between the surface, or outside of the body and the internal organs and functions has been known for thousands of years, and forms the basis for the practice of traditional Oriental diagnosis, or health evaluation. Later we will examine more of these correlations, including those between the facial features and internal organs. But for now the correspondences between the internal organs and the location of pimples and acne are presented in Table 6.

As an example of how these correspondences work, pimples on the upper lip or chin (in the area around the mouth) are often a sign of trouble in the reproductive organs. Women with pimples in this area often suffer from menstrual disorders, including irregular periods, as well as gynecological problems stemming from the buildup of mucus and fat in the reproductive tract. Pimples around the mouth are often a sign of vaginal discharge or sometimes more serious conditions such as fibroid tumors or ovarian cysts. In many cases, the condition of the skin worsens around the time of menstruation. Pimples on the cheeks, which correspond to the breasts, are a sign that fats are accumulating in that part of the body. They sometimes indicate that cysts or other abnormal accumulations of mucus and fat are forming in breast tissue.

Freckles and Aging Spots

Freckles appear most often on the face, hands, arms, shoulders, and other exposed parts of the body. Their tendency to appear on the upper or peripheral parts of the body is due to their cause.

Freckles are caused by the elimination of excess carbohydrates, especially mono- and disaccharides, including refined sugar, honey, fruit, and milk sugar. These more yin substances are attracted to yang sunlight, and therefore freckles tend to come out during the summer. Freckles are produced by melanin, a dark brown pigment formed by *melanocytes*, more yin branch-shaped cells found in the lowest layer of the epidermis. All people have approximately the same number of melanocytes. However, diet and environment play a key role in determining the quality and amount of melanin granules they produce, and hence the pigmentation or color of the skin.

Melanin, a more yin substance, acts as a natural sunscreen by repelling the sun's ultraviolet rays which are also yin. People in northern climates where sunlight is less strong tend to eat a higher volume of more yang animal food. They produce less melanin than people in southern climates where sunlight is stronger and diets are based more on vegetable foods. Less melanin makes the skin lighter in color, while more causes it to be darker. A more yin, vegetable-quality diet causes the melanocytes to produce larger and more distinct melanin granules. In contrast, greater consumption of animal food constricts and inhibits the melanocytes, so that the granules they produce are smaller and tend to clump together. When the body produces melanin only in localized spots, rather than throughout the body as a whole, the result is freckles.

Usually, when people consume a large volume of animal food they also consume a large volume of simple sugars or other yin substances to make balance. The discharge of these sugars, including those in milk, produces the uneven pigmentation that causes freckles to appear.

Exposure to sun stimulates production of melanin. Sunlight, which on the whole is more yang (hot and drying), attracts various yin substances toward the surface of the body where they are converted into melanin. Solar radiation polarizes into more yin and yang wavelengths, with ultraviolet rays occupying the more yin portion of the spectrum and infrared rays occupying the more yang portion. Visible light is in-between, with violet being more yin and red more yang.

Among the ultraviolet (UV) rays, those with shorter wavelengths are more extreme, while those with longer wavelengths are less so. The most yin ultraviolet rays have very short wavelengths and are known as UV-Cs. They cause very serious burning after only a short exposure. Fortunately, UV-Cs are filtered out of natural sunlight by the ozone layer high in the atmosphere. Ozone, a very yin fragile gas made up of three atoms of oxygen, repels these extremely yin rays while letting less yin rays pass through.

Table 7   Solar Radiation According to Yin and Yang

YIN (Short wave) .... *YANG* (Long wave)

Ultraviolet————Visible light————Infrared

UVC——UVB——UVA   Violet——Red

UV-Bs, or middle wave ultraviolet rays, are less extreme than UV-Cs. These short, intense rays are most prevalent at midday between the hours of 10 A.M. and 2 P.M. They are also known as burning rays, since they can cause sunburn. Longer wave ultraviolet rays, or UV-As, are sometimes called tanning rays. They are less intense than UV-Bs and have a subtle, penetrating effect on the skin. Their presence is more or less continual during the day. Because it is more yin, melanin repels or "blocks" more yin ultraviolet rays.

Table 8 Skin Types According to Climate and Diet

Climate: Colder, darker, more northern	
Diet: Higher consumption of animal food	
Type	
I	Burns readily; never tans; fair complexion with light eyes and hair; usually freckles (sensitive)
II	Burns easily; slow to tan if at all; usually fair skin with light eyes (sensitive)
III	Burns moderately; tans to light brown if exposed gradually; usually medium-toned skin with light-brown eyes and hair (normal)
IV	Burns minimally; tans well; usually olive- or yellowish-colored skin with dark brown or black hair and eyes (normal)
V	Usually does not burn; tans deeply; light brown skin (insensitive)
VI	Never burns; deeply pigmented black skin (insensitive)
Climate: Warmer, brighter, more southern	
Diet: Higher consumption of vegetable food	

Dermatologists classify people into six skin types based on their degree of pigmentation and reaction to sunlight. These types can be classified according to the general dietary pattern and type of environment that causes them to develop.

Fair skin with less melanin is generally the result of a diet higher in animal food (with simple sugars and milk often eaten to make balance), in-between skin, the result of a diet higher in complex carbohydrates, and more deeply pigmented skin, a diet higher in simple sugars, such as those in tropical fruits and vegetables. When the diet is high in complex carbohydrates, another pigment, carotene, sometimes gives the skin its characteristic color. Carotenes are found in orange yellow vegetables such as carrots and squash, as well as in a variety of green leafy vegetables. The prevalence of carotene gives the skin a medium toned, olive or yellowish appearance. Sometimes, when people eat too many carrots or squash, their skin may temporarily take on a yellowish or orange color, especially in the hands. This condition, which is easily corrected by adjusting the diet, is a good example of the way that food affects the pigmentation of the skin.

Age spots, smooth brown spots that are larger than freckles, appear most often on the hands, face, and upper chest, are also caused by overconsumption of simple sugars, including refined sugar, honey, and tropical fruits. As excess simple sugars gather toward the surface of the body in order to be discharged, they stimulate production of melanin, and the result can be a large and unsightly brown spot. Although these markings appear at any age, they are most common after fifty.

Freckles and age spots result from the interaction between diet and environment. They can be avoided or minimized by staying away from extremes and basing the diet on centrally balanced grains, vegetables, and other foods. Freckles and age spots often fade once the intake of dietary extremes is changed.

Moles and Skin Growths

Skin growths represent another form of discharge. Among moles, for example, some are raised, hairy, and have a rough texture. Others are smooth and flat. Moles come in a variety of colors ranging from bluish black, black, brown or flesh colored, and arise from the discharge of excess protein. This protein does not necessarily come from the intake of protein itself, but can also be produced by overeating in general, especially of carbohydrates and fats. Because of this, moles were sometimes thought of in Oriental countries as a sign of egocentricity. Moles often turn lighter, dry up, and disappear once a proper diet is started.

Warts are also caused by the discharge of proteins and fats, especially those in milk and other dairy products, and tend to appear when people eat plenty of sugar and fat. Warts are generally more yin, and appear often on the upper parts of the body, although some varieties, such as plantar warts, appear on the feet. Generally, common warts, flat warts, filiform warts—which usually appear on the hands, fingers, face, neck, and chest—are more yin, while plantar warts, which appear on the soles of the feet, are more yang. Genital warts, which are sexually transmissible, arise due to extremes of both yin and yang in the diet, with animal food and sugar as the underlying base for their development.

Warts are also associated with viruses. However, whether or not a virus is able to trigger the discharge of fat and protein in the form of warts depends largely on what a person eats. By changing the composition of cell membranes, a high-fat diet affects the functioning of the immune system and hence the appearance of warts. Writing in *Doctors Look at Macrobiotics*, Martha Cottrell, M.D. states, "A high saturated fat content in the membrane may adversely alter the physical structure and electrical charge of the immunologic receptors on cells, resulting in abnormal recognition of viruses, bacteria, and other antigens." Because of an unbalanced diet, the body's natural immunity loses the ability to neutralize the virus associated with warts. The virus can more easily take root and activate this method of discharge. However, as many people have discovered, warts naturally go away once the intake of milk, cheese, meat, eggs, and sugar is discontinued and more naturally balanced foods are included in the diet, as this allows the immune system to assume a normal, healthy functioning.

Excess protein and fat can also produce skin growths called *seborrheic keratoses*. These pigmented overgrowths of the outer skin layers occur most often on the trunk, face, and scalp. They are most often brownish in color and begin as slightly raised spots that may thicken and take on a rough texture. They sometimes turn black and tend to occur in families due to similarities in dietary patterns and physical constitution. As with moles and freckles, these markings can fade and disappear once the dietary causes are removed and a more balanced dietary pattern adpoted.

Beauty Marks

There are unraised black spots that differ from moles or warts. Known as "beauty marks," they appear in the vicinity of points along the meridians of energy. They also appear at the junction of connecting tissues.

Fig. 6   Beauty Marks

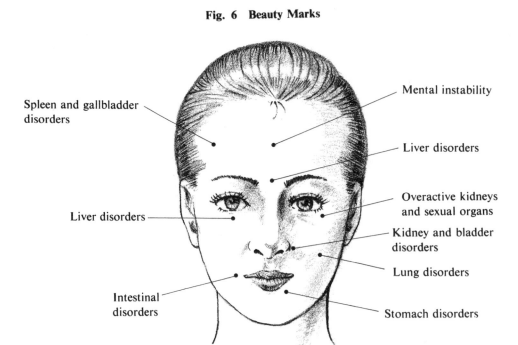

These black spots show the elimination of carbon compounds produced by the burning of excess carbohydrates, proteins, and fats within the body. Unlike freckles, which appear in response to an external source of heat and light—the sun—the source of heat or burning that produces beauty marks is internal. Beauty marks appear after a disease accompanied by a high fever, such as pneumonia, bronchitis, stomach and intestinal fever, and kidney and bladder infections. By observing the location of these spots, and especially the meridian along which they are located, it is possible to determine in which organ the disease occurred. For example, black spots appearing along the lung meridian show that pneumonia or bronchitis occurred in the past, while beauty marks on the stomach or intestine meridians show that a feverish condition once took place in the digestive organs. Beauty marks also appear on regions of the face that correspond to certain organs and functions as shown in Figure 6.

Dilated Vessels

Although red is more yang in comparison to green or purple, when it appears on the face, the cause is an excess of yin. A reddish color is caused by temporary or chronic overexpansion of capillaries that lie just below the surface of the skin. This condition results from overconsumption of sugar, alcohol, tropical fruits, spices, coffee, and other yin extremes. Persons with thinner skin and lighter pigmentation often show this color more readily than those with thicker skin and more ample pigmentation.

In some cases, the red color is more general, so that the face as a whole takes on this hue, while in others it is localized in certain areas, including the sides of the nostrils, cheeks, and near the eyes. When these areas are examined more closely, spidery red lines—caused by overexpanded blood vessels—become visible. These colorations and markings can be corrected by avoiding the intake of dietary extremes, especially the expansive foods and beverages such as those mentioned above.

Stretch Marks

Normal skin is flexible and elastic. As we saw, the strength and elasticity of skin come from the balance between elastin and collagen, or yin and yang, in the connective tissues of the dermis, as well as the softness and flexibility of the fatty layer just below it. However, when the diet is high in cholesterol and saturated fat, as well as in simple carbohydrates such as those in refined sugar, honey, and chocolate, the skin loses this natural resilience as elastin and collagen are depleted and become hard and inflexible.

If skin in this condition is stretched for some reason—as it is during pregnancy—it may not return to normal without leaving behind stretch marks, lined indentations with a reddish or bluish color. Stretch marks tend to appear in parts of the body where skin is repeatedly pulled or expanded, including the buttocks, thighs, adbomen, hips, and breasts. They often occur in the lumbar region of the back. Someone who is overweight and then loses weight may find their skin left with stretch marks. Stretch marks are caused by extremes of both yin and yang. Extreme yin foods expand and stretch the connective tissues (excessive yin also causes blood vessels to become chronically overexpanded, thus resulting in the reddish or bluish color); while excessively yang foods cause a lack of flexibility or "spring."

Stretch marks rarely occur in those who eat a naturally balanced diet. Women who eat macrobiotically, for example, rarely develop these markings on their skin following pregnancy. Stretch marks can be prevented by eating a naturally balanced diet, and they fade more rapidly once a healthfully balanced diet is started.

Varicose Veins

Varicose veins arise when the surface veins of the legs or other parts of the body become chronically blocked and swollen. They sometimes ache and are unsightly, and are caused by overintake of extemes of yin and yang: primarily consumption of excess fluid, including milk, fruit juices, water, tea, coffee, together with fruit, sugar, and other more extremely yin items, and animal-quality fats, especially those in cheese, cream, butter, and other dairy foods. Overconsumption of fluid and yin extremes increases the fluid pressure in the veins and throughout the circulatory system, while the fats found in dairy and other animal foods narrows the passageways in the veins and blood vessels. The combination of pressure and blockage causes the veins to bulge and expand, and become visible on the surface of the body. Varicose veins can be prevented by proper diet. A naturally balanced diet also restores the strength and elasticity of the circulatory system and can lead to gradual disappearance of varicose veins.

Besides proper diet, varicose veins can be treated by alternately applying hot and cold water compresses. First, hold a medium-sized towel under a hot faucet, wring it out and apply hot to the affected area. Leave the towel on until it starts to cool off and then run cold water over it, wring it out, and apply cold to the area for about the same length of time. Repeat with another hot towel, then another cold towel, and so on for about ten minutes.

Loss of Pigmentation

As we saw earlier, melanin is a more yin pigment. A diet higher in plant foods —especially simple carbohydrates—causes more to be produced, while a diet higher in animal products causes less. In some cases, someone with normal pigmentation will experience the progressive loss of pigment, due to the atrophy of pigment producing cells. The result is white or flesh-colored patches that appear "bleached" in comparison to the rest of the skin. They can originate almost anywhere on the body and sometimes spread and cover a wide area.

This condition, known as *vitiligo*, is caused by dietary imbalances, especially overintake of milk and other dairy products (in the case of predominately white patches) and meat, eggs, poultry, and other animal foods (in the case of pink or flesh-colored patches). Vitiligo is especially noticeable in those with darker skin, although fair-skinned people develop it as well.

Loss of pigmentation indicates imbalance in the internal organs, including development of fat and mucus deposits in the lungs, breathing passages, and sexual organs. By disrupting the function of the thyroid, adrenal, pancreatic, and other glands, continual overconsumption of the dietary extremes mentioned above often leads to hormonal imbalances of various types. Endocrine dysfunction (especially of the thyroid and adrenals) is often associated with this condition.

Although it takes time, vitiligo can be corrected through proper diet. It is particularly important to avoid consumption of dairy products and other sources of saturated fat, and to increase the intake of whole grains and vegetables. The intake of vegetable oils is best kept to a minimum, as overconsumption can slow recovery.

Psoriasis

Earlier in this chapter we saw how chronic overconsumption of animal foods can slow the transit of new skin cells. However, in some cases, overintake of cheese, milk, meat, eggs, chicken, and other animal foods has the opposite effect. The overload of protein and fat—beyond the ratio needed for body construction and maintenance—that results from a steady diet of these foods can cause skin cells to start forming and shedding at a highly accelerated pace, sometimes six or seven times the usual rate. When this occurs, new skin cells may take only four or five days to reach the surface of the body. Silvery, scaly skin (something like dandruff) begins to accumulate and the skin underneath becomes hard and red. If the person scratches or rubs these patches, tiny spots of bleeding appear. This condition, known as *psoriasis*, can appear anywhere but develops most often on the elbows, knees, buttocks, lower back, and scalp. In severe cases, it spreads until a wide area of the body is covered.

Like acne and other skin conditions, psoriasis is a form of discharge, primarily of protein and fat. Psoriasis can be improved through proper diet, especially by avoiding animal foods such as those mentioned above, as well as the simple sugars in refined sugar, chocolate, and tropical fruits. During recovery, it is important to keep the intake of vegetable oils, raw fruits and vegetables, baked flour products, and animal food—including low-fat, white-meat fish—to a minimum.

Eczema

The underlying dietary causes of eczema are similar to those of psoriasis, especially the overconsumption of fats and oils, mainly those in dairy and other animal foods, and simple sugars. Among dairy foods, cheese contributes greatly to this condition, as do eggs cooked in butter.

Eczema takes the form of dry, hard, raised areas of skin that may be white, yellow, or reddish in color. It is an indication of imbalance in the internal organs and systems, and the location of the rash shows that certain parts of the body are affected by accumulation of mucus and fat. The cheeks, for example, reflect the condition of the lungs. Eczema on the cheeks shows that mucus is accumulating there. Eczema on the arms and hands or legs and feet normally occurs along the meridians, and reveals dysfunction in the corresponding organs and functions. Eczema on the front or back of the body frequently reflects dysfunction in the organs located in the same general area. The condition is chronic and produces itching. When someone continually scratches the affected area, the skin may become hard and thick.

Overconsumption of dairy and other animal fats and simple sugars often causes allergic reactions in the body, including those of the skin, digestive organs, and lungs and respiratory system. These reactions are the body's attempt to discharge the excessive fats and other factors coming from the diet. Certain items in the home, such as chemicalized soaps, detergents, cosmetics, hairsprays, and deodorants, sometimes act as irritants that trigger a discharge reaction, including an outbreak of eczema. This condition, known as *contact dermatitis*, is common among housewives and others who frequently place their hands in hot soapy water and who use laundry detergents, soaps, and other chemicalized substances on a daily basis.

To minimize exposure to artificial chemicals, we recommend using natural soaps, detergents, and body-care products. However, even if potentially irritating chemicals are largely avoided, eczema can still develop if the person's underlying condition remains unbalanced due to dietary extremes. The fundamental solution to eczema, or any of the other skin conditions described above, is to change the underlying cause by eating a naturally balanced diet.

Callouses

Hard saturated fats are often discharged in the form of callouses on the bottoms of the feet and toes. They are caused most commonly by the overintake of animal foods such as eggs, chicken, cheese, meat, and dairy products. Each toe corresponds to an internal organ. The toes (and fingers) are actually extensions of the energy meridians that charge each of the organs. When callouses develop on the toes, it

Fig. 7 Callouses

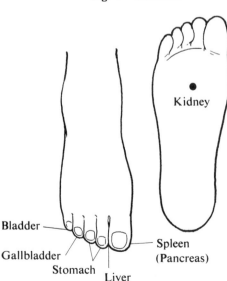

means that the corresponding organ is affected by the accumulation of excess fat and mucus. Moreover, energy normally flows in and out of the toes and bottoms of the feet, serving the purpose of charging the organs and meridians with energy from the environment, and allowing excess energy to be discharged or released. Callouses interfere with the smooth flow of energy through the meridians and contribute to an overall lessening of vitality and aliveness.

In Figure 7, you can see how the toes correlate to the internal organs and meridians. Using these correlations, you can tell by the location of callouses which of your organ/meridians is affected by the accumulation of saturated fats.

Many people have experienced a gradual softening of the palms and soles of the feet after changing to a diet based around whole grains and vegetables. Even hard, rough callouses that have taken years to develop, begin to melt and soften once a naturally balanced diet is started.

Skin Cancer

Today, the sun is being accused of causing cancer and other skin problems, while the role of diet is often overlooked. Many people are afraid to go out in the heat of the day without a chemically manufactured sunscreen. People often have conflicting attitudes toward the sun: on one hand they seek it, while on the other they fear its effects.

The sun is warm, bright, and intense—all more yang characteristics. For thousands of years people living in the sunnier and warmer climates of the world have never appreciably suffered from skin cancer. However, in the less-sunny, northern regions, skin cancer has sharply risen in recent decades, especially among people who work outdoors. We need to consider whether this is the result of some solar phenomenon, such as the effect of ultraviolet rays or depletion of the ozone layer, that affects only industrialized latitudes; whether there is something unique to industrial civilization that is giving rise to this effect; or whether, as many scientists believe, there is something in the pigmentation of the skin or other genetic factors responsible. The solution lies in observing the difference in diet and lifestyle between traditional and modern cultures. People in industrial society eat large amounts of fat, sugar, dairy products, and other greasy and oily foods, as well as soft drinks, drugs, and medications, which create an acidic or extremely yin condition in their blood. Repeated exposure to a strong yang factor such as the sun brings these extreme yin items to the surface, often resulting in a skin tumor or rupture. These refined foods provide the underlying basis for skin cancer, a more yin disorder. The sunlight serves only as a catalyst to localize this toxic excess on the skin. People in tropical society eating a balanced diet of grains, tubers, seeds, vegetables, locally grown fruit, and a small volume of animal food do not get skin cancer no matter how long they are out in the sun because their blood and tissues do not carry the toxic excess.

Researchers have done numerous studies showing that a diet high in fat and protein increases the incidence of skin tumors. They have also done studies showing that vegetable-quality foods inhibit tumor growth. In 1981 a medical doctor from Auburn, California, reported that in conjunction with a natural foods diet, sunlight could inhibit cancer as well as contribute to overall health. Dr. Zane Kime, author of *Sunlight Could Save Your Life*, asserted that when exposed to sunlight, saturated and unsaturated fats in the body turn rancid. Oxidation of these fats damages the tissues, including the fibers of elastin and collagen, stimulates the development of tumors, and ages the skin. However, he found that a diet high in whole grains and leafy green vegetables is rich in antioxidants and will help protect the body from cancer and other ailments.

Other studies have shown that antioxidants, which include vitamins A, C, E, and the B complex, and trace elements such as zinc and selenium, all of which are found in ample amounts in a diet of whole grains, beans, fresh local vegetables, and sea vegetables, help prevent cross-linking of collagen and slow or prevent unnatural aging of the skin. Fats have the potential to break down in the body into free radicals, highly destructive molecules which accelerate the cross-linking process in the skin and other tissues. These stray molecules wedge between strands of collagen and cause chemical reactions that break down and bind the strands together. The result, as we have seen, is a stiffening or hardening of the skin and body as a whole. Once again, the solution to avoiding skin cancer and keeping the skin youthful and healthy lies primarily in eating a naturally balanced diet.

Strong beautiful hair
Reflects vibrant energy
Flowing through each cell

Hair is a symbol of our overall health and vitality. Head hair is closely related to the *microvilli* in the small intestine (tiny, hairlike projections that absorb nutrients), and to the condition of the reproductive organs. Healthy hair shows that digestive ability and sexual vitality are strong. A beautiful head hair is an indication of natural health, and an important part of our sexual attractiveness.

There are two main varieties of hair: more yin hair that grows on the head and more yang hair that appears on the arms, legs, face, chest, and other parts of the body. The predominance of earth's force, which we define in chapter 1, causes the hair on the head to grow upward and outward. Conversely, facial and body hair grow in a downward direction because of the influence of heaven's force. Men normally have more body hair and women have less. In order to understand why this is so, we need to see how heaven and earth influence the development of the sexes.

Male characteristics develop as the result of the predominace of heaven's force during the embryonic period and throughout life. Heaven's descending energy influences the developing embyro in such a way that the sexual organs appear in a downward position and develop outside the body. At puberty, heaven's force stumulates the endocrine glands to begin secreting male hormones, or *androgens*, including testosterone, and this produces more yang characteristics such as a deepening of the voice and the appearance of facial and body hair.

Feminine characteristics develop because of the predominance of earth's expanding energy. During the embryonic period, earth's force causes the female reproductive organs to develop inside the body in a more upward position. Then, at puberty, earth's rising energy stumulates the endocrine glands to produce estrogen and other female hormones. These more yin hormones produce feminine characteristics such as a higher voice and the development of breasts, and also play a role in the onset of menstruation.

The structural differences between men and women are created by the complementarity between heaven and earth. These differences produce attraction between the sexes. However, how these differences develop and to what extent they appear is determined by another important factor: daily food and drink. The forces of heaven and earth provide the invisible blueprint of the human form, while daily food provides the visble substance. For instance, whether or not a woman develops hair on the face and body depends largely on what she eats. If she eats a great deal of animal food, for example, she may offset or neutralize the natural preponderance of more expansive hormones in her body, and develop masculine characteristics as a result.

Strong, healthy hair is a sign that the flow of energy along the primary channel and chakras is generally smooth and active and that life vitality is basically sound. Certain characteristics of the hair, such as the color, thickness of each hair, and texture—whether straight or curly—are part of our constitutional makeup. As we saw in chapter 1, our constitution is determined largely by things such as the dietary practice of parents and ancestors and the type of environment we come from. These factors influence the parental reproductive cells and the genetic information they contain, as well as our condition during the early years of life when our constitution is still being formed. Other characteristics—such as whether the hair is dry or oily, or whether it develops split ends or falls out—are largely conditional, meaning they result from our personal diet and lifestyle. (The underlying pigmentation of the skin is also constitutional, while problems such as the development of oily or dry skin, and markings such as moles, freckles, beauty marks, and age spots, are primarily conditional.) Constitutional factors develop before birth and during the formative years of life, while conditional factors result more from our way of eating and living in the recent past.

Head and body hair (including facial hair) have a complementary relationship, and so does the skin of the scalp and that of the body as a whole. The scalp is more contracted, or yang, while the skin on the body as a whole —with few exceptions—is generally yin or expanded. The subcutaneous layer underlying the scalp is dense and compact in comparison to the subcutaneous layer found in most other places. It includes tissue known as *occipitofrontalis muscle*, *galea*, a flattened, tendonlike structure, and *cranial periosteum*, a fibrous membrane that covers the skull. A similar complementarity exists between the head and the body as a whole, with the head being more yang or compact and the body more yin or expanded. As we will see in chapter 5, the complementary/antagonistic relationship between the head and body forms the basis of the traditional art of Oriental diagnosis, through which we understand the condition of the internal organs by observing the hair and facial features.

Hair Growth

Hair represents the discharge of nutrients that come initially from daily diet. Hair is produced primarily from protein, as well as from fats and minerals, and can also be created from the intake of carbohydrates. In other words, hair is ultimately a transformation of daily food.

The growth of hair reflects the alternation of heaven's and earth's forces in the atmosphere, which also produces the rhythmic expansion and contraction of the heart, lungs, digestive organs, and other organs and glands. Hair growth alternates between a more yin phase of active growth, and a more yang phase of relative stillness or rest. At any given time, about 85 to 90 percent of the hair is in the actively growing phase, and 10 to 15 percent is in the resting phase, with the average ratio between growth and rest being 7 to 1. Moreover, according to scientific studies, for each hair, the more yin period of growth is about 7 times longer than the more yang period of rest. On the earth, the approximate ratio between heaven's and earth's forces is 7 to 1. (Actually, it ranges between 10 to 1 and 5 to 1: the average ratio is 7 to 1.) In order to balance these forces, we tend to eat the inverse of this ratio with the human diet being comprised of approximately 7 parts yin to 1 part yang. This is reflected in the average ratio of minerals to protein to carbohydrate in the human diet, so that on average, the intake of protein tends to be seven times larger than the intake of minerals, and the intake of carbohydrate, seven times larger than the intake of protein. These ratios, which help balance the earth's environment, create the growth cycle of hair.

Hair growth changes with the seasons, in response to natural fluctuations in diet and environmental energy. During the summer, we tend to increase the intake of yin factors in our diets in order to balance warmer temperatures. Also, among the nutrients we consume, a smaller volume is used for active metabolism and the generation of heat and body temperature. One of the ways that we make balance with this is to eat less. Another is to discharge some of the excess in the form of hair. Moreover, in the atmosphere, earth's more yin or rising energy becomes stronger and more predominant during the spring and reaches a peak in the summer. The increase in more yin, upward energy also stimulates the growth of head hair by activating the discharge of excessive nutrients from the peripheral regions of the body.

Conversely, in the autumn and winter, heaven's contracting energy becomes stronger. This slows the rate of hair growth. Moreover, during the winter we tend to increase our intake of more contracting facors in our diets to balance the cold, and more of what we take in is used for active metabolism and the generation of heat. We balance this by eating a little more and by holding more of what we take in inside the body rather than discharging it in the form of head hair. In this way, we naturally conserve heat and energy.

The cycle of hair growth is similar to the cycle of plant growth in nature. Plants become more lush and expanded in summer and more sparse, contracted, and dormant in winter. Just as plants depend on the quality of nutrients in the soil, hair depends on the quality of nutrients supplied by the bloodstream. What we eat and drink is therefore crucial in determining the health and appearance of the hair. Moreover, each hair has a structure that is similar to that of a plant. Each hair consists of a *shaft*, or the part that appears above the skin, and a *root*, or the part that lies below it. The lower part of the root—or *hair bulb*—has an expanded structure. Part of the dermis projects upward into the bulb, and this is known as the *papilla*. Each hair has three layers of cells, including the *cuticle*, or outermost, horny layer, the *cortex*, a more elastic layer of cells that contain pigment which gives color to the hair, and the *central axis*, or *medulla*, through which nourishment is conveyed to the hair.

Just as the roots of plants are enclosed by soil, the roots of each hair are enclosed by hair follicles. Growing and multiplying cells are found in the bulb of the hair root. Blood capillaries in the papilla provide nourishment to the hair through the root. These cells undergo chemical changes, becoming harder, or more yang, in a process that is similar to keratinization of the skin. Hair grows on average 1.5 to 3.0 millimeters per week.

Hair Color

Diet and environment influence the color of the hair in the same way they influence the pigmentation of the skin. The two main hair pigments, melanin and phenomelanin, are secreted by groups of cells known as *melanocytes* located in the upper layer of the dermis. Melanin, which is the more yin of the two, gives hair a darker color. If the melanocytes secrete a more yin form of melanin that is made up of larger granules, the hair is usually black. If the granules are smaller, due to the influence of more yang factors in the diet, the hair tends to be lighter in color. Or, if the diet is high in cheese and other dairy products, eggs, and other animal foods, more yang phenomelanin may predominate, and the hair becomes lighter and may range from brown to yellow. The intake of dairy food especially contributes to the creation of blond hair.

As we saw in chapter 3, sunlight also influences pigmentation. The overall yang influence of the sun stimulates the melanocytes to secrete larger granules of melanin—which are yin—to make balance. When sunlight is weaker, they are more likely to secrete smaller granules, or secrete less melanin and more phenomelanin, giving the hair a lighter color. Red hair, which is the most yang of these colors, results from the influence of iron pigments that come from the intake of a larger volume of meat and other animal foods. Weak sunlight also causes less melanin to be secreted, so that red or blond hair tends to appear in less sunny, northern regions where dairy and other forms of animal food comprise a substantial part of the diet, rather than in bright, sunny regions.

To summarize, light-colored hair is more common when yang factors—including a higher intake of salt and animal food—predominate in the diet, while dark hair is more common when yin factors—including a greater intake of vegetable-quality foods—predominate. At the same time, there are more people with red, blond, or light brown hair in northern climates with less sunshine, while dark hair is more common among people in warm climates with strong sunshine.

Yin and yang can also be used to understand differences in the thickness of hair. In general, head hair is more yin in comparison to body hair. It reflects the flow of earth's upward energy in the body. Thicker head hair (which means that each strand of hair is more thick) is a sign of stronger yin energy, and means that vegetable-quality foods generally have a predominant role in the diet. On the other hand, soft, fine, or thin hair means that more yang foods, especially dairy and other animal products, are predominant. Conversely, body hair is charged by heaven's downward force, and has the opposite quality. Thicker body hair is an indication that heaven's energy is stronger due to the consumption of a larger volume of animal food, while thinner or less body hair means that earth's force is stronger due to the intake of a larger quantity of vegetable foods.

Diet and environment also influence the texture of hair. Curly hair, for example, is generally produced by a diet that is higher in animal food. When viewed under a microscope, the cross-section of curly hair has a more yang, flat-shaped circumference. Straight hair has a more yin, round-shape, and usually results when more yin forms of animal food—such as milk—or a higer percentage of vegetable foods are eaten. Wavy hair is in-between—it has an oval shape—and is generally the product of a diet that is yang but less so than in the case of curly hair. In the case of people in Africa, another strong yang factor causes the hair to curl, namely the heat supplied by the strong sunlight at or near the equator. Exposure to strong sun yangizes the hair, causing it to curl, even though people in these regions traditionally ate vegetable-based diets.

The melanocytes that color hair have a yin, branched or extended structure. The long branches, or *dendrites*, attached to these cells secrete pigments that are absorbed by newly formed hair cells in the hair follicle. Gray hair results when these cells become shriveled or contracted, or when the blood vessels that supply nourishment to the roots of the hair become overly constricted. This causes the secretion of pigments to slow down or stop, and the result is a lack of color in the hair. These conditions are often the result of a diet high in animal food, overly cooked, salty vegetables, or sometimes by a lack of freshness and variety in the diet.

Diet for Healthy Hair

Viewing hair under a microscope reveals a spiral structure that reflects the spiral form found throughout nature. Examples of spirals in nature include the cowlick, or hair spiral, on top of the head, the movement of water down the drain, the movement of hurricanes and ocean currents, the spiral whirls on the tips of the fingers, the spiral shells of the chambered nautilus and other primitive marine creatures, the spiral form of DNA, and the huge, whirling spirals known as galaxies.

Keratin, the protein found in the skin, is a major constituent of hair. The keratin molecules in each hair wind inward around a central axis, creating a seven-stranded spiral pattern. Whether these spiral strands are well-formed and complete, or poorly formed and incomplete depends largely upon the balance of yin and yang in the diet.

Foods that are extremely yin, such as sugar, tropical fruits, chocolate, nightshade vegetables, spices, chemical additives, soft drinks, and others weaken the hair. The crystalline molecules of keratin may start to melt and break down when too many of these items are consumed. As a result, the hair becomes weak and easily damaged. Moreover, the health of hair depends on the proper supply of nutrients. Minerals, for example, give body, strength, and form to the hair. The intake of more extreme yin foods depletes minerals from the body, including calcium from the bones and teeth, and this in turn causes hair to become weaker and less healthy looking. Too many extreme yang foods can produce a similar effect: the hair becomes hard and brittle due to constriction of the blood capillaries that supply it with nutrients.

Similar reactions occur when artificial chemicals are applied externally to wave or color hair. Strong chemical solutions leach minerals from hair, and cause the protein molecules to break down. Their frequent use can result in dry, brittle, and "lifeless" hair.

74

The health of the hair is closely related to the functioning of the microvilli in the small intestine, and to the health of the digestive system as a whole. Whether or not the hair is properly supplied with nutrients depends on how thoroughly foods are digested, how efficiently they are absorbed, and how well the absorbed nutrients flow through the circulatory system to each hair follicle. Therefore, foods that enhance digestion and absorption are essential for strong and healthy hair, as are those that promote smooth functioning of the circulatory system.

The fiber in whole grains is especially helpful in this regard. Fiber is well known for reducing the risk of colon cancer, appendicitis, hemorrhoids, diverticulosis and diverticulitis, and a variety of other digestive disorders. It promotes the rapid transit of the stool through the bowel, and thus allows toxic waste materials to be removed rapidly. This prevents stagnation that can interfere with smooth absorption. Moreover, soluble fiber, such as that contained in brown rice and whole oats, has been found to lower cholesterol. This not only reduces the risk of coronary heart disease, but also benefits the hair by preventing blockage of the blood capillaries that supply it with nutrients. Fiber binds with cholesterol and bile acid and causes excess cholesterol to be eliminated from the body. Because of their structure, the complex carbohydrates in whole grains also benefit the hair. These complex sugars are gradually broken down and not absorbed into the bloodstream until they reach the villi in the small intestine. This contrasts with the rapid absorption of refined sugar, honey, and other forms of simple sugar. Complex carbohydrates strengthen the villi, unlike simple sugars which are rapidly absorbed before they reach the small intestine.

Whole grains contain an ideal balance of minerals, proteins, carbohydrates, and vitamins. The ratio between these major nutrients averages 1 to 7, and matches the ratio between active growth and rest in the hair-growth cycle. That is, in whole grains, the ratio of minerals to protein is about 1 to 7, and the ratio of protein to carbohydrate is also 1 to 7. This makes grains ideal as principal foods that match, in terms of their yin and yang energeis, the natural growth cycle of hair. Eating whole grains such as brown rice, millet, barley, whole wheat, and others promotes smooth, even growth of hair.

Foods that are naturally fermented such as *miso*, *tamari* soy sauce, pickled vegetables, and other traditionally processed foods also facilitate smooth digestion and absorption. Miso, the dark purée made from soybeans, unrefined sea salt, and usually, fermented barley or brown rice, contains living enzymes that facilitate digestion, strengthen the quality of the blood, and provide a nutritious balance of complex carbohydrates, essential oils, protein, vitamins, and minerals. Miso soup prepared with fresh local vegetables, sea vegetables, and sometimes whole grains or noodles is an ideal food for strengthening digestion and contributing to strong, beautiful hair. Natural soy sauce, which is often sold under the name *tamari* has similar beneficial effects and can be used in moderate amounts to season soups, broths, and certain dishes.

Pickled vegetables, including naturally processed sauerkraut, also strengthen digestion. Throughout history, people in all parts of the world made pickles from a variety of root, ground, and leafy green vegetables, and from certain varieties of sea vegetables, fruits, fish and seafood. Pickles stimulate the appetite, strengthen the intestines, and aid digestion. They are especially helpful in aiding assimilation of whole grains and are often eaten together. A small volume of non-spicy, naturally processed pickles can be included daily along with other dishes.

In Japan and other traditional cultures, sea vegetables were used to strengthen the hair. Varieties such as *kombu*, wakame, nori, hijiki, *arame*, and others were valued for their properties in making the hair strong and beautiful. Not only were sea vegetables eaten on a daily basis, they were also used to make shampoo and other natural beauty-care products. Sea vegetables have qualities that match the quality of healthy hair. They have an ideal combination of firmness (provided by their high mineral content) and flexibility or softness, which results from growing underwater. For strong, soft, and beautiful hair, we recommend eating sea vegetables on a daily basis.

Whole natural foods contain vitamins and minerals that are essential for strong, healthy hair. Vitamin A, for example, is important for the health of the skin, hair, and nails. Deficiencies of vitamin A can contribute to a thickening of the scalp and to accumulation of oil and perspiration below its surface. This produces dry hair and the buildup of dandruff. As we saw in chapter 3, the best sources of vitamin A are carrots, winter squash, rutabaga, and other yellow or orange vegetables, along with broccoli, kale, and other dark leafy vegetables. Nori, which we suggest eating daily, is also a good source.

The B vitamins, found in abundance in whole grains, beans, seeds, and in land and sea vegetables, are also important in healthy hair. Deficiencies of B vitamins have been linked to problems such as excessively oily hair, dandruff, baldness, and premature graying. Minerals also play an important role in the health and appearance of the hair and skin. The human body contains various kinds of minerals such as calcium, phosphorus, potassium, sulfur, chlorine, sodium, magnesium, and iron, as well as minute amounts of trace elements such as iodine, manganese, copper, nickel, arsenic, bromine, silicon, selenium, and others. Approximately 80 percent of the body consists of water, in which these minerals and trace elements are found, and our bloodstream and other bodily fluids are similar in composition to the primordial ocean in which life began.

Minerals and trace elements are essential to form bones, muscles, hair, and other body structures. According to some nutritionists, for example, copper is contained in an enzyme that gives structure to the hair. If it is deficient, hair may not be properly formed or have a strong, healthy quality. Copper also plays a part in hair color. Calcium, which is supplied in foods such as leafy green vegetables, beans and bean products such as *tofu*, tempeh, and miso, sea vegetables, seeds and nuts, and fish and seafood, is important in the formation of collagen, the connective tissue found in the skin and throughout the body.

Like seawater that neutralizes various toxins streaming into the ocean from the land, the minerals in our circulatory system serve to maintain smooth metabolism by harmonizing the influx of excessive dietary factors. For example, excessive sugar intake results in the condition of acidosis in the blood, which is neutralized by using minerals such as calcium, and is ultimately eliminated from the body in the form of carbon dioxide and water. Therefore, a constant supply of minerals in the form of good-quality unrefined sea salt, whole grains, and vegetables, and especially

Table 9   Iron Content of Various Foods

Foods noted for their iron content include liver and other organ meats, spinach, and molasses. However, whole grains, beans, green leafy vegetables, and seeds generally contain comparable amounts of iron, and sea vegetables contain about two to four times the amount found in animal food. The U.S. RDA varies from 10–18 mg/day. (Figures per 100 grams, unit mg. 100 g=3.5 ounces, a typical serving unless otherwise noted.)

Whole Grains	Buckwheat	3.1
	Millet	6.8
	Oats	4.6
	Soba	5.0
	Whole wheat, various	3.1–3.3
Beans	Azuki beans	4.8
	Chick-peas	6.9
	Lentils	6.8
	Soybeans	7.0
Green Leafy Vegetables	Beet greens	3.3
	Dandelion greens	3.1
	Mustard greens	3.0
	Parsley	6.2
	Spinach	3.1
	Swiss chard	3.2
Seeds*	Pumpkin seeds	11.2
	Sesame seeds	10.5
	Sunflower seeds	7.1
Sea Vegetables*	Arame	12.0
	Dulse	6.3
	Hijiki	29.0
	Kombu	15.0
	Nori	23.0
	Wakame	13.0
Fish and Seafood	Herring	1.1
	Sardines	2.9
	Abalone	2.4
	Oyster	5.5
Meat and Poultry	Beef	3.6
	Chicken	1.6
	Egg yolk	6.3
	Beef liver	6.5
	Calf liver	8.7
	Chicken liver, various	7.9
Refined Sugar	Molasses	6.0

* A typical serving will usually be from one-fourth to one-half this amount.
Source: U.S. Department of Agriculture and Japan Nutritionist Association.

Table 10   Calcium Content in Various Foods

Dairy foods are known as a source of calcium, but many other foods are also rich in this element and often contain more than dairy foods. Calcium needs vary with age and other factors. The U.S. RDA varies from 800–1,200 mg/day. (Figures per 100 grams, unit mg. 100 g=3.5 ounces, an average serving unless otherwise noted.)

Leafy Green Vegetables	Beet greens	100
	Collard greens	203
	Daikon greens	190
	Kale	179
	Mustard greens	183
	Parsley	200
	Spinach	98
	Watercress	90
Beans and Bean Products	Broad beans	100
	Chick-peas	150
	Kidney beans	130
	Soybeans	226
	Miso	140
	Natto	103
	Tofu	128
Grains	Buckwheat	114
*Sea Vegetables**	Agar-agar	400
	Arame	1,170
	Dulse	567
	Hijiki	1,400
	Kombu	800
	Nori	400
	Wakame	1,300
*Seeds and Nuts**	Sesame seeds	1,160
	Sunflower seeds	140
	Sweet almonds	282
	Brazil nuts	186
	Hazelnuts	209
Fish and Seafood	Carp	50
	Haddock	23
	Salmon	79
	Shortneck clams	80
	Oyster	94
Dairy Food	Cow's milk	118
	Eggs	65
	Goat's milk	120
	Cheese, various	250–850
	Yogurt	120

* A typical serving will usually be from about one-fourth to one-half this amount.
Source: U.S. Department of Agriculture and Japan Nutritionist Association.

mineral-rich sea vegetables is necessary and highly recommended for natural health and beauty.

Refined table salt is not a good source of essential minerals. It is nearly pure sodium chloride, to which trace amounts of mineral compounds, *dextrose* (a form of refined sugar), and usually potassium iodide have been added. This product is unsuitable for meeting metabolic requirements and is a primary reason why many people take nutritional supplements. Another reason is to supplement minerals and vitamins lost from foods grown in mineral-poor soil that has been depleted by chemical fertilizers, pesticides, and other sprays. Scientific tests show that organic fruits and vegetables contain up to three times more minerals and trace elements than inorganic produce. Unrefined sea salt, the traditional type of salt used in macrobiotic cooking and food preparation, retains all the natural mineral compounds and trace elements (about sixty in number) found in the sea.

It is commonly believed that milk and other dairy products can supply more calcium than other foods and that the best sources of iron are liver and other animal foods. However, many other foods contain these nutrients and often in proportionately greater amounts than meat or dairy foods.

When selecting protein sources, it is important to choose those that are low in cholesterol and saturated fat. This means that vegetable-quality proteins, such as those in whole grains, beans, seeds, and sea vegetables, are better than those derived from animal sources. As we saw in chapter 3, the cholesterol and saturated fat contained in meat, eggs, chicken, and dairy foods accumulate in the blood vessels, including those that provide the hair and skin with nourishment. This can deprive the hair of adequate nourishment and can lead to weakness and dry hair. If animal food is consumed in a temperate, four-season climate, low-fat, white-meat fish is the preferred variety. It can be eaten several times per week on average.

Eating a natural, ecologically balanced diet is the most fundamental way to create strong, healthy, and beautiful hair. However, as everyone now knows, modern diets are often extreme and excessive. An unnatural way of eating contributes to many problems with the hair and scalp, several of which are discussed below.

Dandruff

The main symptoms of dandruff are peeling and flaking of the scalp. Normally, when skin cells reach the surface of the body, they are sloughed off. When someone has dandruff, these cells are not discharged as a fine powder but clumped together to form large, flaky scales. In severe cases, redness and flaky skin appear on other parts of the body, including the eyebrows, eyelids, chest, sides of the nose, navel, around the groin, and on the upper back. This disorder is similar to psoriasis, and is known as *seborrheic dermatitis*.

Although they appear dry, dandruff flakes are actually made up of oil and protein. Applying oily or greasy preparations to the scalp does not help the problem, nor does it change the underlying cause. Like other conditions of the skin and hair, the cause of dandruff is dietary. Dandruff is an elimination of excess, especially proteins and fats. It can be caused by overeating in general, or by the overintake of animal food or oily and fatty foods from either animal or vegetable sources. Although medicated shampoos may temporarily suppress symptoms, they also do not change the underlying condition that produces dandruff. Moreover, they contain chemicals such as tar, sulfur, zinc pyrithione, or other antibacterial agents that deplete nutrients from the hair and scalp. The solution to dandruff is simple, and is based on avoidance of dietary extremes, especially the overconsumption of animal fats and proteins.

A naturally balanced diet of whole grains, fresh local vegetables, beans, sea vegetables, and other whole natural foods helps eliminate dandruff. The use of oil in cooking is best kept moderate until the condition clears up. High-quality sesame oil is the preferred variety, and a small amount can be used to sauté vegetables or other foods several times per week. Raw oil and deep-fried dishes are best avoided until the dandruff goes away, while nuts and nut butters—which contain plenty of fat and oil—are best avoided or kept to a minimum. Overeating, even of high-quality natural food, creates excess in the body that can delay improvement. Chewing well helps prevent this, so during the recovery period, chew each mouthful until it becomes liquid. Also, try not to eat for several hours before going to sleep, as food eaten prior to bed is often improperly digested and absorbed and is turned into excess in the body.

Excess Facial and Body Hair

As we saw at the beginning of this chapter, head and body hair are complementary and antagonistic. Head hair grows primarily under the influence of earth's rising energy, while body hair is created more by heaven's downward force. These primary forces affect the sex hormones, and these in turn affect the hair.

When a woman develops noticeable hair on the face or body, it means that heaven's more yang energy has become excessive. The source of this excessive energy is the overintake of strong yang foods, especially meat, eggs, cheese and other dairy products, poultry, shellfish, and other foods of animal origin. In many cases, strong yang foods stimulate the adrenal glands to secrete excessive amounts of androgen, or male hormone, which is also present in the female body. In severe cases, the adrenals may malfunction, producing the condition known as *hirsutism*, or the excessive overgrowth of facial and body hair. This condition is frequently accompanied by underdeveloped breasts and erratic menstrual periods, both of which also indicate an overabundance of heaven's contracting energy.

The area between the nose and mouth, where men develop a moustache, corresponds in the body to the reproductive organs. This area changes in response to the body's secretion of sex hormones. Normally, women do not develop hair here, and when they do, it means that the overconsumption of animal food has altered their hormonal balance and affected their reproductive organs. Meat, eggs, cheese, chicken, red-meat fish, and other animal-quality foods are the most common causes of this condition.

Current approaches to excess hair are directed toward removing the unwanted hair, not changing the underlying cause. The most common methods of hair removal include shaving, rubbing with pumice, waxing, plucking, softening hair with chemicals, and electrolysis. Among these, shaving and rubbing with pumice have the least harmful effects, although rubbing is often too rough for delicate skin. Plucking with tweezers or spreading warm wax on the skin and pulling hair out from the roots damages hair follicles. Plucking sometimes leads to inflammation and the appearance of coarse new hair. The strong chemicals in the creams, sprays, and lotions used to melt away hair, damage the skin—causing irritation—and are absorbed into the bloodstream. In *electrolysis*, a tiny needle is inserted into the hair follicles and electric current is used to destroy the papilla. This destructive procedure distrupts the flow of electromagnetic energy along the meridians, and affects the organs nourished by these meridians. Methods of hair removal that destroy the roots or cause them to atrophy deprive the body of channels of discharge. If follicles are damaged or closed as the result of these practices, toxins that would normally discharge through them start to accumulate in the bloodstream and throughout the body.

If a woman avoids extremes (especially too much animal food) and eats a naturally balanced diet, her hormones will be naturally balanced as well. Women who avoid overeating and base their diets on whole grains and vegetables normally do not develop excess facial or body hair. Changing to a balanced diet can even help unwanted hair to naturally fall out. Macrobiotic eating is the key to smooth, delicate skin free of excess hair and skin markings.

Dry Hair/Oily Hair

Dry and oily hair often have similar dietary causes. Dry hair is brittle at the ends and has a hard, strawlike texture. It lacks the natural gloss of normal, healthy hair, and may have many split ends. Oily hair is often dry at the ends, but looks and feels oily at the roots, and is frequently accompanied by dandruff. As we saw earlier, when plenty of animal food is consumed, hard, saturated fat accumulates in blood vessels that supply the skin and hair, as well as in the pores and hair follicles. Initially, the body tries to discharge these fats through the oil glands and pores. When this occurs, the result can be oily skin or hair, or acne. The over-consumption of fried foods, commercial salad dressings, and vegetable-quality oils —including those in nuts and nut butters—contributes to this condition.

Often, however, the intake of hard saturated fat continues beyond the body's ability to discharge excess. This process occurs gradually and it takes time before the body's abilities are overtaxed. In youth, when excess is still actively discharging, an extreme diet often results in acne or oily skin. The ability to discharge declines sharply after age 35, and that is when results of accumulation start to become visible. The skin often becomes harder and drier at this time and the hair dry and brittle. The accumulation of fat clogs sweat glands and oil ducts so that hair and skin do not receive enough moisture, resulting in dehydration at the surface of the body.

Overintake of salt and high-sodium foods contributes to this problem, as does insufficient consumption of fluid. However, most cases of dry hair are caused by the overintake of saturated fat. Of course, chemical dyes, permanent-wave solutions, chemical shampoos or conditioners, and other artificial products weaken hair and can leave it dry and brittle. Synthetic bleaches, for example, destroy melanin, the natural coloring pigment of hair, while waving solutions alter the chemical structure of keratin, diminishing the strength and elasticity of hair. Moreover, synthetic dyes contain chemicals that irritate the skin, some of which have been found to be carcinogenic.

The solution to dry hair is to discontinue the use of synthetic products such as these and change one's diet away from the reliance on animal foods that contain saturated fat. Even the intake of vegetable oils is best kept moderate, and oily, greasy, or fried dishes are best avoided until normal moisture is restored. The intake of baked flour products, roasted seeds and nuts, rice cakes, and other foods that can cause dryness when eaten excessively, is best kept to a minimum. It is important to have plenty of variety in the diet by including a wide range of grain, bean, vegetable and other dishes, and to keep the use of sea salt, as well as condiments or seasonings that contain it, moderate. High-quality sesame oil can be used for sautéing several times per week in moderate amounts, while quickly steamed and lightly blanched vegetables can be eaten daily. Similar recommendations also apply for oily hair, especially the avoidance of saturated fat and oily or greasy dishes. A naturally balanced macrobiotic diet, based on whole cereal grains, beans and bean products, fresh local vegetables, sea vegetables, and other whole natural foods is the most fundamental way to restore fullness, body, and natural gloss to the hair.

Split Ends

When the bonds that hold the strands of protein in hair together break down, split ends are the result. The breakdown of hair results from several causes, especially the consumption of yin extremes, including drugs and medications, in the diet. Overintake of sugar, soft drinks, ice cream, chocolate, and spices weakens the molecular bonds in hair, and often causes the hair shaft to split or fragment. These foods deplete minerals that hold hair together. External influences also play a role in this condition. Dyes, shampoos, and waving solutions contain chemicals, many of which are extremely yin, and their overuse also weakens hair and can result in split ends. The accumulation of hard fats in the capillaries that supply hair with nourishment can also cause splitting. If the capillaries contract enough to deprive the hair of adequate nourishment, it becomes brittle, weak, and may split at the ends.

A naturally balanced diet, plus the use of natural, nonchemical beauty-care products, is the best way to avoid split ends. Strong, healthy hair begins growing as soon as a natural diet is started, so that in time, the hair will become strong, smooth, and beautiful.

Hair Loss

Hair loss is becoming increasingly common today, even among women. Every year, millions of dollars are spent on chemical creams and shampoos that are promised to grow hair. People also undergo a variety of unnatural procedures, including hair transplants, in order to restore lost hair. However, as we will see, diet and lifestyle play a primary role in the development of baldness. Baldness is a preventable condition, regardless of the prevalence of it in one's family. A primary reason why baldness tends to occur in families is because of similar dietary and lifestyle patterns that families share. Hair loss occurs in one of three general patterns:

1. *Yin hair loss*—begins on the front of the head. It often starts with a receding hairline and continues until much of the hair on the front is gone. It is caused by overexpansion and looseness in the cells of the hair follicles, so that the hair becomes loose and falls out. The primary cause is overconsumption of liquid, as well as the intake of too many yin extremes, including tropical fruits, juices, soft drinks, sugars, sweets, stimulants, chemicals, drugs, medications, raw vegetables, tomatoes, potatoes, eggplant, and vegetables of tropical origin. This type of hair loss is sometimes associated with more yin health conditions such as diabetes, epilepsy, and anemia, and with the use of drugs such as amphetamines and cholesterol-reducers, both of which are extremely yin.

2. *Yang hair loss*—occurs in the center of the head, and is caused by overconsumption of yang extremes, including meat, poultry, eggs, dairy foods, and in some cases, fish and seafood. Too much animal protein, saturated fat, and salt is the main cause, together with overintake of dried, roasted, or baked foods.

   This type of hair loss is sometimes referred to as *androgenic baldness*, and is on the rise among women primarily because of rising meat, cheese, and poultry consumption. It is associated with too much testosterone in the blood. As we saw in the discussion of acne, free testosterone is attracted toward the hair follicles so that the body can discharge it. Specialized cells in the hair follicles convert testosterone into a more potent form known as *dihydrotestosterone*. This more yang hormone tends to stimulate the growth of facial hair (which is more yang) while suppressing the growth of head hair (which is more yin). It causes hair follicles on the scalp to shut down.

   As we saw in the discussion of facial hair, production of excess testosterone is stimulated by overintake of meat, eggs, cheese, poultry, and other animal foods. Often, when a woman eats plenty of these foods, her body will react by producing excess male hormone. This can trigger an episode of thinning hair. Moreover, about 140 pharmaceuticals currently in use today, including certain varieties of birth control pills, stimulate production of androgens in the body. These are referred to as *androgenic drugs*, and contribute to hair loss.

3. *Combination hair loss*—usually covers a large area of the front, sides, and

central regions of the head, and may occur in the form of thinning hair. Normally, between 50 to 100 hairs are shed and replaced daily. When replacement of old hairs becomes too slow, noticeable thinning takes place. This type of hair loss is caused by the combination of extremes, including too much animal food and extreme yin items such as sugar, fruits, chemicals, and drugs. An extreme or imbalanced diet lacking in balanced nutrients from whole grains, beans, vegetables, and sea vegetables frequently leads to conditions such as psoriasis, severe dandruff, boils, and other skin disorders, and these often cause hair to fall out.

Modern approaches to hair loss, including hair transplants, hair weaving, hair implantation, and fiber implants sidestep the underlying cause and have serious drawbacks, including potential long- and short-term side effects. Chemical preparations touted to stimulate hair growth also miss the underlying cause and also have potentially negative effects. Researchers are also developing drugs that block the conversion of testosterone into its more potent form, as well as drugs that prevent the hormone from entering the hair follicles. However, using powerful drugs for baldness is an unnecessarily extreme measure. A naturally balanced diet is the safest and most sure way to prevent hair loss. A macrobiotic diet based on proper proportions of whole grains, fresh local vegetables, beans, sea vegetables, occasional low-fat, white-meat fish, and other whole foods helps restore normal hormone levels without side effects. It corrects the underlying casue of baldness. Moreover, as one's condition and overall health improves as the result of eating well, it is possible to stimulate or repair dormant follicles, although this process takes time.

Natural Hair Care

As much as possible, use natural and organic hair-care products. Many commercial shampoos, conditioners, and rinses contain chemicals that in the long term are damaging to hair. Daily or regular shampooing, rinsing, and conditioning with natural products (available in natural food stores) helps keep hair healthy and beautiful. When applying shampoo, be sure to massage the scalp, as this activates circulation and energy flow, and stimulates hair at the roots. As much as possible, avoid using electric hair dryers or other devices on the hair as these disturb the flow of energy along the meridians and, over time, can cause drying and depletion of the hair.

Nails

Like hair, nails are created from the discharge of excess nutrients, especially minerals, proteins, and fats. Their compostion is very similar to that of hair. Nails are composed largely of keratin, the form of protein found in the skin and hair.

The nails have a more condensed, hard structure that counterbalances the softer, more flexible structure of hair.

The hard, visible part of the nail is referred to as the *nail plate*, and the skin under it as the *nail bed*. The nail grows from a matrix, which is located in the lower part of the bed. Here, living cells produce the nail plate, which is not composed of living cells. The uppermost portion of the matrix is visible on the lower part of the nail in the form of the half-moons, or *lunula*. The skin that grows on the base of the nail is called the *cuticle*. Blood vessels are found in the nail bed, and as we will see, the quality of the blood is reflected in the color and condition of the nails. Nails depend on the bloodstream for nourishment, and the quality of nourishment determines their condition and appearance. Therefore, care of the nails begins with a naturally balanced diet.

The fingers and toes—and hence the fingernails and toenails—are part of the body's energy system. In chapter 2 we saw how energy from the environment flows deep within the body through the chakras and primary channel. The meridians are branches of this main channel, and each meridian subdivides into numerous smaller branches that connect with and charge the body's cells and tissues. Each hair follicle receives energy from these meridian branches. This constant charge of life-force makes hair grow. The energy that supplies the hair follicles is minutely differentiated in comparison to that flowing along the meridians. Hence when nutritional factors discharge in the form of hair, they are carried along these tiny branches and take a more yin, differentiated form. In contrast, the nails are created by the more consolidated stream of energy that flows through the meridian as a whole, and have a more solid, dense structure.

Fig. 8

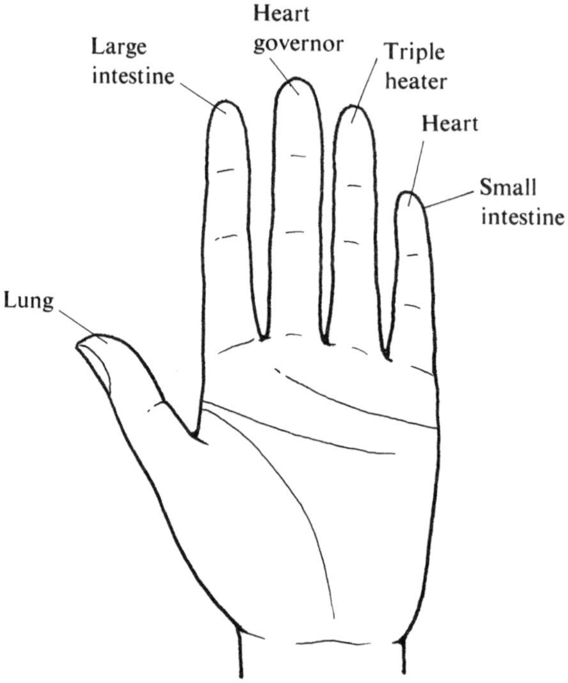

Nails are influenced not only by the quality of blood and body fluids, but also by the charge and quality of energy supplied from the chakras, organs, and meridians. They are reflections of our total health.

In Figure 8, you can see how the fingernails correspond to the internal organs, body functions, and meridians. (Please see Fig. 7 of the foot on p. 66 for correlations between the toes and toenails and organ/meridians.) When a particular nail shows some problem or abnormal condition, it is a sign that the flow of energy in the corresponding meridian is unbalanced. Using these correlations, you can begin to see how our external appearance reflects our internal condition.

Nail Colors

The color of the nails reflects the condition of the blood that circulates in the nail bed. Different colors are caused by differences in condition that come about because of the influence of diet, activity, and other aspects of daily life. The more common nail colors are presented below, together with what they mean about our condition.

- Pinkish red is the color of normal, healthy nails. It shows that the blood is in generally sound condition and that the person's health is on the whole more balanced.
- Nails that are reddish-purple result from overintake of yin extremes, including dairy foods, sugar, concentrated and artificial sweeteners, tropical fruits and juices, nightshade vegetables, fats and oils, chemicals and drugs, as well as coffee and other stimulants. They show that the internal condition has become weaker and that the person may be experiencing fatigue and lowered resistance to illness.
- Dark red nails indicate the accumulation of fatty acids, cholesterol, and/or minerals in the blood, resulting from too many animal foods, including meat, eggs, cheese, poultry, and salt. They are an indication that the flow of energy through the body is stagnated or blocked, and often appear together with dry hair and skin.
- Whitish nails are usually an indication of weak circulation, low hemoglobin, and general anemia. These conditions result primarily from overintake of refined flour, fruit, juices, sugar, concentrated sweeteners, and raw foods, which, when eaten excessively, thin and weaken the blood. In some cases, however, this condition results from an opposite cause, especially the constriction of blood vessels and capillaries resulting from overintake of salt, dried, roasted, or baked foods, and animal foods. If we are in good health, this color does not appear on the nails, although it may be present when the fingers are stretched, especially on the thumb and index finger.

Other Nail Conditions

A variety of conditions appearing on or around the nails reveal certain things about a person's overall condition and dietary habits. Several of these correspondences are listed below:

- Small white dots on the nails show the elimination of sugars, including cane sugar, honey, syrups, fruit sugars, milk sugars, alcohol, chocolate, and other simple sugars. Simple sugars cause an acid reaction in the bloodstream, and this requires minerals to maintain a healthy alkaline quality in the blood. Depletion of calcium from the bones and teeth is a common result of this imbalance—especially when simple sugars are consumed regularly—and this is a primary cause of tooth decay and, in later life, osteoporosis. One of the signs of potential mineral depletion and possible deficiency is the appearance of white dots on the fingernails. They show that zinc and other minerals are possibly deficient due to the intake of simple sugars. This condition can be remedied fairly quickly by restoring a natural balance in the diet and by avoiding the regular consumption of simple sugars.

  The location of the white dot shows approximately when the excess sugar was eaten. On average, fingernails take about four to six months to grow, with the speed of growth being more rapid in children and slower after age fifty. (Toenails take about twice as long as fingernails to grow.) So, if the white dot appears on the middle of the nail, the excess sugar was eaten about two-and-a-half months before.
- Vertical ridges on the nails result from nutrient imbalances especially the over-intake of carbohydrates and salt and the underintake of protein and fats. These irregularities take time to appear.
- Horizontal indentations in the nails show a recent change in diet or living place. For example, if a person moves to a different climate, such as from Chicago to Miami, and changes from a diet high in animal foods and well-cooked dishes to one based around salad and fruit, a horizontal groove may start to appear on the fingernail. A reverse change, from a warmer to a colder climate can also produce these indentations. If the person did not move in the recent past, then horizontal grooves show a change in their way of eating.
- If the ends of the nails become split or uneven, it indicates an overintake of yin extremes. *Hangnails*, in which the skin on either side of the nail starts to peel, are also indications of too much yin, including sugar, tropical fruits, milk and ice cream, chocolate, and drugs and medications. In Oriental diagnosis, these conditions were understood to show problems in the reproductive organs, including the possibility of menstrual disorders, fibroids and other types of cysts or tumors, infertility, and other conditions.
- Long nails are the result of a more yin diet, often including plenty of raw vegetables and fruits, with other yin items such as sugar and sweets, chocolate and spices, and ice cream and soft drinks also eaten in excess. Throughout history, long, decorated nails were associated with a more luxurious lifestyle

with a minimum of physical exertion, and with a diet rich in more yin, exotic foods. Long nails often indicate that a person's physical vitality has become weaker.

Diet for Beautiful Nails

As you can see, diet has a direct effect on the health and appearance of the nails. Foods and beverages influence the nails in a way that is similar to the way they influence the skin and hair. As with the hair, the formation of keratin in the nails depends upon the balance of yin and yang in the diet. If too many animal foods and salt are consumed, for example, the nails may become hard and brittle, or they may contract and shrivel. Blockage in the arteries and blood vessels caused by too many saturated fats deprives nails of nutrients needed for proper formation. In many cases, dietary imbalance causes the toenails, especially the nail on the large toe, to become hard, thick, and discolored. Malformation and/or yellowish discoloration of the large toenail shows that overconsumption of cheese, chicken, eggs, and other animal foods has affected the organs in the central part of the body, including the pancreas, gallbladder, liver, and spleen.

Overconsumption of yin extremes can also cause the nails to develop improperly. As explained above, splitting of the ends of the nails, hangnails, or nails that peel at the tips result from too many yin extremes, as do discolorations stemming from changes in the quality of blood that flows under the nail bed and throughout the body.

A naturally balanced diet of whole grains, beans and bean products, sea vegetables, local vegetables and other whole natural foods is the best way to grow strong, healthy nails. Whole natural foods contain an ideal balance of vitamins, minerals, proteins, carbohydrates, and essential natural oils, and contribute to the health and appearance of the nails. At the same time, as part of a natural approach to daily care, it is best to minimize or avoid using strong chemical products on the nails. Products such as nail polish, nail-polish removers, and cuticle removers contain strong chemicals that are best avoided for optimal natural health. As your health and overall condition start to improve through balanced diet, your nails will become strong, healthy, and beautiful.

Chapter 5 *Natural Facial Care*

The best cosmetics
Are foods selected daily
From nature's pantry

Care of the face begins with daily food. The appearance of the face depends on our overall state of health, including the condition of the internal organs. And this, in turn, is determined largely by what we eat and drink.

The numerous complementary regions of the body—outside and inside, front and back, periphery and center, and upper and lower sections—are parts of the whole and reflections of yin and yang. They are mirror images of one another. When something changes on the inside, for example, it triggers a response or reaction on the outside. If we know what to look for, we can understand what visible, external signs are telling us about our condition. What is hidden inside is thus revealed on the surface.

The relationship between the upper body—especially the face and head—and the lower body—especially the internal organs—illustrates the mirror-image principle. Comparing the size and structure of the two, the head is small, compact, and more yang, while the rest of the body is large, expanded, and more yin. The head is actually a compact version of the body, and the body an expanded version of the head.

During pregnancy, human life in the womb develops simultaneously in numerous opposite yet complementary directions. In one, energy and nutrients gather toward the inside and lower regions, eventually forming the internal organs, glands, bones, and tissues. In a counterbalancing movement, energy and nutrients gather toward the upper and peripheral regions, and eventually form the head, face, skin, arms and legs. These complementary spirals of development occur together, so that as organs develop internally, facial and other features appear on the surface to make balance. Each feature develops in tandem with a particular organ, and after birth, mirrors the health and condition of the organ it corresponds to.

Yin and yang provide the context out of which these relationships emerge. If we know them, we can discover what specific lines, wrinkles, markings, and discolorations reveal about our condition, as well as what is causing a particular problem or imbalance. They also help us discover how to correct problems by showing, in terms of energy balance, how foods affect the body and mind. In this chapter, we examine each of these aspects, beginning with correspondences between the facial features and internal organs.

The art of seeing the condition of our health in the face is derived from the traditional practice of Oriental diagnosis or health evaluation. This ancient art was practiced widely in China, Japan, and other Asian countries and formed an integral part of the centuries-old system of Oriental medicine, which includes such practices as acupuncture and shiatsu massage. Readers who would like to study Oriental diagnosis in greater depth may consult books such as *How to See Your Health* (Japan Publications, Inc., 1980) and *Your Face Never Lies* (Avery Publishing Group, 1983) by Michio Kushi.

Reading the Face

The relationship between the head (or face) and body is complementary and antagonistic. As the organs develop inwardly during pregnancy, the facial features expand outwardly. Organs in the lower body, such as the bladder and intestines, appear in the upper region of the face, while organs in the upper body, such as the heart and lungs, appear in the lower part of the face. Centrally located organs, such as the liver and pancreas, appear in the middle region of the face. Below we explain the correspondences between the internal organs and facial features, and discuss what certain lines, wrinkles, and discolorations reveal about our condition.

Fig. 9 Face-Organ Correlations

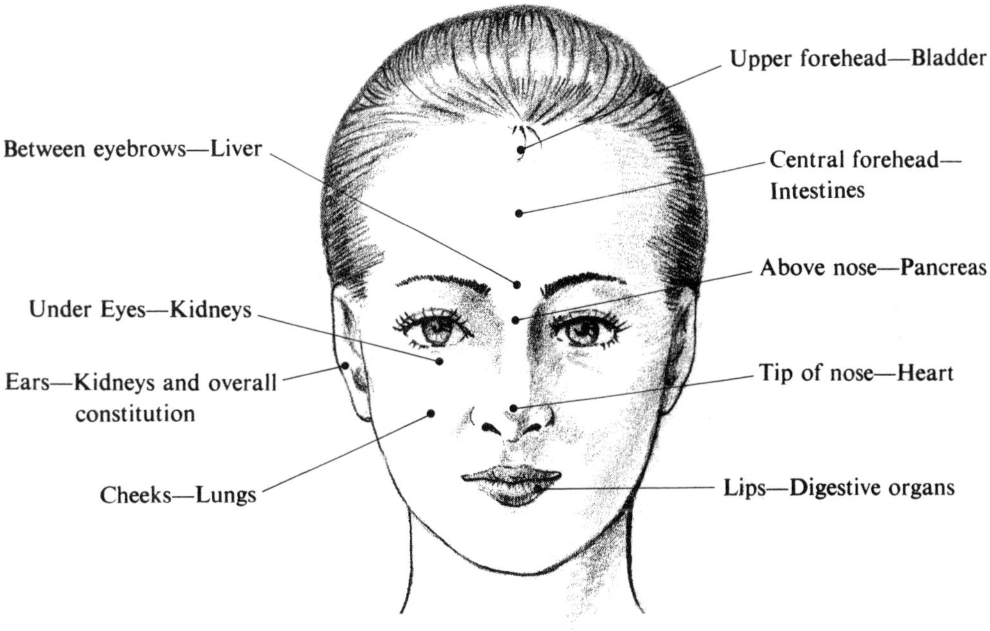

Upper forehead—Bladder

Between eyebrows—Liver

Central forehead—Intestines

Above nose—Pancreas

Under Eyes—Kidneys

Ears—Kidneys and overall constitution

Tip of nose—Heart

Cheeks—Lungs

Lips—Digestive organs

Upper Forehead—Bladder

The upper forehead, or hairline, corresponds to the bladder. If you frequently perspire from the forehead, it is a sign that your bladder is overexpanded due to the intake of too much liquid. Pimples show that mucus and fat are accumulating in the bladder.

Central Forehead—Intestines

The middle part of the forehead corresponds to the small and large intestines. Numerous horizontal lines here show that the intestines are overexpanded, largely because of the overconsumption of saturated and unsaturated fats, sugars, fruits, and other yin extremes, plus the chronic overintake of liquid, including soft drinks, orange juice, milk, alcohol, and coffee. Pimples show accumulation of fat and mucus in the intestines.

Between the Eyebrows—Liver

The region between the eyebrows shows the condition of the liver. One or several deep vertical lines here are usually an indication of liver trouble. They show that the liver has become overexpanded and possibly hard due to the intake of too many animal foods that contain saturated fat, as well as too many simple sugars, including refined sugar, tropical fruits, chocolate, ice cream, and alcohol. Pimples in this region show possible accumulation of fat and mucus in the liver. Hardness or tightness in the liver often produces negative emotions such as short temper, irritability, and anger.

Above the Nose—Pancreas

Today, many people develop a horizontal crease or wrinkle above the nose. This mark corresponds to tightness in the pancreas caused by the overintake of animal foods, especially chicken, cheese, and eggs, and shrimp, lobster, crab, and other types of shellfish. It is an indication that hard fats are accumulating in the pancreas and disrupting the normal secretion of insulin and anti-insulin. It is often a sign of *hypoglycemia*, or chronic low blood sugar.

Underneath the Eyes—Kidneys

The region below the eyes corresponds to the kidneys. Eyebags are indications of trouble in the kidneys caused by overconsumption of fluids, simple sugars, or fatty foods. They are signs that fat and fluid are starting to pool throughout the body. Bluish or purplish discolorations are also signs of fat and mucus accumulation, while a whitish color shows that overconsumption of dairy foods, including milk, yogurt, and ice cream, has contributed to the buildup of fats. These signs show that our vitality is becoming weaker. Eyebags and discolorations in this region also indicate that fat and mucus are accumulating in the ovaries, with the potential to develop ovarian cysts in the future.

Ears—Kidneys/Overall Constitution

Large, thick, and well-developed ears with a detached lobe are indications of a strong and well-balanced constitution, together with natively strong kidneys. The ears develop during pregnancy and well-developed ears show that the mother ate a balanced diet of minerals, protein, and complex carbohydrate. Smaller and thinner ears with an attached lobe indicate a less-vital constitution and result from over-intake of protein, especially from animal sources, during pregnancy. Larger ears tend to be more common among people born before World War II due to the simpler diet (with less animal food) and more physically challenging daily life experienced by people until the middle of this century.

Tip of the Nose—Heart

The tip of the nose corresponds to the heart. Enlargement or puffiness in the tip of the nose shows overexpansion of the heart due to too many extreme yin foods and beverages, including sugar, tropical fruits, soft drinks, ice cream, chocolate, coffee, and alcohol. Hardening at the tip shows that saturated fats are accumulating in the blood vessels that supply the heart. Overconsumption of cheese is the most common cause of hardening, although the overintake of other types of animal food can also cause it to appear.

Overintake of yin extremes causes blood capillaries under the skin to become overexpanded. If the reddish color that results appears on the tip of the nose, it is an indication of overexpansion of the heart and circulatory vessels, and the tendency toward high blood pressure. Pimples on the nose are a sign that fats are being discharged and may be accumulating in the bloodstream, arteries, and blood vessels.

Cheeks—Lungs

The condition of the lungs can be seen in the cheeks. In adults, reddish or "rosy" colored cheeks indicate capillary expansion and the possibility of mucus deposits in the lungs. Pimples on the cheeks are caused by too much fat and sugar, and show that fat and mucus are accumulating in the lungs and respiratory passages. Puffy, swollen, or sagging cheeks also show the possibility of mucus and fat accumulation, as well as overall weakness in the lungs.

Lips—Digestive Organs

In the mouth we can read the condition of the digestive and reproductive systems. The upper lip reveals the condition of the upper section of the digeitive system, especially the stomach, while the lower lip corresponds to the small and large intestines. If the lips become swollen or puffy, the digestive organs have become overexpanded and loose, and the ability to digest and absorb nutrients has become weak. An expanded upper lip means that the trouble is primarily in the stomach, while a swollen or protruding lower lip means that the intestines are not functioning optimally. A puffy or expanded lower lip is often a sign of chronic constipation.

Facial Color ————————————————————————————

Reddish color in the face is the result of capillary expansion and is a sign that too many strong yin foods and drinks are being consumed. It shows that the heart and circulatory system are overworked, and may be a sign of high blood pressure. A pale white color is often a sign of overintake of milk and other dairy products, and shows that mucus and fat have accumulated throughout the body. A pink complexion results from the combination of too much milk and too much sugar. A yellowish complexion is often an indication of trouble in the liver, gallbladder, spleen, and pancreas, due to the intake of hard fats such as those in chicken, cheese, and eggs. Greenish discolorations on the face or other parts of the body show the tendency to develop cancer, especially in the part of the body that corresponds to the external discoloration.

Daily Foods as Cosmetics

As you can see, dietary excesses are the primary causes of these conditions. Imbalances in the facial features or skin color can be prevented by staying away from extremes and basing your diet on centrally balanced foods. Well-prepared natural foods are the best cosmetics. A naturally balanced diet makes it easier to keep your condition healthy and your face young looking and beautiful. In order to be able to use daily foods as cosmetics, we need to see how their energies affect the internal organs, facial features, and body as a whole.

As we saw in chapter 2, the body receives a constant supply of energy from heaven and earth. Heaven's more yang, downward force and earth's more yin, upward force both run along a central line deep within the body. These forces charge the body and all of its functions, and it is along this central line that seven highly charged energy centers, or chakras, arise. Lines of energy, or meridians, radiate outward from this central line toward the surface of the body in the way that the ridges of a pumpkin branch outward from its central core. The meridians charge each of the organs and subdivide into smaller streams that provide energy to each cell.

Heaven and earth do not charge both sides of the body equally; heaven's force is stronger on one side, and earth's force on the other side. So, although both sides of the body appear to be similar, they often function in an opposite, yet complementary way. When we walk or run, for example, we put the right foot forward and the left foot backward, and vice versa, in an alternating pattern. As we move our right arm to the front, our left moves to the rear, and vice versa.

How then, can we tell which of these forces is stronger on the left and which is stronger on the right side of the body? Most people use their right hand for more active, outward, and expansive movements, and their left for supportive, stabilizing, or contractive movements. When writing, for example, the right hand moves outward as the pen glides across the page, while the left counterbalances by keeping still and applying pressure to the paper. When throwing a ball, the right arm thrusts forward away from the body, while the left moves in the opposite direction toward the rear. The right hand is used for throwing, and the left for catching and receiving. When swinging a bat, most people use their right arm to push the bat forward, and the left to pull it in the opposite direction. These basic tendencies often appear among left-handed people as well. When a left-handed person uses a pen or pencil, for example, they often do so by curling the left wrist inward in the form of a contracting spiral as they write.

Another clue is found in the structure of the large intestine. The large intestine moves up the right, across the middle, and then down the left side of the body. Clues such as these point to the predominance of earth's rising, active energy on the right side of the body, and heaven's downward, stabilizing force on the left.

Fig. 10 The Energy Balance of Foods

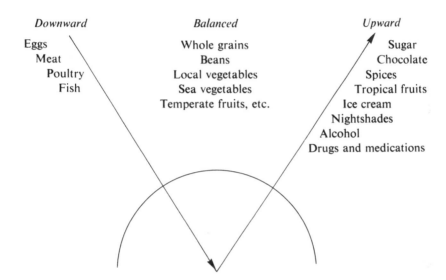

Daily foods can also be understood in terms of these primary forces. In chapter 1, we classified foods into three categories: extreme yin, extreme yang, and centrally balanced. Extreme yang foods are strongly charged by heaven's downward force. These extreme "downward" foods include eggs, meat, poultry, shellfish, and red-meat or blue-skinned fish such as salmon, tuna, and bluefish. Extreme yin foods are strongly charged with earth's rising energy. Strong "upward" foods include sugar, chocolate, spices, tropical fruits, soft drinks, ice cream, nightshade vegetables, and drugs and medications. Centrally balanced foods, including grains, beans, and fresh local vegetables, are neither strongly "upward" or strongly "downward." Although they receive energy from heaven and earth, on the whole they are more evenly balanced than the extremes indicated above.

Foods from either extreme disrupt the smooth flow of energy in the body. Eating plenty of meat, cheese, chicken, or other foods with strong downward energy, for example, blocks or suppresses the flow of earth's upward force on the right side of the body, including the energy that nourishes the liver. Moreover, as the fats and other excessive factors contained in these foods accumulate, they cause the liver to become hard, tight, and enlarged. In this condition, the liver blocks the flow of upward energy. This produces tension throughout the body, especially in the liver and the region of the face that corresponds to it. And, as saturated fats cause collagen to harden, lines and wrinkles that appear because of tension become more permanent, unless, of course, the underlying condition is corrected through balanced diet.

Energy blockages like these affect not only our physical health and appearance, but our mood and emotions as well. When upward energy on the right side of the body becomes blocked because of strong "downward" foods, we start to feel impatient and frustrated. We may become irritable and short-tempered, and feel as if we are being "blocked" or prevented from actively doing what we want. If blocked energy continues accumulating, it may burst forth in a sudden, uncontrollable explosion, similar to the eruption of a volcano. We call these volcanic eruptions "anger."

The pancreas is located more on the left side of the body where the opposite, downward flow of heaven's force is stronger. Overconsumption of strong upward foods—especially simple sugars—offsets this energy and weakens cells in the pancreas that secrete insulin. *Insulin*, a more yang hormone that lowers blood sugar, is strongly charged with heaven's force. Eating too many strong upward foods can dilute the quality of insulin to the point that it lacks the power to lower blood sugar. This condition is known as *diabetes*.

Overconsumption of strong downward foods produces the opposite effect. If the diet contains plenty of cheese, chicken, eggs, and shellfish, downward energy begins to accumulate in the pancreas. Hard fats also build up in the organ, causing tightness and stagnation. These conditions weaken the pancreas' ability to secrete *anti-insulin*, the hormone that performs a function that is opposite to that of insulin. Anti-insulin causes the blood sugar level to rise. Normally, both hormones function together to keep the level of blood sugar within a normal range. However, if anti-insulin is deficient, the person may begin to experience chronic low blood sugar, or hypoglycemia. This widespread disorder produces symptoms such as fatigue, depression, and the craving for sweets.

How, then, can we use daily food to restore balance in the internal organs, facial features, and our condition as a whole? The key to this is the understanding of "energetic compatibility," or being able to match the quality of energy in foods with that of the organs, meridians, and chakras. For example, foods such as leafy greens, barley, and naturally fermented products reflect earth's upward energy in a moderate way, and promote the smooth flow of upward energy in the body. Eating these items helps restore health and harmony in the liver and other parts of the body that are especially charged by this energy. On the other hand, foods such as millet, squash, and cabbage are moderately charged with downward energy. Eating them promotes the smooth flow of heaven's force in the body, and helps restore the pancreas to a healthy condition. As health is restored to the internal organs, imbalances in the facial features also start to change. So, for example, as the intestines become strong and flexible, swelling or puffiness in the lower lip gradually disappears and the lips return to their normal thickness. Or, as excess fluid and fats are discharged from the kidneys, eyebags and discoloration below the eyes gradually fade. Of course, in order to restore balance to any organ or part of the body, it is necessary to avoid extremes and provide the body as a whole with a wide range of energies by including a variety of high-quality natural foods in the diet. Then, within the range of centrally balanced foods, we include those that match the energy of the particular organ we are considering. Below we describe how foods affect the internal organs and how to select centrally balanced foods to restore harmony to the inside and outside of the body.

In the classification presented below, we list the organs in pairs—with more yang, solid or compact organs discussed together with more yin, hollow or expanded ones. The organs in each pair complement each other, and function as a complete energy unit.

Rebalancing the Liver and Gallbladder

Foods with mildly upward, or expanding energy help restore balance to the liver and gallbladder. Among the grains, barley, a more light, expansive grain, is especially charged by earth's rising energy, as is whole wheat. Varieties that are planted in winter and harvested in spring are especially good. Whole barley or wheat can be included several times per week in your menus. So, for example, you can cook 15 to 20 percent barley or wheat berries together with brown rice in your main grain dishes. Barley can also be used to make delicious soups, and can be included in a variety of other dishes. Natural, unyeasted sourdough bread, *udon* noodles, *seitan* (wheat-meat), and other products made from whole wheat flour can also be included from time to time. However, be careful not to overdo baked flour products, as overconsumption can cause dryness or tightness that restricts the smooth flow of upward energy in the body.

Natural fermentation, a process in which foods break down and decompose, arises because of the predominance of earth's rising or expansive energy. The mildly expansive and naturally sour taste of fermented foods matches the energy in the liver and gallbladder. Naturally processed *mugi*, or barley miso, is made from barley and soybeans, and is especially good for stimulating upward energy, as are foods such as *umeboshi* plum, sauerkraut, pickled vegetables, and naturally processed umeboshi and brown rice vinegar. However, please note that these foods are naturally processed with sea salt (a strong contracting influence that helps balance the expanding energy of fermentation), and as a result are best used in moderate amounts as seasonings or condiments.

Certain vegetables also activate the flow of upward energy in the body. As you can see in Figure 11, vegetables are nourished by both heaven and earth. Roots grow down, below the soil under the influence of heaven's force. Leafy greens branch upward, above the soil. The leafy green portion of vegetables such as daikon, carrots, turnips, and dandelion generally match the upward energy that nourishes the liver and gallbladder, and can be included daily as a part of a balanced macrobiotic diet. Light, barley miso soup, in which leafy greens are included, is an excellent food for the liver and gallbladder.

Fig. 11 Balance of Energy in Vegetables

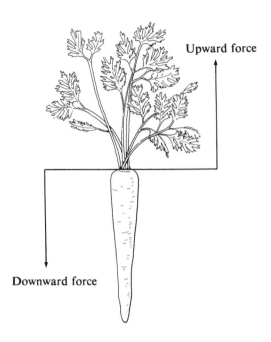

Upward force

Downward force

Interestingly, until modern times, many traditional cooks picked fresh dandelions and other wild greens in the spring and included them in their menus. Spring is the season in which earth's rising energy starts to become active, and is the time when we naturally seek lighter and fresher dishes to balance the changing environment. Eating dandelions and other fresh greens at this time helps release stagnation in the liver and gallbladder caused by months of heavy winter cooking.

Fruits with a naturally sour taste, such as plums and sour apples, can also be used on occasion to release tension and stagnation in the liver. Because of their strong expansive nature, fruits are best cooked with a pinch of sea salt before being eaten. Fire and salt are contracting influences, and help counterbalance the strong upward energy in fruits. However, a small volume of fresh, temperate-climate fruits may be eaten on occasion by those in good health. A small volume of high-quality natural barley malt may also be used from time to time to release tightness in the liver.

Rebalancing the Heart and Small Intestine

Foods with extreme energies are ultimately detrimental to the circulatory and digestive systems. Normally the arteries and blood vessels are open and flexible. Eating too many animal foods can cause them to become clogged with deposits of fat and cholesterol. If the blood vessels become narrow and constricted because of these accumulations, blood no longer flows smoothly through them. When this happens in the blood vessels that supply the heart, the result can be a heart attack. When it occurs in the blood vessels that supply the brain, the result is often a stroke. Both conditions are common today because people eat plenty of eggs, cheese, meat, and other fatty animal foods. As you can see, eating foods with extreme contractive energy restricts or suppresses the heart's natural function in distributing blood outward to the body. An overly constricted condition in the heart and circulatory system often appears as hardening at the tip of the nose. This condition is often accompanied by a hardening of the collagen that produces arthritis-like symptoms throughout the body, together with hard, dry skin.

The other major type of heart disease arises because of too many strong upward foods in the diet. Sugar, alcohol, chocolate, soft drinks, ice cream, and drugs and medications weaken the heart muscle and blood vessels. This can produce a wide variety of conditions including mitral valve prolapse, high blood pressure, enlargement of the heart, and others. An overly expanded condition in the circulatory system often appears externally as enlargement or swelling at the tip of the nose, or sometimes as a reddish color—caused by the dilation of capillaries—on the tip of the nose or face as a whole.

As an example of how overconsumption of more yin foods or beverages effect the body, a study in the *New England Journal of Medicine* published in February, 1989 revealed that long-term overconsumption of alcohol was damaging to the heart and other muscles of the body. In the study of 50 alcoholic men conducted at the University of Barcelona, almost half the subjects had deteriorating muscle strength that was directly related to the total amount of alcohol consumed. Sugar, chocolate, tropical fruits, soft drinks, and other extremely yin foods or beverages have a similar long-term effect.

The heart and circulatory vessels are especially charged by actively expanding energy, similar to that which predominates in the atmosphere in summer. The heart is located near the central line of energy deep within the body and nourished by the active flow of heaven's and earth's forces along this channel. The rhythmic pulse of heaven's and earth's forces in the heart chakra produces the rhythmic expansion and contraction of the heartbeat.

The small intestine is energetically compatible with the heart. The small intestine chakra is also situated along the active, central channel of energy, and is charged directly by the pulse of heaven's and earth's forces along this line.

Our digestive tract is well suited to digesting plant foods. Human intestines are longer than those of carnivores such as lions and tigers. Our long, convoluted intestines provide ample opportunity for animal foods to break down into toxic bacteria and compounds such as ammonia. The toxic by-products generated by the decomposition of animal foods often accumulate in the intestines and deplete the stock of beneficial bacteria found there, while the saturated fats in animal foods clog the capillaries in the villi and diminish their powers of absorption.

Strong expansive foods cause the villi to become chronically dilated, and this also weakens their ability to absorb digested food particles. These conditions can lead to a situation in which someone must continually eat larger and larger amounts of food in order to obtain nutrients. They wind up eating more and using less. The common result is overweight combined with nutritional deficiency. For many people, being overweight is the primary obstacle to looking and feeling good.

Among the grains and their immediate relatives, corn helps restore balance to the heart and small intestine. Corn that is freshly picked in summer is especially beneficial. It can be eaten on the cob (without butter of course), or used in soups, vegetable, sea vegetable, and a variety of other dishes. Summer vegetables, including cucumber, broad leafy greens such as mustard greens and Chinese cabbage, and other fresh, farm and garden produce, also help dissolve deposits of fat and cholesterol.

Sea vegetables embody qualities of flexibility and strength that are ideal for toning the heart and circulatory vessels. Their flexibility comes from growing in a watery environment where they gently sway back and forth under the influence of tides and ocean currents. Their strength comes from their high mineral content. When eaten regularly as a part of a balanced diet, sea vegetables such as wakame, kombu, arame, and hijiki impart strength and resilience to the circulatory system as a whole.

Plants from the sea are also good for the intestines. The villi in the small intestine are like single-celled amoeba or primitive sea plants that suck in and absorb nutrients. Sea vegetables, which are more primitive than land plants, strengthen the villi. Naturally fermented foods also have a primitive quality, due to the bacteria and enzymes they contain. Eating them helps strengthen the beneficial bacteria that inhabit the small intestine. (These bacteria are often depleted by antibiotics.) When used properly, fermented foods such as pickles, sauerkraut, umeboshi plum, and fermented soyfoods like miso and tamari soy sauce are all beneficial to the intestines. Miso soup, in which wakame is included, is especially good for strengthening the small intestine.

Rebalancing the Pancreas, Spleen, and Stomach

The pancreas and spleen have a more solid and compact structure and are energized by the downward flow of heaven's force on the left side of the body. The hollow and expanded stomach is compatible with these organs and is also nourished by downward energy on the left side.

Complex carbohydrates, which are charged by downward energy, have a stabilizing effect on these organs. Good sources of complex carbohydrate include whole grains, beans, naturally sweet vegetables such as cabbage, fall squash, carrots, and onions, and sea vegetables. Complex carbohydrates help the pancreas maintain proper levels of glucose in the blood.

Among cereal grains, millet is especially good for restoring the balance of energy in these organs. It can be cooked along with brown rice in your main grain dish, and also makes a delicious soup, especially when combined with naturally sweet vegetables such as squash or carrots. Soft millet makes a delicious porridge that is especially nourishing and soothing in the morning. Sweet brown rice, which is more glutenous and higher in fat and protein than regular brown rice, also provides a natural sweetness that harmonizes the energy in these organs. It can be included as a special grain from time to time. Sweet brown rice is especially delicious when cooked along with dried chestnuts, which are also a good source of complex carbohydrates. Pounded sweet brown rice, known as *mochi*, is also an excellent source of natural sweetness, and can be eaten often as a snack. Mochi and other sweet-rice dishes also help the skin become smooth, full, and naturally beautiful.

Naturally sweet vegetables are also good for the energy balance in these organs. The desire for sweetness is natural and instinctive. Everyone is attracted to sweets to balance the naturally salty bloodstream and because of the body's constant requirements for energy. Newborn babies, for example, are automatically attracted to the natural sweetness in mother's milk, and this enables them to grow. However, the key issue in life is what quality of sweet we select to satisfy this natural attraction. If we choose wisely, meaning the high-quality, naturally sweet flavor of whole grains, beans, sweet-tasting vegetables, and other complex carbohydrate foods, we can enjoy natural health and beauty throughout life. If we choose unwisely, meaning the processed, artificially sweet flavor of simple sugar, we risk losing natural health and beauty. We consider complex carbohydrates "natural" because their sweetness is readily available as is. Whole grains harvested from the field or sweet vegetables taken from the garden require no processing, other than cooking and thorough chewing, to extract their naturally sweet flavor. On the other hand, refined and processed sugars require a great deal of processing to extract their sweetness. Tropical fruits, which also contain simple sugars, are not native to temperate climates, and are available in those regions only because of modern methods of transportation and refrigeration, as well as chemically intensive agriculture.

Fig. 12   The Circle of Tastes

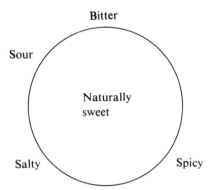

For maximum health and enjoyment, it is important to base each meal around the naturally sweet flavor of whole grains, beans, sweet-tasting vegetables, and other complex carbohydrate foods. The other flavors—sour, bitter, spicy, and salty—are best kept mild and used to contrast and bring forth the naturally sweet flavor of these foods. In macrobiotic cooking, the sour taste is provided by foods such as umeboshi plums, sauerkraut and other pickled vegetables, sour fruits like apples, plums, and occasionally lemon, and naturally fermented umeboshi and brown rice vinegar. The bitter taste is provided by leafy green vegetables such as watercress, parsley, daikon, carrot, turnip, mustard, and other greens, and by condiments and other foods that are lightly roasted. A mild spicy flavor comes from chopped raw scallions, grated raw daikon, and occasionally natural mustard or ginger. A salty flavor is provided by the moderate use of condiments, seasonings, pickles, and other foods that are naturally processed with sea salt. Again, these supplementary flavors are best kept mild and used to highlight, rather than overwhelm or cover up, the natural sweetness of complex carbohydrates.

Naturally sweet grains and vegetables also restore balance to the stomach and spleen. Chewing well is also essential, as saliva, a mildly alkaline substance, helps neutralize strong acid in the stomach. Umeboshi plums, which have an alkalizing effect in the body, are especially helpful in rebalancing and strengthening the stomach and digestive organs. They can be used as condiments several times per week or in making *ume-sho-kuzu*, a traditional home remedy for neutralizing an overacid stomach and strengthening the digestive organs as a whole.

Rebalancing the Lungs and Large Intestine

The lungs are densely packed with blood vessels and tiny air sacs known as *alveoli*. They have a more dense or compact structure and are counterbalanced in the body by the large intestine, which is a long (about 1.5 meters) hollow tube that is squeezed like an accordion into a tight space. Both organs span the left and right sides of the body, and on the whole represent more dense or contracted energy.

Because of their more condensed energy, the lungs and large intestine are particularly sensitive to yang extremes, including meat, eggs, cheese, poultry, and other animal foods. As we saw earlier, our long and convoluted digestive tract is well suited to the breakdown and absorption of plant fibers. Energetically, there is a tremendous difference between plant and animal foods. The minerals, proteins, carbohydrates, and fats in plants are very stable, while the proteins and other nutrients in animal foods are highly unstable. Whole grains, for example, retain their life energy and nutritive value for hundreds or even thousands of years, and as macrobiotic cooks around the world have discovered, grains, beans, sea vegetables, and other vegetable foods can be stored without refrigeration or artificial preservation. On the other hand, animal foods decompose very quickly, and a great deal of effort and expense is required to slow the speed at which they break down into toxic compounds and bacteria. This unstable quality creates numerous problems in the large intestine.

It is well known that the rates of colon cancer are highest among people in the modern, industrialized countries who consume a great deal of meat, poultry, and dairy food, and lowest among people in Asian, African, and Latin American countries where animal food is eaten much less often. Conversely, the rates of colon cancer are highest among people who consume little dietary fiber and lowest among those for whom fiber is a major part of the diet. Interestingly, the relationship between consumption of animal food and consumption of vegetable fiber tends to be complementary and antagonistic. People who eat a great deal of animal food consume less fiber, while those who eat plenty of fiber tend to consume less animal food. In the past, dietary fiber formed a much greater part of people's diets worldwide, but as the intake of animal food increased in the twentieth century, consumption of fiber went down. According to some estimates, the intake of fiber is now about one-fifth of what it was a hundred years ago, mostly as the result of a steep drop in grain consumption. It was during this time that the rates of colon, breast, and other cancers, heart disease, and other degenerative conditions became epidemic.

Overintake of sugar, chocolate, ice cream, tropical fruits, tomatoes, potatoes, and other nightshade vegetables, drugs and medications, and other yin extremes can cause the intestine to become swollen and loose. In this condition, peristalsis becomes too weak to move waste products through with regularity, and chronic constipation is the result. Milk and milk products also contribute to this problem by causing irritation and allergic reactions in the digestive tract. Allergy to cow's milk often begins in infancy and takes the form of frequent digestive upsets, irritation, diarrhea, and other problems in the digestive tract that continue throughout life. Milk, milk products, and simple sugars also cause sticky mucus to accumulate in the lungs and large intestine, resulting in a lessening of the capacity to absorb oxygen and discharge carbon dioxide and other waste products. A lack of oxygen in the bloodstream contributes to anemia and stale, unhealthy looking skin, hair, and nails.

The fiber and nutrients in brown rice are ideal for restoring health to these organs. Brown rice matures and is harvested in the autumn, a season of downward or condensed energy in the atmosphere that matches the energy of the lungs and large intestine. Brown rice also has an ideal balance between minerals, proteins, and carbohydrates, making it suitable for use as a principal grain throughout the year. Brown rice is also easy and delicious to eat in its whole form. There is no need to crush it into flour or process it in some way. Moreover, the fiber in rice bran (contained in the outer coat of brown rice) has been found to be highly effective in reducing cholesterol. Recent studies conducted by the U.S. Department of Agriculture found that a diet including 10 percent dietary fiber from rice bran reduces cholesterol by more than 15 percent.

Of course, other whole grains also contain fiber that lowers cholesterol. However, care must be taken when eating grains in the form of flour. Too many baked flour products—even those made from whole grains—can cause stagnation in the intestines and digestive tract.

Figure 11 (p. 96) can help us understand how to use daily food to rebalance the energy in the lungs and large intestine. The root portion of the vegetable, which grows below the ground under the influence of heaven's force, activates and energizes the lower body, including the intestines. Roots absorb nutrients from the soil, similar to the way that the intestines absorb nutrients from daily food. Conversely, the leafy green portion, which grows upward due to the influence of earth's expanding energy, nourishes the upper body, including the lungs. Leafy greens perform a respiratory function for plants, just as the lungs do in our bodies. In order to receive a balanced mix of upward and downward energy, try to obtain carrots, daikon, turnips, and other root vegetables along with their leafy green tops. Both sections can be cooked in the same dish or separately. Contracted greens such as these match the condensed energy of the lungs and large intestine more closely than those with broader and more expanded leaves. Among these vegetables, carrots and their tops are especially good for the lungs and large intestine.

Burdock, a long brown root that grows wild throughout North America and other parts of the world, is excellent for vitalizing the intestines. It grows deep in the soil and is strongly charged with heaven's force. Burdock is good for strengthening digestion and reducing fatigue. It can be included several times per week in a variety of dishes, including *kinpira*. In this dish, burdock is cut into thin shavings and sautéed with thinly sliced carrots in a small amount of sesame oil or water.

Kuzu, a white starch powder made from the root of the kuzu plant, also strengthens the digestion. Like burdock, kuzu root grows deep into the soil and is charged with strong heaven's energy. In the southern United States where the plant is plentiful, it is referred to as kudzu. It can be used in making soups, sauces, gravies, and desserts, and in preparing ume-sho-kuzu.

Lotus root (the edible root of the lotus flower plant) grows underwater in segmented lengths and has been valued for centuries in traditional medicine for its properties in dissolving mucus and restoring health to the lungs and respiratory organs. Lotus root is light brown in color and contains thin, hollow chambers. It is available fresh (in season) and dried in Oriental and natural food markets. Both varieties can be used often in preparing vegetable and other dishes. Lotus root is also used to prepare a tea that is especially good for clearing mucus from the lungs and respiratory passages.

As we mentioned earlier, sea vegetables restore strength and flexibility to the small and large intestines, and can be included daily in soups, side dishes, grains, beans, and condiments. One variety, known as agar-agar, is a good natural laxative. Agar-agar is processed into light translucent bars, flakes, or powder, and is used in making a delicious gelatinlike dish known as *kanten*. These products are dissolved in hot water and then poured over fruit, vegetables, beans, or nuts. Kanten is a delicious natural dessert that is especially refreshing in summer.

Rebalancing the Kidneys and Bladder

The kidneys have a more solid and compact structure that is counterbalanced by the hollow and expanded bladder. The left kidney is charged by heaven's downward force, and the right, by earth's expanding energy. On the whole, the energy that charges these organs "floats" between heaven and earth in the way that water does.

Dietary extremes cause a variety of imbalances in these organs. Too many animal fats clog the fine network of capillaries and specialized cells, or *nephrons*, in the kidneys that filter and cleanse the blood. Moreover, uric acid and other toxic by-products produced by the breakdown of animal proteins can often build up in the kidneys and damage these delicate cells. Excess sugar turns into fat that accumulates in the kidneys, and so the intake of cake, candy, chocolate, ice cream, and soft drinks can also interfere with the functioning of these cells.

Drinking too much also taxes the kidneys and bladder. People often drink more than they need. For example, a habit such as exercising in the hot sun and then drinking plenty of cold liquid stresses the kidneys and circulatory system. The result can be fatigue, tiredness, or the development of eyebags and other signs of expansion in the face. Theories that recommend drinking a certain amount of fluid each day to "flush" and cleanse the system also contribute to the tendency to overdrink. However, if we eat a naturally balanced diet and drink according to actual need, our system will not be toxic to begin with, and will not require "flushing" to remove waste products. The kidneys are also sensitive to cold. The intake of iced or chilled drinks and foods like ice cream accelerates the hardening and calcification of fat in these organs, and this can lead to the formation of kidney or bladder stones.

The kidneys are also very sensitive to salt. When used properly, high-quality, mineral-rich sea salt has a milder, less-harsh effect on the kidneys than refined table salt. However, it is best to use salt—even the best quality natural sea salt—in moderation. The overuse of sea salt or condiments or seasonings that contain it can lead to tightness in the kidneys and throughout the body, along with fluid retention that contributes to a puffy or swollen appearance.

Among whole natural foods, beans are especially good for strengthening the kidneys and bladder. Low-fat varieties such as azuki, chick-peas, lentils, and black soybeans can be included daily, as can naturally processed soybean foods such as tofu, dried tofu, and tempeh. A variety of other beans—such as pinto, navy, and kidney—can also be eaten on occasion.

A variety of macrobiotic drinks and home health-care practices also help restore health and vitality to the kidneys and bladder. Azuki bean tea, which is easy to make at home, is especially good. To prepare, boil one cup of azuki beans in three cups of water and simmer for twenty minutes. Strain off the juice and drink a cupful or two hot. Azuki bean tea can be enjoyed several times per week for about a month. The leftover beans can also be recycled and added to other dishes.

Hot ginger compresses also energize and activate the kidneys. To make a ginger compress, prepare a pot of hot ginger water as you would for the ginger body scrub discribed in Part III. Then fold a medium-sized cotton towel several times lengthwise, so that it becomes long and thin. Hold it from both ends and dip the center into the hot ginger water. Wring it out tightly, and if it is too hot to place on the skin, shake it slightly. Place the hot towel across the center of the back so that it covers both kidneys. Then place a dry towel on top of it to hold in the heat.

While the hot towel is still on the skin, prepare another ginger towel in the same manner. Apply it as soon as the first towel cools, and repeat this procedure, replacing towels every two to three minutes until the skin becomes red and warm. You can apply ginger compresses several times a week for several weeks. The ginger compress is fine for use by normally healthy adults as a part of home health care. However, it should not be used in cases of fever or inflammation. Persons with cancer or serious illness should use a milder application, such as a hot towel compress, unless otherwise advised by a qualified macrobiotic teacher.

Callouses on the ball of the foot where the kidney meridian begins (Fig. 7 on page 66) contribute to stagnation in the kidneys. Soaking the feet in hot water or ginger water can be very helpful in softening these deposits and releasing blocked energy in the meridian. It also stimulates the toes, including the fifth toe, which corresponds to the bladder meridian. Soaking the feet in hot ginger water is an excellent way to soften callouses and can be done whenever you do a ginger compress. A nightly foot soak in plain hot water is also recommended for those who would like to soften callouses on the bottoms of the feet. It is also helpful to walk barefoot on the grass, beach, or soil whenever the weather permits. This allows earth's force to charge the meridians on the toes and bottoms of the feet without the interference of shoes, and activates and stimulates their corresponding organs.

Beauty Cycles

The energy that nourishes the body is not static. It is dynamic and moving, and constantly cycles back and forth between upward and downward, inward and outward, and rapid and slow movement. These fluctuations occur together with cycles of energy in the earth's atmosphere and throughout the universe as a whole.

In the cycle of the seasons, for example, spring represents the beginning of expansion. New vegetation appears and green (a more yin color) begins to predominate. Summer is the period of peak expansion, as strong sunlight and high temperatures stimulate rapid and abundant growth in the vegetable world and plenty of activity in the human world. As summer draws to a close, vegetation becomes more contracted as red, yellow, and brown (more yang colors) gradually appear. Contracting energy becomes strongest in autumn, as trees and other forms of vegetation shed their leaves and enter a dormant state. Our activities also become more inward and mental in comparison to the activities of spring and summer. After the winter solstice, increasing sunlight slowly reactivates the vegetable world. This process is gradual and is offset somewhat by continuing cold temperatures, so that the atmosphere tends to float between expansion and contraction, or upward and downward movement. Then, with the arrival of spring, energy bursts forth in the plant and animal world and a new cycle begins.

A similar cycle occurs every day. In the morning, upward energy is stronger as the sun rises and we get up and become active. Upward energy reaches a peak at noon, after which energy starts to become more downward and contracted. Afternoon is a time of downward energy, and as the sun sets in the evening, energy in the atmosphere becomes very condensed. Condensed energy begins to disperse as morning approaches, and at night, the atmosphere "floats" between heaven and earth.

The movement of energy in the body changes in accord with these cycles. During periods when upward and expanding energy are stronger, for example, organs that are especially nourished by these energies become active. Conversely, during periods when downward and contracting energy are stronger, the organs charged by these forces become active. The flow of energy in the body correlates with the cycle of the seasons and the daily cycle of energy as follows:

Energy	Season/Time of Day	Organ Pair
Upward	Spring/Morning	Liver/Gallbladder
Expanding	Summer/Noon	Heart/Small Intestine
Downward	Late Summer/Afternoon	Spleen, Pancreas/Stomach
Condensed	Autumn/Evening	Lungs/Large Intestine
Floating	Winter/Night	Kidneys/Bladder

The facial features, skin, and other aspects of our appearance are influenced by these cycles. Body fluids tend to "float" up toward the head and out toward the periphery of the body at night. As a result, skin tends to look more full and fresh early in the morning after a good night's sleep. Wrinkles and other irregularities in the face often become less visible in the morning. However, if we are consuming too many liquids or fatty foods, eyebags and stretching caused by the pooling of fats or fluid may become more pronounced. The evaporation of fluid caused by perspiration during the day tends to make the skin and other cells in the body more contracted by afternoon. Dry skin may become more noticeable at this time, and if we have been consuming too many extreme yang foods, our face may start to look tight and drawn.

This tendency is made worse by the drop in blood sugar that many people experience in the afternoon. Chronic hypoglycemia, or low blood sugar, produces fatigue, anxiety, and stress, together with cravings for chocolate, ice cream, soft drinks, coffee with sugar, or other foods that cause a rapid rise in blood sugar. The outcome of giving in to these cravings is often excessive weight gain that undermines our self-image and appearance.

The emotional stress triggered by hypoglycemia also underlies a host of skin disorders, including eczema, hives, and others. Tension and anxiety cause the body to release androgens that activate oil-producing glands in the skin. The result is often an outbreak of acne, pimples, or oily skin. Other hormones secreted in response to changes in mood and emotions influence such external features as the color, elasticity, and tone of the skin, the activity of the oil glands, the circulation of blood to the capillaries below the skin, and the formation of new skin and hair cells. As you can see, diet and emotions have a direct effect on the way we look.

If we ignore these daily cycles, our health and appearance start to suffer. Normally, the downward movement of heaven's force causes us to seek relaxation and sleep at night. Skin and other body cells draw in energy from the environment that recharges and refreshes each cell. Foods with strong upward energy counteract and disturb this cycle. Coffee, for example, accelerates upward energy in the body. It causes the most yin portion of the brain—the forebrain—to become hyperstimulated. Drinking coffee makes it difficult to fall asleep when we should. If this happens often, the result is chronic fatigue that takes a toll on the way we look. Forcing ourselves to stay awake at night causes blood and energy to be diverted away from the face and skin and toward the muscles and internal organs. Chronic lack of sleep produces a strained, hollowed-out look and often causes dark circles to appear under the eyes that are signs of fatigue in the kidneys, adrenal glands, and body as a whole.

The cycle of the seasons also affects our health, appearance, and moods. Higher temperatures in spring and summer cause us to drink more, and the strong upward energy of these seasons accelerates the movement of fluid toward the surface of the body. As a result, more moisture reaches the skin and we perspire more readily. Conversely, downward energy and cold temperatures during the fall and winter often make the skin drier and more contracted. Oil glands become more sluggish during these seasons. Central heating also contributes to dry skin. Modern heating systems cause the air to become very dry. Many homes and apartments have humidity levels that range between 5 and 15 percent. If the humidity in the air drops below 30 percent, the atmosphere will rob moisture from the skin. Using heat moderately but not excessively helps to counteract this, as does opening the windows for short periods to allow outside air to remoisturize the air inside. Keeping green plants in the house, especially fast-growing varieties that require frequent watering, also helps remoisturize the atmosphere in your house or apartment.

Taking long hot baths or showers also causes the skin to become drier. The cells in the upper layer of skin readily absorb water, and the more they absorb, the more they contract and dry out once the water evaporates. Swimming in chlorinated swimming pools has a similar effect. Spending a lot of time in air conditioning also dries the skin, as modern cooling systems remove moisture from the air.

The changes in diet and activity that occur as the seasonal cycle progresses also influence our appearance. During the summer, for example, people often increase consumption of liquid, soft drinks, ice cream, raw fruits, and other yin extremes. These cause the heart and circulatory system to expand and overwork. The result can be redness in the face or tip of the nose, due to capillary expansion, or swelling at the tip of the nose. Overconsumption of yin extremes in summer also dilates and weakens the stomach, small intestine, and other digestive organs. The result is often the appearance of swelling or puffiness in the lips.

In winter, the intake of animal foods, fats, and other more contracted foods increases. If consumption becomes excessive, the skin may become drier and harder. These foods also block the flow of upward energy, including energy that nourishes the liver. As a result, liver lines may become more deep and pronounced in winter or early spring. Overintake of salt and fat during the winter can weaken the kidneys and make dark circles or bags under the eyes appear more noticeable. At the same time, eating more of these foods increases tightness and hardness in the pancreas and makes chronic hypoglycemia become worse. As a result, many people experience recurring depression during winter. This condition, known as *seasonal affective disorder*, or SAD, is the result of an excess of downward energy in the pancreas caused by dietary imbalances.

Transitioning to Natural Beauty

Eating a naturally balanced diet in harmony with the seasons and daily cycle of energy provides the basis for a natural, chemical-free approach to health and beauty. It is important to include a variety of foods in your diet. Including a wide range of whole grains, beans, vegetables, sea vegetables, soybean foods, seasonings, and condiments makes it easier for you to enjoy a wide range of energies in your meals. In Part II, we help guide you in this direction by presenting the full range of foods included in the standard macrobiotic diet. Although it is not necessary to use all of these foods at once, try to have as much variety as you can when implementing these guidelines.

Using a variety of cooking methods also helps you receive a varied and well-balanced mix of energies. Cooking has a tremendous influence on our health and appearance. In general, modern high-tech cooking devices, including electric stoves and microwave ovens, produce chaotic effects on the body's energy flow, and are not recommended for optimal health. On the other hand, more natural methods of cooking, including cooking with a gas flame, vitalize and harmonize the flow of energy in the body. In macrobiotic cooking, we use a wide range of cooking methods, including quick boiling and steaming to accelerate upward energy, and an equally wide range of styles, including slow boiling and pressure cooking, to accelerate downward energy. Learning to cook macrobiotically is an essential first step in making the transition to natural beauty.

A naturally balanced diet strengthens our condition and helps prevent imbalances from developing. As you continue eating well, you will look and feel more fresh, healthy, and alive. And just as each season and time of day has its own special beauty, you will look your natural best from morning until night and from season to season throughout the year.

PART II
Diet for a Beautiful You

Chapter 1 *Macrobiotic Guidelines*

Macrobiotics
Is as flexible and free
As nature itself

In Part I, we saw how diet influences our health and appearance, either positively or negatively. We discussed how foods common in the modern diet contribute to problems with the skin, hair, nails, and face, and how more centrally balanced foods such as whole grains and vegetables help prevent these conditions and contribute to a beautiful natural appearance. In this chapter, we present a complete diet plan for natural health and beauty. This way of eating, known as the standard macrobiotic diet, includes an incredible variety of whole natural foods. These guidelines are broad and flexible and help us to eat in harmony with nature. Thousands of people around the world now practice macrobiotics and have experienced improvements in the way they feel and how they look.

The standard macrobiotic diet is also in accord with the latest thinking in preventive nutrition. Dietary guidelines issued by the American Heart Association, the American Cancer Society, the U.S. Surgeon General, and other public health agencies are generally in accord with macrobiotic principles. It is becoming increasingly clear that a diet based on complex carbohydrates and high in fiber and low in fat, cholesterol, and processed foods can lower the risk of chronic illness. In many respects, the teaching of macrobiotics anticipated these guidelines and the current emphasis on preventive nutrition. For over thirty years, macrobiotic education has emphasized the importance of cooking with low-fat, high-fiber foods. The macrobiotic way of eating offers thousands of delicious and time-tested recipes.

The guidelines in this chapter are for persons who live in temperate climates. Modifications are necessary if you live in a far-northern or tropical zone. Of course, each of us has different dietary needs. An active working mother needs to select her foods differently from a retired grandmother. Children need to eat differently from adults. Individual guidance is always helpful when changing your diet. For this reason we suggest that you attend macrobiotic cooking classes or meet with a qualified macrobiotic advisor. Programs such as the Macrobiotic Way of Life Seminar and the Macrobiotic Residential Seminar presented by the Kushi Institute in Brookline and Becket are especially recommended for this purpose. Thousands of people from around the world have found these programs invaluable when beginning macrobiotics. There are also a wide variety of books that discuss the nutritional and health aspects of macrobiotics, as well as many fine cookbooks. For your convenience, these are listed in the bibliography.

The percentages of foods presented below are for an entire day's consumption and not necessarily at every meal. Breakfast, for example, is often more simple, while lunch and dinner are more elaborate. The percentages are calculated by volume and not by weight. It is not necessary to include all of these foods at once when changing to a more naturally balanced diet. However, it is important to have a wide variety of foods and dishes in your daily menus. The recipes in the following chapter can help you translate these guidelines into delicious and nourishing meals. Principal foods (the macrobiotic "four food groups") are eaten daily and include whole grains and their products, beans and bean products, vegetables, and sea vegetables. Supplementary foods such as low-fat, white-meat fish, seasonal fruits, nuts, and natural sweeteners are eaten from time to time, while condiments, snacks, pickles, seasonings, and beverages are used daily but in small amounts.

Standard Macrobiotic Diet

Whole Cereal Grains

Whole cereal grains are the staff of life and an essential part of a way of eating for health and beauty. For people in temperate climates, they may comprise 50 to 60 percent of daily intake. Below is a list of the whole grains and grain products that are recommended:

Fig. 1   The Standard Macrobiotic Diet

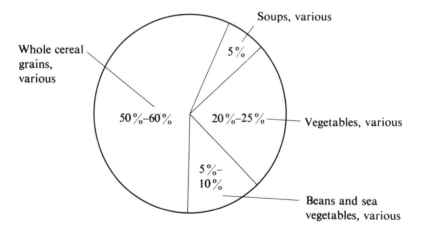

Plus occasional supplementary foods:
    Fish and seafood, using less fatty varieties
    Seasonal fruits, cooked, dried, and fresh
    Nuts and seeds, various
    Natural nonaromatic and nonstimulant
      beverages, various
    Natural processed seasonings and condiments,
      various

Regular Use
Short grain brown rice
Medium grain brown rice
   (in warmer areas or seasons)
Barley
Pearl barley (*hato mugi*)
Millet
Corn
Whole oats
Whole wheat berries
Buckwheat
Rye
Other traditionally used whole
   grains

Occasional Use
Long grain brown rice
Sweet brown rice
Mochi (pounded sweet rice)

Cracked wheat (bulgur)
Steel-cut oats
Rolled oats
Corn grits
Cornmeal
Rye flakes
Couscous
Other traditionally used whole
   grain products

Occasional Use Flour Products
Whole wheat noodles
Udon (wheat) noodles
Somen (thin wheat) noodles
Soba (buckwheat) noodles
Unyeasted whole wheat bread
Unyeasted whole rye bread
Fu
Seitan

Soups

Soups may comprise about 5 to 10 percent of daily intake. For most people, this means one or two cups or bowls of soup per day, depending on their desires and preferences. Soups can include vegetables, grains, beans, sea vegetables, noodles or other grain products, bean products like tofu, tempeh, or others, or occasionally, fish or seafood. Soups can be moderately seasoned with either miso, tamari soy sauce, sea salt, umeboshi plum or paste, or occasionally, with ginger.

Light miso soup, with vegetables and sea vegetables, is recommended for daily consumption, on an average of one small bowl or cup per day. Mugi (barley) miso is recommended for regular consumption, followed by soybean (*Hatcho*) miso. A second bowl or cup of soup may also be enjoyed, preferably seasoned mildly with tamari soy sauce or sea salt. Other soup varieties include:

Bean and vegetable soups
Grain and vegetable soups
   (i.e., brown rice, millet, barley, pearl barley, and so on)
Puréed squash and other vegetable soups

Vegetables

Roughly one quarter to one third (25 to 30 percent) of each person's daily intake can include vegetables. Nature provides an incredible variety of local vegetables to choose from. Those recommended for regular use include:

Regular Use
Acorn squash
Bok choy
Broccoli
Brussels sprouts
Burdock
Butternut squash
Cabbage
Carrots
Carrot tops
Cauliflower
Chinese cabbage
Collard greens
Daikon
Daikon greens
Dandelion leaves
Dandelion roots
Hokkaido pumpkin
Hubbard squash
Jinenjo
Kale
Leeks
Lotus root
Mustard greens
Onion
Parsley
Parsnip
Pumpkin
Radish
Red cabbage
Rutabaga
Scallions
Turnip
Turnip greens
Watercress

Occasional Use
Celery
Chives
Coltsfoot
Cucumber
Endive
Escarole

Green beans
Green peas
Iceberg lettuce
Jerusalem artichoke
Kohlrabi
Lambsquarters
Mushrooms
Patty pan squash
Romaine lettuce
Salsify
Shiitake mushroom
Snap beans
Snow peas
Sprouts
Summer squash
Wax beans

Avoid (for optimum health and vitality)
Artichoke
Bamboo shoots
Beets
Curly dock
Eggplant
Fennel
Ferns
Ginseng
Green/Red pepper
New Zealand spinach
Okra
Plantain
Potato
Purslane
Shepherd's purse
Sorrel
Spinach
Sweet potato
Swiss chard
Taro (albi) potato
Tomato
Yams
Zucchini

Vegetables can be served in soups, or with grains, beans, or sea vegetables. They can also be used in making rice rolls (homemade sushi), served with noodles or pasta, cooked with fish, or served alone. The cooking methods used for vegetables include boiling, steaming, pressing, sautéing (both waterless and with oil), and pickling. A variety of natural seasonings, including miso, tamari soy sauce, sea salt, and brown rice or umeboshi vinegar are recommended. To ensure adequate variety in the selection of vegetables, it is recommended that three to five vegetable side dishes be eaten daily.

Beans and Bean Products

Beans and bean products may be eaten daily or often, so that they comprise about 5 to 10 percent of daily intake. The following may be used in cooking:

Regular Use	Navy beans
Azuki beans	Pinto beans
Black soybeans	Soybeans
Chik-peas (garbanzo beans)	Split peas
Lentils (green)	Whole dried peas

Occasional Use	*Regular Use Bean Products*
Black-eyed peas	Dried tofu
Black turtle beans	Fresh tofu
Great northern beans	Natto
Kidney beans	Tempeh
Mung beans	

Beans and bean products can be cooked in the following ways: (1) with kombu (about 10 percent); with carrots and onions (about 20 percent); with acorn/butternut squash; with chestnuts (about 20 to 30 percent); in soup with vegetables; and with whole grains (about 10 to 15 percent beans). It is best to cook beans with a small strip of kombu. The minerals in the kombu soften the hard outer shell of the beans, making them more digestible. It also enhances their flavor.

Sea Vegetables

Sea vegetables may be used daily in cooking. Side dishes can be made with arame or hijiki and included several times per week. Wakame and kombu can be used daily in miso and other soups, in vegetable and bean dishes, or as condiments. Toasted nori is also recommended for daily or regular use, while agar-agar can be used from time to time in making a natural jelled dessert known as kanten. Below is a list of the sea vegetables used in macrobiotic cooking.

Regular Use (almost daily)
Arame
Hijiki
Kombu
Wakame
Toasted nori

Occasional or Optional Use
Agar-agar
Dulse
Irish moss
Mekabu
Sea palm
Other traditionally used sea vegetables

Condiments

A variety of condiments may be used, some daily and others occasionally. Small amounts may be used on grains, soups, vegetables, beans, and other dishes. Condiments allow everyone to freely adjust the taste and nutritional value of foods, and stimulate and contribute to better appetite and digestion. The most frequently used varieties include:

Main Condiments
Gomashio (a half-crushed mixture of roasted sesame seeds and roasted sea salt)
Sea vegetable powder
Sea vegetable powder with roasted sesame seeds
Tekka (selected root vegetables sautéed with dark sesame oil and seasoned with soybean, or Hatcho, miso)
Umeboshi plum (pickled plums)

Other Condiments
Cooked miso with scallions or onions

Nori condiment (nori cooked with tamari soy sauce)
Roasted sesame seeds
Shiso leaf powder
Shio kombu (kombu cooked with tamari soy sauce)
Green nori flakes
Brown rice vinegar (used mostly as a seasoning)
Umeboshi plum and raw scallions or onions
Umeboshi vinegar (used mostly as a seasoning)
Other traditionally used condiments (not highly stimulating ones)

Pickles

A small amount of natural vegetable pickles can be eaten daily or often as a supplement to main dishes. They stimulate appetite and help digestion. Some varieties —such as pickled daikon, or *takuan*—can be bought prepackaged in natural food stores. Others—such as quick pickles—can be prepared at home. Certain varieties take just a few hours to prepare, while others require more time.

Regular Use
Rice bran pickles
Brine pickles
Miso bean pickles
Miso pickles

Pressed pickles
Sauerkraut
Tamari soy sauce pickles
Takuan pickles
Amazaké pickles

Avoid (*for optimum health*)
Dill pickles
Herb pickles
Garlic pickles

Spiced pickles, vinegar pickles
(commercial apple cider
vinegar or wine vinegar
pickles)

Supplementary Foods

A variety of supplementary foods can be enjoyed occasionally. Some items can be eaten several times per week, and others—such as seasonings and beverages—are used daily but in smaller amounts than the foods listed above. Supplementary foods include:

• White-meat Fish

For variety, enjoyment, and nourishment, fish and seafood may be enjoyed on occasion by those in ordinary good health. The frequency of eating fish and seafood varies according to climate, age, sex, and personal needs and can range from once in a while to more regularly, the standard being about once or twice per week in a temperate climate.

Ocean Varieties
Cod
Flounder
Haddock
Halibut
Herring
Ocean trout
Perch
Scrod
Shad
Smelt
Sole
Other varieties of white-meat
   ocean fish

Freshwater Varieties
Bass
Carp
Catfish
Pike
Trout
Whitefish
Other varieties of white-meat,
   freshwater fish

Dried Fish
Bonito flakes (dried bonito,
   freshly shredded)
Chirimen iriko (very small dried
   fish)
Dried white-meat fish

Note: Shellfish such as lobster, crab, and shrimp are best limited or avoided for optimum health as they are high in cholesterol.

• Fruit and Dessert

In general, fruit can be enjoyed on occasion by those in normal good health. Frequency of consumption varies according to climate, season, age, level of activity, and personal need and health considerations. The average is about two to four times per week.

Among fruits, locally grown or temperate-climate varieties are preferred, especially for persons living in these regions. As much as possible, it is best to avoid consumption of tropical fruit. Below, the varieties of fruit that can be eaten in a temperate climate are presented according to season of availability or optimum season for use:

Spring
Cherries
Dried fruit
Plums
Strawberries

Summer
Apricots
Blackberries
Blueberries
Cantaloupes
Cherries
Dried fruit
Grapes
Peaches
Raisins
Raspberries
Strawberries
Tangerines
Watermelon

Autumn
Apples
Dried fruit
Grapes

Pears
Raisins

Winter
Pears
Raisins
Dried fruit

Dried Fruit (unsulfured)
Apples
Apricot
Cherries
Peaches
Pears
Plums
Prunes
Raisins

Avoid in a Temperate Climate
Banana
Dates
Figs
Pineapple
Other tropical fruits

• Nuts

Nuts can be eaten from time to time as snacks and garnishes. It is best to keep their consumption occasional and to eat them in small amounts. Nuts that are roasted and lightly salted (with natural sea salt) or a small amount of tamari soy sauce are preferred. Among the many types of nuts, nontropical varieties that are lower in fat are recommended. Below are several varieties of nuts for use:

Occasional Use
Almonds
Peanuts
Pecans
Walnuts

Nuts to Avoid (tropical varieties) for Optimum Health
Brazil nuts
Cashews
Hazel nuts
Macadamia nuts
Pistachio nuts

• Seeds

A variety of seeds may be eaten from time to time as snacks. They can be lightly roasted with or without salt. Varieties of seeds include:

Pumpkin seeds
Sesame seeds
Sunflower seeds
Other traditionally consumed seeds

• Snacks

A variety of natural, high-quality snacks can be eaten from time to time. They can be made from grains, beans, nuts or seeds, sea vegetables, and temperate-climate fruits. The following foods can be used as snacks:

Leftovers
Noodles
Popcorn (homemade and un-
  buttered)
Puffed whole cereal grains
Rice balls
Rice cakes

Seeds
Homemade sushi (without
  sugar, seasoning, or MSG)
Mochi (pounded, steamed sweet
  brown rice)
Steamed sourdough bread

• Sweets

The naturally sweet flavor of cooked vegetables is preferred for optimum health. One or several of the vegetables listed below can be included in dishes on a daily basis:

Cabbage
Carrots
Daikon
Onions

Parsnips
Pumpkin
Squash

In addition, a small amount of concentrated sweeteners made from whole cereal grains may be included when craved. Dried chestnuts, which also impart a sweet flavor, may also be included on occasion, along with occasional consumption of hot apple juice or cider. Additional sweeteners include:

Amazaké (fermented sweet
  rice drink)
Barley malt
Brown rice syrup
Chestnuts (cooked)
Hot apple cider (with a pinch

of sea salt)
Hot apple juice (with a pinch
  of sea salt)
Mirin (fermented sweet brown
  rice liquid)

• Seasonings

A variety of naturally processed seasonings are fine for regular use. Unrefined sea salt is used regularly in cooking whole grains, beans, and many vegetables. Tamari soy sauce, miso, and umeboshi plums, which have been salted and pickled, are also used frequently, but in general, the use of seasonings is best kept moderate. Rather than using them to add a salty flavor to your dishes, it is better to use them to being forth the natural light sweetness of the whole grains, vegetables, beans, and sea vegetables and other ingredients you are cooking with. The use of salt is a highly individual matter, and is based on factors such as age, sex, activity, and the climate in which we are living.

The following seasonings are used most often in macrobiotic cooking:

Regular Use:
Miso, especially barley (mugi)
   and soybean (Hatcho)
Tamari soy sauce
Unrefined white sea salt

Occasional Use:
Ginger
Horseradish
Mirin
Rice vinegar

Umeboshi vinegar
Umeboshi plum or paste
Sesame oil (dark)

*Avoid (for optimum health and
   vitality):*
All commercial seasonings
All stimulating and aromatic
   spices and herbs
All irradiated spices and herbs

• Beverages

A variety of natural beverages can be included for daily, regular, or occasional consumption. The frequency and amount of beverage intake vary according to the individual's personal condition and needs as well as the climate, season, and other environmental factors. Generally, it is advisable to drink comfortably and when thirsty and to avoid icy cold drinks. The following beverages are used most often in the practice of macrobiotics:

Regular Use:
Bancha twig tea (*Kukicha*)
Bancha stem tea
Roasted barley tea
Roasted brown rice tea
Natural spring water (suitable
   for daily use)
High-quality natural well water

Occasional Use:
Grain coffee (100 percent
   roasted cereal grains)

Sweet vegetable broth
Dandelion tea
Kombu tea
Umeboshi tea
Mu tea
Freshly squeezed carrot juice
   (if desired, about 2 cups per
   week)

Infrequent Use:
Green leaf tea
Green magma

Vegetable juice
Northern climate fruit juice
Beer (natural quality)
Saké (natural quality)
Wine (natural quality)

Avoid (for optimum health and vitality):
Distilled water
Coffee
Cold or iced drinks

Hard liquor
Aromatic herbal teas
Mineral water and all bubbling waters
Chemically colored tea
Stimulant beverages
Sugared drinks
Tap water
Artificial, chemically treated beverages
Tropical fruit juices

Natural Lifestyle Suggestions

Together with eating well, there are a number of practices that we recommend for natural health and beauty. Practices such as keeping physically active and using natural cooking utensils, fabrics, home furnishings, and body-care products are especially recommended. The suggestions presented below complement a balanced natural diet and can help you enjoy more satisfying and harmonious living.

- Live each day happily without being preoccupied about your health. Keep active mentally and physically. Sing a happy song every day to uplift your spirits.
- Greet everyone and everything with gratitude, particularly offering thanks before and after each meal.
- Try to get to bed before midnight and get up early in the morning.
- Try not to wear synthetic clothing or woolen articles directly against the skin. Wear cotton instead. Keep jewelry and accessories as simple, graceful, and natural as possible.
- Whenever possible, go outdoors in simple clothing. When the weather permits, walk barefoot on grass, beach, or soil. Go on regular outings, especially to beautiful natural areas. A half-hour walk each day activates circulation and energy flow and helps keep the hair and skin fresh and beautiful. Moderate exercise such as walking also lowers the risk of cardiovascular disease, cancer, and other illnesses according to a study published in the *Journal of the American Medical Association* in November 1989. The eight-year, 13,344-subject study was conducted by researchers at the Institute for Aerobics Research in Dallas reinforces the evidence that moderate exercise increases longevity and that it can help ward off cancer, a relationship discovered only in the past few years.
- Keep your home clean and orderly. Make the kitchen, bathroom, bedrooms, and living rooms shiny clean. Keep the atmosphere of your home bright and cheerful.
- Maintain an active correspondence. Express love and appreciation to parents,

children, brothers and sisters, relatives, teachers, and friends.

- Try not to take long hot baths or showers unless you have been consuming too much salt or animal food.
- Every morning and every night, scrub your body with a hot, damp towel until your circulation becomes active. When a complete body scrub is not convenient, at least do the hands, feet, fingers, and toes.
- Use natural cosmetics, soaps, shampoos, and other body-care products. Brush your teeth with natural preparations or sea salt.
- Keep as active as possible. Daily activities such as cooking, scrubbing floors, cleaning windows, washing clothes, and others are excellent forms of exercise. If desired, you may also try systematic exercise programs such as yoga, martial arts, aerobics, and sports.
- Try to minimize time spent in front of the television. Color television especially emits unnatural radiation that can be physically draining. Turn the television off during mealtimes. Balance television time with more productive activities.
- Heating pads, electric blankets, portable radios with earphones, and other electric devices can disrupt the body's natural energy flow. They are not recommended for regular use.
- Put many green plants in the living room, bedroom, and throughout the house to freshen and enrich the air.
- Chew each mouthful of food thoroughly, at least until it becomes liquid. Chewing serves as a form of meditation in which we are able to concentrate and appreciate our foods and the life-giving properties they contain. Chewing well also helps us to avoid overeating and maximizes the digestion and absorption of foods. Chewing releases tension and stress and helps us get more from less. It is especially important when complex carbohydrates are the mainstay of the diet.
- Whenever possible, try to avoid eating before bed, ideally for three hours. Eating before sleeping leads to the improper digestion and absorption of foods, and when it takes place regularly, to a gradual weakening of the digestive organs.
- The highest quality fire for cooking is that produced by wood; next, charcoal; followed by gas. Electric and microwave cooking are best avoided for maximum health. If you have an electric stove, convert to gas at the earliest opportunity.
- The best quality of water for cooking or drinking is clean well, spring, or mountain-stream water. City water can be used for washing foods or utensils. Distilled water is best avoided.

The art of cooking
Is the art of creating
Natural beauty

The recipes in this chapter make use of many of the whole natural foods introduced in the previous chapter. They offer you a sample of the hundreds, and even thousands of dishes used every day by macrobiotic cooks around the world. Additional recipes and guidance on shopping, meal planning, washing and preparing foods, and setting up your kitchen can be found in the macrobiotic cookbooks listed in the bibliography. We also recommend attending macrobiotic cooking classes in your area or programs such as the Macrobiotic Way of Life Seminar for personal guidance and training.

Unless otherwise noted, the recipes below yield four to five servings. Please adjust the quantities when cooking for more or fewer people.

Whole Grain Dishes

Pressure-cooked Short Grain Brown Rice

Brown rice is a staple in most macrobiotic households. We recommend including it on a daily basis.

>**2 cups organic short grain brown rice**
>**2½–3 cups water**
>**pinch of sea salt per cup of rice**

Wash rice by placing it in a bowl, pouring cold water over it to cover, and gently stirring with your fingers. Pour off water. Repeat once to remove any dust and broken or damaged grains. Then place the rice in a colandar and rinse once more under cold water. Once rice has been washed, place it in the pressure cooker and add water. Place the cooker, uncovered, over a low flame for about 10 minutes. Then add sea salt, cover, and turn the flame to high. Bring the cooker up to pressure. Reduce the flame to medium-low and place a metal flame deflector under the cooker. Cook for 50 minutes. After this time, remove the cooker from the flame and allow the pressure to come down. When the pressure is down, remove the cover and let the cooker sit for 4 to 5 minutes. Remove the rice and place it in a wooden serving bowl. Garnish and serve.

For variety: Cook the rice with 15 to 20 percent millet, barley, wheat berries, azuki or other beans. Wash millet separately as you would brown rice, and add it to the cooker along with the rice. Beans, barley, and wheat berries are best washed and soaked before you add them to the rice. Wash the beans, barley, or wheat berries in the same manner as brown rice. Then soak them in cold water for 6 to 8 hours and combine with brown rice, sea salt, and water. Cook as above.

Boiled Brown Rice

Boiled rice is lighter and fluffier than pressure-cooked rice. It can be enjoyed from time to time, especially in warm weather.

> **2 cups organic brown rice**
> **4 cups water**
> **pinch of sea salt per cup of rice**

Wash the rice and place it in a heavy pot. Add water and place on a low flame for about 10 minutes. Then add sea salt, cover, turn the flame to high, and bring to a boil. Reduce the flame to medium-low, and place a flame deflector under the pot. Simmer for 1 hour or until all water has been absorbed. Remove, place in a wooden bowl, garnish and serve.

For variety: Cook with 15 to 20 percent millet, barley, wheat berries, or beans. Prepare as described above.

Soft Brown Rice (Rice *Kayu*)

Soft brown rice makes a deliciously creamy breakfast cereal.

> **1 cup cooked brown rice**
> **3–4 cups water**

Place leftover cooked rice in a pressure cooker and add water. Cover, turn the flame to high, and bring up to pressure. Reduce the flame to low and cook for 25 to 30 minutes. Remove from the flame, allow the pressure to come down, and then remove the cover. Spoon into individual serving bowls, garnish with chopped scallions, and serve. Soft brown rice is delicious when eaten with a pinch of gomashio or umeboshi plum.

For variety: Add different combinations of grains or vegetables to the rice and cook as above. Winter squash cut into bite-sized chunks is especially delicious and sweet. Sliced daikon or turnips are also very nice. Once the rice is cooked, you may even season with a little puréed miso, simmer another 2 to 3 minutes, serve, and garnish.

Brown Rice with Chestnuts

Chestnuts are rich in complex carbohydrates. They make rice dishes incredibly sweet.

> **1½ cups organic short grain brown rice**
> **½ cup dried chestnuts**

2½–3 cups water
pinch of sea salt per cup of rice and chestnuts

Wash the rice and chestnuts separately as explained previously. Place in pressure cooker and add water. Let the rice and chestnuts soak 6 to 8 hours. Then add sea salt, place the cover on the cooker, and place the cooker on a high flame. Reduce the flame to medium-low, place a flame deflector under the cooker, and cook for 45 to 50 minutes. Remove from flame, allow the pressure to come down, and remove the lid. Place in a wooden serving bowl, garnish, and serve.

For variety: Cook brown rice with white or red lotus seeds in place of chestnuts. Wash the seeds, soak for 6 to 8 hours together with washed rice, and cook as above.

Rice Balls

Rice balls are an excellent food for lunch boxes or when traveling. Toasted nori helps keep the hair shiny and beautiful.

2 cups leftover cooked brown rice
1 umeboshi plum
1 sheet nori

Moisten your hands in a dish of water. Place 1 cup of cooked rice in your hands and mold it into a ball. Press your finger into the center to make a hole, and insert half an umeboshi plum in the hole. Pack the ball again until the hole is closed.

Roast the nori over a gas burner by holding it about 10 inches above the flame. Roast it for several seconds until the color changes from black to green. Fold the sheet of nori in half lengthwise, and tear in half. Fold in half once more and again tear. You should now have 4 equal sized squares of toasted nori.

Place the nori squares one piece at a time on the rice ball until it is completely covered with nori. Two squares of nori are sufficient for one rice ball. The nori will stick to the rice ball. It may be necessary to moisten your fingers occasionally to keep the rice and nori from sticking to them. Do not use too much water. The less water used in making rice balls, the better they taste and the longer they will stay fresh. Repeat with the remaining rice and nori. You should now have two rice balls. (To make more rice balls, simply increase the quantity of ingredients listed above.)

Fried Rice with Vegetables

The high-quality sesame oil used in this dish is fine for those in good health. It helps soften and beautify the skin.

4 cups leftover cooked brown rice
1 medium onion
1 medium carrot
1 bunch scallions
1–2 Tbsp dark or light sesame oil

1–2 Tbsp tamari soy sauce

Wash and peel the onion and then dice it. Wash the carrot and cut it into matchsticks. Place the sliced vegetables on a plate. Wash the scallions and chop finely. Place in a bowl.

Lightly brush a skillet with sesame oil, place on a high flame, and heat up. Place the onions in the skillet, and sauté for 1 to 2 minutes. Layer the carrots on top of the onions. Next, place the cooked rice on top of the onions and carrots, cover, and reduce the flame to low. If the rice is dry, add several drops of water to moisten when frying. Cook for about 10 to 15 minutes. Add the tamari soy sauce and scallions. Cover and cook for another 5 to 7 minutes. Do not mix until the last several seconds of cooking. Mix, place in a wooden serving bowl, garnish, and serve.

Millet with Squash and Cabbage

This dish helps satisfy the craving for sweets.

2 cups organic millet
1 cup buttercup or butternut squash
1 cup green cabbage
3 cups water
pinch of sea salt per cup of millet

Place millet in a bowl and pour cold water over it. Stir with your hands. Pour off the water and repeat twice. Then place the millet in a fine mesh strainer, rinse under cold water, and drain. Take a stainless steel skillet, and place it on a high flame to heat up. When hot, add the drained millet. Dry-roast by moving the millet back and forth with a bamboo rice paddle until it releases a nutty fragrance and becomes slightly golden. Be careful not to scorch or burn it. Remove the millet and place it in a pressure cooker.

Wash the squash and cabbage. Cut the squash into bite-sized chunks, and cut the cabbage into 1-inch pieces.

Place the vegetables in the pressure cooker with the millet. Add the water and salt, cover, and place on a high flame. Bring up to pressure, reduce the flame to medium-low, and place a flame deflector under the cooker. Cook for 15 minutes. Remove from the flame, and allow the pressure to come down. Remove the cover, and let sit for 4 to 5 minutes to loosen the bottom grains. Remove the millet and vegetables, place in a wooden serving bowl, garnish, and serve.

For variety: Boil the millet and vegetables instead of pressure cooking. Combine with 6 cups of water and a pinch of sea salt and boil for 30 to 35 minutes. Millet is also good with vegetables such as carrots, parsnips, turnips, rutabaga, or daikon.

Pearl Barely with Vegetables

Pearl barley (hato mugi) helps dissolve hardened fat deposits caused by eating animal food. It can be eaten regularly to help keep the skin smooth, soft, and beautiful.

2 cups pearl barley (hato mugi)
5 shiitake mushrooms
5½–6 cups water
1 strip kombu, 3–4 inches long
3 stalks celery
2 medium carrots
¼ cup scallion roots
1 medium onion

Place the shiitake mushrooms in a small bowl, cover with warm water, and soak for 10 to 15 minutes. Remove and squeeze out the water with your hands. Save the soaking water, and include it as part of the water measurement above. Remove and discard the stems. Dice the shiitake and set on a plate. Wipe the kombu with a clean, damp sponge, and place in a small bowl. Cover with cold water and soak for 3 to 5 minutes. Remove and dice. Set diced kombu on a plate. Save the soaking water and include as part of the water measurement above.

Dice the celery and the carrots. Finely mince the scallion roots. Dice the onion.

Wash the pearl barley as you would brown rice. Place the barley, vegetables, and water in a pressure cooker, cover, and place on a high flame. When the pressure comes up, reduce the flame to medium-low, and place a flame deflector under the cooker. Cook for 35 to 40 minutes. Remove from the flame and allow the pressure to come down. Remove the cover, place in a serving bowl, garnish, and serve.

Brown Rice with Barley

Barley adds a nice light quality to your main rice dish.

1½ cups organic brown rice
½ cup barley
2½–3 cups water
pinch of sea salt per cup of rice and barley

Wash the barley, place in a bowl, cover with cold water, and soak for 6 to 8 hours.

Wash the rice and place in a pressure cooker. Add the soaked barley. Add the water, including the barley soaking water. Place the uncovered pressure cooker on a low flame for about 10 minutes. Add the sea salt and cover. Turn the flame to high, and bring up to pressure. When the pressure is up, reduce the flame to medium-low, place a flame deflector under the cooker, and cook for 50 minutes. Remove from the flame, and allow the pressure to come down. When the pressure is down, remove the cover, and let sit for 4 to 5 minutes. Remove, place in a wooden serving bowl, garnish, and serve.

Sweet Brown Rice with Black Soybeans

Sweet brown rice is more glutenous than regular rice and rich in protein. It helps keep the skin and hair full and soft.

1½ cups organic sweet brown rice
½ cup organic black soybeans

2½–3 cups water
pinch of sea salt per cup of rice and beans

Wash and drain the black soybeans. Heat a stainless steel skillet. When the skillet is hot, place the damp beans in it, and dry-roast by pushing them back and forth with a bamboo rice paddle. Roast until the skin becomes tight and slightly splits in half. Remove the roasted beans and place in a pressure cooker.

Wash the sweet rice as you would plain brown rice, rinse, and add to the beans in the pressure cooker. Add water and place on a low flame for about 10 minutes. Add sea salt, cover, and turn the flame to high. When the pressure is up, reduce the flame to medium-low, and place a flame deflector under the cooker. Cook for 50 minutes. Remove from the flame and allow the pressure to come down. When the pressure is down, remove the cover, and allow to sit for 4 to 5 minutes. Remove the rice and beans, and place in a wooden serving bowl. Garnish and serve.

Mochi

Mochi, or pounded sweet brown rice, helps provide strength, suppleness, and flexibility to the skin and body as a whole. It is available ready-made at most natural food stores and usually comes in one pound packages or pre-cut into smaller pieces.

Slice mochi (if uncut) into several 2-inch by 2-inch pieces. (You should be able to get 6 to 8 pieces from a one pound package of uncut mochi.) Heat up a skillet, reduce the flame to medium-low, and place the mochi in it. Cover and cook for 3 to 4 minutes. Remove the cover, turn the mochi over, and brown the other side for 3 to 4 minutes, or until each piece puffs up slightly. Remove and place on a serving plate. Garnish with a couple drops of tamari soy sauce and chopped scallions, and serve with a teaspoonful of fresh grated daikon.

For variety: Place several pieces of toasted mochi in your miso soup for a very sweet, warming treat.

Corn on the Cob

Fresh corn is a wonderful summer treat. It has a nice light energy that calms and relaxes the body.

4 ears of sweet corn
1 quart water
small pinch of sea salt

Remove the husks from the corn and rinse under cold water. Place water in a pot, add sea salt, and bring to a boil. Place the corn in the pot, cover, and simmer 5 to 7 minutes, or until the corn is tender and sweet. Remove and place on a serving platter. Rub an umeboshi plum on corn for a delicious sweet and salty flavor.

Whole Oat Porridge

This traditional porridge is especially delicious on cool winter mornings. The soluble fiber in whole oats helps lower cholesterol.

> 1 cup organic whole oats
> 5 cups water
> pinch of sea salt

Place whole oats, water, and sea salt in a pot. Bring to a boil. Reduce the flame to very low and cook overnight. (This porridge can be made more quickly by dry-roasting the oats and pressure cooking them for 60 minutes.) Remove from the flame, place in serving bowls, and garnish with your favorite condiments, unsulfured raisins, or on occasions, a small amount of barley malt or rice syrup.

Soups

Basic Miso Soup

Miso soup is valued in traditional cultures for its cleansing and purifying qualities. It contributes to smooth and healthy skin and hair.

> $\frac{1}{4}$ cup wakame (approximately $\frac{1}{2}$ oz dry weight)
> 4–5 cups water
> 1 medium onion
> $1\frac{1}{2}$–$2\frac{1}{2}$ Tbsp puréed barley miso

Rinse wakame twice under cold water. Place in a small bowl and cover with cold water. Soak for 3 to 5 minutes. Slice the wakame into $\frac{1}{4}$-inch pieces.

Place water in a pot, cover, and bring to a boil. Place the sliced wakame in the boiling water, cover, and reduce the flame to medium. Simmer for 2 to 3 minutes.

Peel the onion, wash, and slice in thin half-moons. Place the onion in the water with the wakame, cover, reduce the flame to medium-low, and simmer for 5 to 7 minutes, or until the onion and wakame are soft. Reduce the flame to very low.

Place miso in a bowl and spoon a small amount of hot broth over it. Mix until it becomes a thick paste. Place the diluted miso in the hot vegetable broth in the pot, cover, and let sit for 2 to 3 minutes without boiling.

Take a soup ladle and place individual servings in bowls. Garnish with sliced scallions, chives, or chopped parsley.

For variety: Try different ingredients for a variety of textures and flavors, including:

> Wakame and daikon
> Wakame, shiitake mushrooms, and daikon
> Wakame, carrot, and onion
> Wakame, carrot, onion, and tofu
> Wakame, onion, and winter squash

Wakame, onion, cabbage, and carrot
Wakame, onion, carrot, and mochi

Millet and Squash Soup

This delicious soup helps relieve sweet cravings. It is especially good in the autumn.

$\frac{1}{2}$ cup organic millet
1 cup buttercup or butternut squash ($\frac{1}{4}$ medium squash)
1 strip kombu, 2–3 inches long
1 medium onion
1 stalk celery
1 piece daikon, 2–3 inches long
4–5 cups water
$\frac{1}{4}$–$\frac{1}{2}$ tsp sea salt

Wipe kombu with a clean, damp sponge. Place it in a small bowl, cover with cold water, and soak for 3 to 5 minutes. Remove and dice. Place the diced kombu in the bottom of a pot.

Peel, wash, and dice the onion. Place the diced onion on top of the kombu.

Dice the celery and place it on top of the onion. Quarter the daikon and slice into $\frac{1}{4}$-inch thick pieces. Place the sliced daikon on top of the celery. Cube the squash and place it on top of the daikon.

Wash and drain the millet. Then layer it on top of the vegetables. Add water, cover, and bring to a boil. Reduce the flame to medium-low, and simmer for 30 to 35 minutes. Add the sea salt, cover, and simmer another 10 minutes. Mix, place in individual serving bowls, and garnish with chopped scallions, chives, parsley, or celery leaves.

For variety: Cook squash with brown rice or barley. Barley needs to be soaked for 6 to 8 hours before cooking. Cook rice for 50 to 60 minutes; barley for 1 to $1\frac{1}{2}$ hours. The soup can also be lightly seasoned with tamari soy sauce or puréed miso instead of sea salt.

Azuki Bean Soup

Azuki beans help strengthen the kidneys. Eating them helps reduce puffiness and discoloration, especially underneath the eyes.

1 cup organic azuki beans
1 strip kombu, 2–3 inches long
1 medium onion
1 cup buttercup or butternut squash
1 stalk celery
1 leek
$\frac{1}{4}$ cup green beans
4–5 cups water
$\frac{1}{4}$–$\frac{1}{2}$ tsp sea salt

Wash azuki beans, place in a bowl, and cover with water. Soak for 6 to 8 hours.

Wipe kombu with a clean, damp sponge, place in a small bowl, and cover with cold water. Soak for 3 to 5 minutes. Remove and dice. Peel, wash, and dice onion. Cube the squash, and dice the celery. Wash and slice the leek into $\frac{1}{4}$-inch thick rounds. Wash the green beans and remove their ends. Slice the beans into pieces 1 inch long.

Place the kombu on the bottom of a heavy pot. Layer the onion, celery, leeks, green beans, and squash on top of the kombu. Then place the azuki beans on top of the vegetables. Add water, cover, and bring to a boil. Reduce the flame to medium-low, and simmer for about $1\frac{1}{2}$ to 2 hours or until the beans are soft. Add sea salt, cover, and simmer for another 20 to 30 minutes or until the beans are very soft. Remove from flame and ladle into individual serving bowls. Garnish and serve.

Puréed Squash Soup

This soup is incredibly sweet and delicious.

> **5 cups buttercup squash (1 medium size)**
> **4–5 cups water**
> **$\frac{1}{8}$ tsp sea salt**
> **sliced scallions for garnish**

Wash the squash and remove the seeds. Peel off the skin and cut the squash into chunks. Place the chunks in a pot, add water and a pinch of sea salt. Cover, bring to a boil, reduce the flame to medium-low, and simmer about 10 to 15 minutes or until the squash is soft. Remove from flame, pour the liquid and squash into a hand food mill, and purée until creamy and smooth. Place in a pot and add the remaining sea salt. Cover, bring to a boil, reduce the flame to medium-low, and simmer for another 10 minutes. Remove from flame, spoon into individual serving bowls, and garnish each with a few sliced scallions.

For variety: Try chopped broccoli, cauliflower, or summer squash instead of winter squash. Prepare as above.

Vegetable Stew

This dish is especially hearty and warming.

> **1 strip kombu, 2–3 inches long**
> **4 shiitake mushrooms**
> **2 sliced round fu**
> **4 slices dried tofu**
> **1 small onion**
> **1 stalk celery**
> **1 ear sweet corn (when in season)**
> **1 small leek**
> **2 medium carrots**

    1 cup green cabbage
    1 small piece burdock
    4–5 cups water
    1–2 Tbsp tamari soy sauce
    ½ tsp grated ginger
    sliced scallions for garnish

Wipe kombu with a clean, damp sponge, and place in a bowl. Cover with water and soak for 4 to 5 minutes. Remove, dice, and set aside. Reserve water. Place the shiitake mushrooms and fu in separate bowls, cover with warm water, and soak for about 10 minutes. Remove the shiitake, squeeze out liquid with your hands, and cut away the stems. Quarter the shiitake, set aside, and reserve the soaking water. Remove the fu, squeeze out liquid with your hands, and slice into bite-sized pieces. Reserve the soaking water, and set the fu pieces aside. Place the dried tofu in a small bowl, cover with warm water, and soak for about 5 minutes. Remove and squeeze out liquid. Discard soaking water. Rinse under cold water, squeeze again, and slice into 1-inch squares. Set aside.

    Wash the vegetables. Slice the onion into ½-inch thick wedges and set aside. Slice the celery on a ½-inch diagonal and set aside. Remove the corn from the cob, and set aside. Slice the leek into ½-thick slices, and set aside. Cut the carrots into bite-sized, irregularly shaped pieces. Cut the cabbage into 1-inch pieces, and set aside. Slice the burdock on a ¼-inch thick diagonal, and set aside.

    Layer ingredients in a pot in the following order: kombu, shiitake, celery, onion, burdock, fu, dried tofu, corn, cabbage, and carrots. Add water, cover, and bring to a boil. Reduce the flame to medium-low, and simmer 15 to 20 minutes or until the vegetables are tender. Add the tamari soy sauce and the leeks, cover, and cook for another 5 to 7 minutes. Squeeze ginger juice into soup, and simmer 1 minute more. Remove, spoon into individual serving bowls, and garnish with sliced scallions.

Vegetables

Steamed Greens (Kale)

Quickly steamed greens are rich in vitamins and minerals. We suggest including them daily. Substitute other greens for kale for variety.

    1 medium bunch of kale
    water

Wash the kale, remove the stems, and slice on a thin diagonal. Then slice the leafy green portion.

    Place about ½ to 1 inch of water in a pot, set a metal steamer basket down inside the pot, or a bamboo steamer basket on top of the pot. Place on a high flame and bring to a boil. Place the hard stems in the steamer basket, cover, and steam 1 minute. Set the sliced leafy green portion on top of the stems, cover, and steam until tender. For most greens this takes about 3 to 5 minutes, depending on the thickness or hardness of the vegetable. The greens should be bright green in color and slightly crisp when done.

If you do not have a vegetable steamer basket, place about ¼ inch of water in the bottom of a pot, cover, and bring to a boil. Place the stems in the boiling water, cover, and cook ½ to 1 minute. Set the leafy green portion on top of the stems, cover, and steam for 3 to 5 minutes.

Notes: Greens such as watercress, mustard greens, parsley, and carrot tops may become more bitter when steamed. It is often better to boil bitter tasting greens.

Boiled (Blanched) Salad

Boiled salads (quickly blanched vegetables) are rich in vitamins and minerals. They can be enjoyed daily or often.

This dish usually contains a variety of vegetables that may be sliced before or after cooking. Use the same water to boil each of the vegetables separately. Boil those with the mildest flavors first, and those with stronger or more bitter flavors last.

> **water**
> **¼ cup red onion, sliced in ¼-inch wedges**
> **½ cup carrots, sliced on a thin diagonal**
> **1 cup broccoli flowerettes**
> **½ cup cabbage, sliced in 1-inch squares**
> **1 cup cauliflowe flowerettes**
> **¼ cup celery, sliced on a thin diagonal**

Place about 2 to 3 inches of water in a pot, cover, and bring to a boil. Add the red onions, cover, and cook 1 to 2 minutes. Remove, drain, and allow to cool. Place the cooked onions in a bowl. Add the carrots to the boiling water, cover, and cook 1 to 2 minutes. Remove, drain, cool, and place in the bowl with the onions. Next, place the broccoli in the boiling water, cover, and cook 2 to 3 minutes. Remove, drain, cool, and place in bowl. Place the cabbage in the boiling water next, cover, and cook for 2 minutes. Remove, drain, cool, and place in bowl. Next add the cauliflower, cook for 2 to 3 minutes. Remove, drain, cool, and place in bowl. Last add the celery, cover, and cook 1 to 2 minutes. Remove, drain, cool, and add to the bowl with the other vegetables. Mix the vegetables with cooking chopsticks and serve.

Nishime Vegetables

This very sweet dish helps relieve the craving for sweets caused by hypoglycemia. *Nishime* is the Japanese word for the style of cooking used in this dish.

> **1 strip kombu, 4–6 inches long, soaked, and sliced in 1-inch squares**
> **4 shiitake mushrooms, soaked 10 minutes, de-stemmed, and quartered**
> **¼ cup celery, sliced in ¼-inch thick diagonals**

1 cup daikon, cut in ½-inch thick rounds
½ cup buttercup or butternut squash, sliced in large, bite-sized pieces
1 cup carrots, sliced in bite-sized irregular shapes
water
pinch of sea salt
tamari soy sauce

Place the kombu in the bottom of a heavy pot. Layer the vegetables on top of the kombu in the following order: shiitake mushrooms, celery, daikon, squash, and carrots. Add about ½ inch of water to the pot and a pinch of sea salt. Cover, bring to a boil, reduce the flame to medium-low, and simmer for about 30 minutes. Remove the cover, add a few drops of tamari soy sauce, cover, and cook another 5 to 7 minutes. Remove the cover, turn the flame up slightly and cook uncovered until there is very little liquid left in the pot. Mix the vegetables in the pot to coat them with remaining sweet cooking liquid. Remove and place in a serving dish.

Daikon, Daikon Greens, and Kombu

Combining roots and greens in one dish is an especially nutritious way to eat vegetables.

2 cups daikon, sliced in ½-inch thick rounds
1 cup daikon greens, chopped
1 strip kombu, 4–5 inches long, soaked, and cut into 1-inch squares
water
small pinch of sea salt
tamari soy sauce

Place the kombu in the bottom of a heavy pot. Set the daikon rounds on top of the kombu. Add enough water to half-cover the daikon. Add a pinch of sea salt, cover, and bring to a boil. Reduce the flame to medium-low, and simmer for about 30 minutes. Season with a few drops of tamari soy sauce, and set the daikon greens on top of the daikon rounds. Cover and cook another 4 to 5 minutes until the greens are tender but still bright green. Remove and place in a serving bowl with any remaining cooking water.

Kinpira Burdock and Carrots

This dish is especially good for restoring vitality and reducing fatigue. The word *kinpira* refers to the style of cooking used in this dish.

1 cup burdock, shaved or sliced in matchsticks
1 cup carrots, sliced in matchsticks
dark sesame oil
water
tamari soy sauce

Brush a small amount of dark sesame oil on the bottom of a skillet and heat up. Add the burdock and sauté 2 to 3 minutes. Place the carrots on top of the burdock, but do not mix. Add enough cold water to just cover the burdock but not the carrots. Bring to a boil, cover, and reduce the flame to medium-low. Simmer about 10 minutes or until the burdock is tender. Season lightly with a small amount of tamari soy sauce, cover, and cook another 5 to 7 minutes. Remove the cover and turn the flame to high, continuing to cook until there is almost no liquid left in the pot. At this point, mix the vegetables and place in a serving bowl.

Dried Daikon and Kombu

This dish helps dissolve deposits of hard fat and contributes to making the skin smooth and soft.

> 2 cups dried daikon, rinsed, soaked 5 minutes, and sliced
> 1 strip kombu, 4–5 inches long, soaked and sliced in very thin matchsticks
> water
> tamari soy sauce

Place the kombu in the bottom of a heavy skillet. Set the dried daikon on top of it. Add enough water to about half-cover the daikon (the soaking water from the daikon and kombu can be used as part or all of your water measurement). Cover, bring to a boil, reduce the flame to medium-low, and simmer for about 30 to 35 minutes. Remove the cover, season with a few drops of tamari soy sauce for a mild taste, cover, and cook another 5 to 7 minutes. Remove the cover, turn the flame up, and cook off any remaining liquid. When there is almost no liquid left, mix the daikon and kombu. Remove and place in a serving bowl.

Sautéed Chinese Cabbage

Vegetables are delicious when sautéed in a small amount of high-quality sesame oil. Sesame oil helps keep the skin smooth, soft, and flexible.

> 4 cups Chinese cabbage, sliced on a wide diagonal
> dark sesame oil
> tamari soy sauce

Place a small amount of sesame oil in a skillet and heat up. Add the sliced cabbage and sauté, gently pushing the cabbage around the skillet with cooking chopsticks until half done. Add a small amount of tamari soy sauce and continue to sauté until done.

Water-sautéed Vegetables

Vegetables can be sautéed in water if you need to limit your intake of oil.

> water
> $\frac{1}{2}$ cup onions, sliced in thin half-moons
> $\frac{1}{4}$ cup celery, sliced on a thin diagonal
> $\frac{1}{2}$ cup cabbage, sliced in 1-inch squares
> 2 cups buttercup or butternut squash, seeds removed and sliced thin
> tamari soy sauce

Place enough water in a skillet to just cover the bottom. Bring the water to a boil. Place the onions in the boiling water and sauté by gently moving them back and forth with a wooden spoon or chopsticks. Sauté 1 to 2 minutes. Next, place the celery, cabbage, and squash on top of the onions. Do not mix. Add enough water to just cover the onions. Bring to a boil, reduce the flame to medium-low, cover, and simmer until the vegetables are soft (approximately 10 minutes). Remove the cover, season with a few drops of tamari soy sauce, cover again, and simmer for another 4 to 5 minutes. Remove the cover, raise the flame to high, and cook off any remaining liquid. When the liquid is just about gone, mix the vegetables. Remove and place in a serving bowl.

Pressed Salad

Pressed vegetables retain vitamins, minerals, and enzymes. The easiest way to press vegetables is with a specially made jar known as a "pickle press" that can be found in most natural food stores.

> 1 cup Chinese cabbage, thinly sliced
> $\frac{1}{4}$ cup celery, sliced on a thin diagonal
> $\frac{1}{2}$ cup onion, sliced in thin half-moons
> $\frac{1}{4}$ cup red radishes, sliced in thin rounds
> $\frac{1}{4}$ cup cucumber, quartered and thinly sliced
> $\frac{1}{4}$–$\frac{1}{2}$ tsp sea salt
> 2 tsp brown rice vinegar

Place all the vegetables in a bowl and thoroughly mix sea salt and brown rice vinegar with them. Remove from the bowl, place in a pickle press, and tighten the lid and pressure plate. Let sit for about an hour before removing the cover. Then remove the vegetables, squeeze out any remaining liquid with your hands, and place in a serving bowl. If the vegetables are too salty for your taste, rinse them quickly under cold water, squeeze out liquid, then serve.

Fresh Garden Salad

Fresh salads add vitamins, minerals, fiber, and a fresh, light quality to meals.

> 2 cups fresh lettuce, washed and torn or sliced in bite-sized pieces
> $\frac{1}{2}$ cup carrot, coarsely grated
> $\frac{1}{2}$ cup cucumber, halved, and thinly sliced
> $\frac{1}{4}$ cup red onion, sliced in thin rings
> $\frac{1}{4}$ cup raisins
> $\frac{1}{4}$ cup roasted pumpkin seeds
> $\frac{1}{4}$ cup celery, sliced on a thin diagonal

Place all ingredients in a bowl, mix, and serve with one of the natural dressings explained below.

Cucumber and Wakame Salad

Besides being quite delicious, sea vegetables add calcium and other minerals to your salads.

2 cups cucumber, sliced in thin rounds
½ cup wakame, washed, simmered in plain water for 10 minutes, and sliced
1 cup iceberg lettuce, torn in bite-sized pieces
¼ cup roasted black sesame seeds

Place all ingredients in a mixing bowl and toss to mix. Spoon one of the following dressings over each serving. (For additional natural salad and dressing recipes, refer to *Aveline Kushi's Wonderful World of Salads*, Japan Publications, Inc., 1989.)

Umeboshi Dressing

This all-natural dressing has a wonderfully refreshing salty-sour taste.

2 umeboshi plums, pits removed
2 Tbsp roasted tan sesame seeds
1 tsp parsley, scallions, or chives, minced
¾ cup water

Place the roasted sesame seeds in a suribachi and grind until about half-crushed. Add the umeboshi and parsley and grind until smooth. Add the water and mix thoroughly. Spoon 1 or 2 tablespoonfuls of dressing over each serving of fresh or boiled salad.

Umeboshi-Brown Rice Vinegar Dressing

Naturally fermented brown rice or umeboshi vinegars are also wonderful in salad dressings.

2 Tbsp umeboshi vinegar
1 tsp brown rice or sweet brown rice vinegar
1 Tbsp chopped parsley, scallions, or chives
1 tsp mirin (sweet cooking saké)
¾ cup water

Place the parsley, scallions, or chives in a *suribachi* and grind for several seconds. Add the remaining ingredients and stir to mix thoroughly. Spoon 1 to 2 tablespoonfuls of dressing over fresh or boiled salad.

Tofu Dressing

Fresh tofu can be used to make a thick, creamy dressing for salads.

1 cake (1 lb) fresh firm-style tofu
1 tsp umeboshi paste or 3 umeboshi plums (remove pits)
1 Tbsp chopped scallions
2 Tbsp finely grated onion

½ **cup water**

Place umeboshi paste or plums in a suribachi and grind until smooth. Add the scallions and grind again until smooth. Add the onion. Purée the tofu in a hand food mill and place it in the suribachi with the plum, scallions, and onion. Purée until smooth. Add water and mix thoroughly. Spoon 1 to 2 tablespoonfuls of dressing over each serving of fresh or boiled salad.

Beans and Bean Products

Azuki Beans with Kombu and Squash

This deliciously sweet dish helps satisfy the desire for sweets. It can be enjoyed several times per week.

    1 cup azuki beans, washed and soaked 6–8 hours
    1 strip kombu, 3–4 inches long
    1 cup winter squash (buttercup, butternut, etc.), washed, and sliced into bite-sized chunks
    water
    ⅛–¼ tsp sea salt

Place the kombu on the bottom of a heavy pot. On top of the kombu, place the squash. Next, place the azuki beans on top of the squash. Add enough water to just cover the squash, but not the beans. Bring to a boil, cover, and reduce the flame to medium-low. Simmer for about 1½ to 2 hours or until the beans have softened. While the beans are cooking, you may need to add small amounts of water from time to time as water evaporates and the beans absorb moisture. Add only enough water to just cover the beans. Once the beans have softened, add the sea salt, cover, and cook for another 30 minutes or until they are completely soft. Remove and place in a serving bowl.

Chick-peas with Kombu and Carrots

Chick-peas become very sweet when cooked with carrots. They can be served in a variety of ways on a regular basis.

    2 cups chick-peas, washed and soaked for 6–8 hours
    1 strip kombu, 4–5 inches long, soaked, and sliced in 1-inch squares
    2 cups carrots, sliced in bite-sized chunks
    2½–3 cups water
    ⅛–¼ tsp sea salt

Place the kombu, carrots, and chick-peas in a pressure cooker. Add water, cover, and bring up to pressure. Reduce the flame to low, and cook for about 1½ hours. Remove from the flame and let the pressure come down. Remove the cover from the cooker when all pressure is out. Add the sea salt, place the uncovered cooker on a medium flame, and simmer for another 20 to 30 minutes until the beans are very soft. Allow any remaining liquid to cook off. Remove and place in a serving bowl.

Japanese Black Soybeans

Japanese black soybeans have been traditionally valued for their restorative properties, and were considered especially strengthening for the reproductive organs. Eating them helps keep the hair smooth and shiny.

> **2 cups Japanese black soybeans, washed and soaked 6–8 hours with a 4–5-inch strip of kombu**
> **water**
> **$\frac{1}{8}$ tsp sea salt**
> **tamari soy sauce**

Place the beans, kombu, and enough soaking water to completely cover the beans in a heavy pot. Do not cover. Bring to a boil. Reduce to medium-low, and simmer for 2 to 2½ hours. While the beans are cooking, you may need to add water to just cover them from time to time as liquid evaporates and the beans absorb water. Also, during the first half-hour of cooking, a gray foam will float to the surface of the beans. Skim this off and discard it. When the beans have softened (after about 2 hours of cooking), add the sea salt and cook for another 30 minutes or until the beans are completely tender. At the very end of cooking, when there is almost no cooking liquid left in the pot, add a few drops of tamari soy sauce. Mix the beans and cook another 4 to 5 minutes. Remove and place in a serving bowl.

Scrambled Tofu

This dish is a satisfying alternative to high-cholesterol scrambled eggs.

> **1 cake fresh tofu (1 lb)**
> **dark sesame oil**
> **$\frac{1}{4}$ cup onion, sliced in thin half-moons**
> **$\frac{1}{2}$ cup fresh sweet corn, removed from cob**
> **$\frac{1}{2}$ cup carrots, sliced in matchsticks**
> **tamari soy sauce**
> **$\frac{1}{4}$ cup sliced scallions or chopped parsley**

Brush a small amount of dark sesame oil on the bottom of a skillet and heat up. Add the onions, and sauté for 1 to 2 minutes. Layer on top of the onions, without mixing, first the sweet corn and then the carrots. Use your fingers to crumble the tofu over the vegetables. Cover, reduce the flame to medium-low, and simmer for several minutes until the vegetables are tender and the tofu is light and fluffy. Season with a small amount of tamari soy sauce, cover, and cook for another 4 to 5 minutes. Add the scallions, cover, and cook for another minute. Mix the tofu and vegetables and place in a serving bowl.

Tempeh and Leeks

Tempeh, a traditional Indonesian soybean food, is cholesterol-free yet rich in protein.

1 package fresh tempeh (10 oz), sliced in ½-inch cubes
2 leeks, washed and sliced into ½-thick diagonals
water
tamari soy sauce

Place the tempeh in a pot. Add enough water to cover, bring to a boil, cover the pot, and reduce the flame to medium-low. Simmer for 20 to 25 minutes. Add a small amount of tamari soy sauce, cover, and cook for another 5 minutes. Set the leeks on top of the tempeh, cover, and steam the leeks for 2 to 3 minutes. Remove the cover, turn the flame up, and cook off any remaining liquid. Remove and place in a serving bowl.

Sea Vegetables

Arame with Onion and Carrots

Arame is rich in calcium and other essential minerals. It helps keep the hair smooth, shiny, and strong.

2 cups arame (1¼ oz), washed, rinsed, drained, and sliced
½ cup onions, sliced in thin half-moons
½ cup carrots, sliced in matchsticks
dark sesame oil
water
tamari soy sauce

Brush a small amount of dark sesame oil in the bottom of a skillet and heat up. Place the onions in the hot skillet, and sauté 1 to 2 minutes. Layer the carrots and then the arame on top of the onions. Do not mix. Add enough cold water to just cover the onions and carrots but not the arame. Bring to a boil, cover, and reduce the flame to medium-low. Simmer for 30 to 35 minutes. Season with several drops of tamari soy sauce for a mild flavor, cover, and simmer for another 5 to 7 minutes. Remove the cover, turn the flame up, and cook until almost no liquid remains in the skillet. Mix the arame and vegetables and cook untill all liquid is gone (approximately 1 to 2 minutes). Remove and place in a serving dish.

Hijiki with Lotus Root and Onions

Hijiki is also rich in calcium and minerals. It combines well with vegetables, tofu, or tempeh.

2 oz hijiki (approximately 1¼ oz dry weight), washed, soaked 3–5 minutes, and sliced
½ cup fresh or dried lotus root
1 cup onions, sliced in thin half-moons
water
tamari soy sauce

If you are using fresh lotus root, wash, quarter, and slice in thin pieces. If you use dried lotus root, wash, soak in warm water for 30 minutes, and slice.

Place enough water in a skillet just to lightly cover the bottom and bring to a boil. Add the onions and sauté for 1 to 2 minutes. Layer the lotus root then the hijiki on top of the sautéed onions. Add enough cold water (include the soaking water from the lotus root as part of your water measurement) to just cover the onions and lotus root but not the hijiki. Bring to a boil, cover, and reduce the flame to medium-low. Simmer for 40 to 45 minutes or until the hijiki is tender. Add several drops of tamari soy sauce for a mild flavor, cover, and continue to cook for another 5 to 7 minutes. Remove the cover, turn the flame up, and cook until there is very little liquid remaining. Mix the hijiki and vegetables together, and continue to cook another minute or so until all liquid is gone. Remove and place in a serving bowl.

Wakame and Vegetables

Wakame is delicious in soups, salads, or cooked with vegetables. It strengthens and beautifies the hair and skin.

> 2 cups wakame, washed, soaked 3–5 minutes, and sliced
> 1 cup onions, sliced in thick wedges
> 1 cup carrots, sliced in bite-sized chunks
> $\frac{1}{2}$ cup parsnips, sliced in bite-sized chunks
> water
> tamari soy sauce

Place the onions, carrots, and parsnips in a heavy pot. Set the wakame on top of the vegetables. Add about $\frac{1}{2}$ inch of water to the pot. Bring to a boil, cover, and reduce the flame to medium-low. Simmer for about 30 minutes. Season with several drops of tamari soy sauce, cover, and cook another 5 to 7 minutes. Remove the cover, cook off most of the remaining liquid, mix, and cook 1 to 2 minutes longer until no liquid remains. Remove and place in a serving dish.

Kombu with Dried Tofu and Carrots

Kombu was used in the Orient to make shampoo. It strengthens and nourishes the roots of the hair.

> 1 strip kombu, soaked 3–4 minutes, and sliced in 1-inch squares
> 1 cup dried tofu, soaked 5 minutes, rinsed, and sliced in 1–2-inch pieces
> 2 cups carrots, sliced in bite-sized chunks
> water
> tamari soy sauce

Place the kombu in a heavy pot. Set the dried tofu and carrots on top of the kombu. Add enough water to half-cover the vegetables. Bring to a boil, cover, and reduce the flame to medium-low. Simmer for 30 to 35 minutes. Season with several drops of tamari soy sacue for a mild flavor, cover, and cook another 5 to 7 minutes. Remove the cover, turn the flame up, and continue to cook until almost all liquid is gone. Mix and cook 1 to 2 minutes more until all liquid evaporates. Remove and place in a serving dish.

Green Vegetable Sushi

These bite-sized vegetable rolls are perfect for lunch boxes or as a side dish.

> **2 bunches of watercress (or other leafy greens), washed**
> **2 sheets nori, toasted**
> **water**
> **4–6 shiso leaves, 4–5 inches long**
> **2 Tbsp tan sesame seeds, toasted**

Place about 2 inches of water in a pot and bring to a boil. Add the watercress and cook for 45 seconds to 1 minute. Remove, place in a colander, rinse under cold water, and drain. With both hands, squeeze excess water from the watercress. Place a sheet of toasted nori on top of a bamboo sushi mat. Take half of the watercress and spread it evenly to cover the lower half of the sheet of nori closest to you. Take 2 to 3 shiso leaves and lay them in a straight line across the width of the watercress and nori. Sprinkle 1 tablespoon toasted sesame seeds on top of the watercress. Tightly roll up the nori and watercress in the sushi mat as you would if making brown rice sushi. Before unrolling the mat from around the sushi, squeeze gently to remove any excess liquid, and to seal the nori tightly around the watercress. Remove the mat. Place the watercress roll on the cutting board and slice in half. Then slice each half in half, and each quarter again in half. You will now have 8 pieces of sushi. Place attractively on a platter. Repeat the same process with the remaining watercress and nori.

Condiments

Gomashio

Gomashio contains an ideal balance between sea salt, which is yang, and sesame oil, which is yin. It helps keep the skin and body as a whole strong yet flexible.

> **1–1¼ tsp sea salt**
> **1 cup tan or black sesame seeds**

Place the sea salt in a hot stainless steel skillet, and dry-roast for 2 to 3 minutes until the color changes from white to off white. Remove and pour the sea salt into a suribachi, or Japanese clay grinding bowl. Grind the salt with a wooden pestle (*surikogi*) until it becomes a very fine powder.

Wash the sesame seeds, place in a fine mesh strainer, rinse under cold water, and drain. Roast the damp seeds in a dry stainless steel skillet over a medium flame. Stir continuously with a bamboo rice paddle, pushing the seeds back and forth and shaking the skillet occasionally to evenly roast the seeds. When the seeds give off a nutty fragrance, darken in color, and begin popping, take a seed and crush it between your thumb and pinky. If it crushes easily, it is done. If not, continue to roast.

Place the roasted seeds in the suribachi with the ground sea salt, and grinds together until the seeds are about 80 percent crushed. Allow the gomashio to cool off completely before placing it in a tightly sealed glass container for storage. To use, sprinkle lightly over grains, vegetables, or other dishes.

Sesame-Sea Vegetable Powder

Sea vegetables also combine nicely with sesame seeds to make delicious and nourishing condiments.

  1½ oz dry wakame, dulse, or kombu
  1 cup tan sesame seeds

Place unwashed wakame, dulse, or kombu on a baking sheet, place in a 350° F oven, and roast for approximately 20 minutes or until dark and crisp, but not burnt.

Wash the sesame seeds, rinse, drain, and dry-roast in a stainless steel skillet as described in the recipe for gomashio.

Crumble the baked sea vegetable into a suribachi, and grind with a wooden pestle until it is a fine powder. Then place the roasted sesame seeds in the suribachi, and grind together with the sea vegetable powder until the seeds are about 80 percent crushed. Use as you would gomashio.

Miso Scallion Condiment

This condiment has a strong salty flavor. A small amount can be used from time to time as a relish.

  1 Tbsp barley miso
  2 cups scallions (green onion), chopped (chop the bulbs and roots very finely and keep them separate from the green stems)
  1 tsp dark sesame oil
  3 Tbsp water

Place sesame oil in a skillet and heat up. Sauté the scallion roots for 1 to 2 minutes. Add the chopped scallion greens. Do not mix. Place the miso in a cup, add the water, and purée. Place the puréed miso in the center of skillet on top of the scallions. Place on a very low flame, cover, and cook for about 5 to 7 minutes. Mix the miso and scallions and sauté 1 to 2 minutes more. Remove, allow to cool, and place in a sealed glass container until ready to use. Serve 1 to 2 teaspoonfuls occasionally with grain, noodle, or vegetable dishes. Store in the refrigerator.

For variety: Try chives, parsley, leeks, or carrot tops instead of scallions for a different flavor and texture.

Kombu Powder

This condiment is rich in minerals and helps strengthen the body's natural immunity.

4 strips kombu, 6–8 inches long, dusted off with a clean damp sponge

Heat up a heavy skillet and place the strips of kombu in it. Cover the skillet, reduce the flame to low, and dry-roast the kombu until dark and crisp, but not burnt. This may take 30 minutes or more. Remove the kombu, place in a suribachi, and grind to a very fine powder. Allow to cool and place in a sealed glass container to store. To use, sprinkle lightly over grain, noodle, or vegetable dishes.

Shio Nori

This condiment is rich in iron. It can be used from time to time as a relish.

> **1 package untoasted nori (10 sheets)**
> **2 cups water**
> **2 Tbsp tamari soy sauce**

Tear the nori into small pieces and place them in a saucepan. Add the water, bring to a boil, reduce the flame to medium-low, and cover. Simmer about 10 minutes. Add the tamari soy sauce, and cook for another 10 minutes or so until the nori becomes a thick paste and there is almost no liquid left.

One or 2 tablespoonfuls of shio nori may be eaten from time to time with grain, noodle, or vegetable dishes. To store, place in a sealed glass container and keep in a cool place.

Umeboshi and Shiso

Umeboshi plums are imported from Japan and are available ready to eat at most natural food stores. They grow in the warmer southern regions of Japan and are related to the apricot. Traditionally fermented with sea salt and pickled with shiso leaves, umeboshi plums combine a sour and salty taste. They strengthen digestion, help neutralize impurities in the blood, and keep the skin smooth and clear. They can be used in making rice balls and sushi, or in soups, dips, and salad dressings, rubbed on sweet corn, or served as a condiment with rice or other grains. The dark, red leaves that come with the umeboshi plums are known as shiso leaves. These salty-sour leaves can be used in preparing condiments and as seasonings in certain dishes. They have many beneficial properties, and are particularly helpful in keeping the hair strong and shiny.

Pickles

Pickles can be eaten frequently as a supplement to main dishes. They stimulate appetite and help digestion. Some varieties, such as pickled daikon, or takuan, can be bought prepackaged in natural food stores. Other quick pickles can be made at home. Below are recipes for delicious easy-to-make pickles.

Onion Tamari Pickles

> **2 cups onions, sliced in thin half-moons**

¼ cup tamari soy sauce
1 cup water

Mix the tamari soy sauce and water. Place the sliced onions in a quart glass jar and pour the tamari-water mixture over them. Mix and let sit for 2 to 3 days or up to 1 week. Refrigerate when done. When serving, rinse under cold water to remove any excessive salt taste.

For variety: Try pickling thinly sliced pieces of raw rutabaga, turnip, daikon, or carrot for variety.

Umeboshi Pickles

7–8 umeboshi plums
2 quarts water
3–4 cups sliced daikon, turnip, cabbage, or whole red radishes

Place the umeboshi in a large glass jar and add 2 quarts of cold water. Shake and let sit for 2 to 3 hours. Place the vegetables in the salty water, cover the top of the jar with clean cotton cheesecloth, and let sit in a cool place for 2 to 3 days. To store finished pickles, cover the jar and place in the refrigerator. When serving rinse under cold water and slice if whole.

Quick Umeboshi Pickles

1 package red radishes, washed and sliced in thin rounds
1–2 Tbsp umeboshi vinegar

Place the radish slices and umeboshi vinegar in a pickle press and mix. Fasten the top on the press and apply pressure. Let sit for 1 to 2 hours. Remove, rinse, and serve.

Brine Pickles

10–12 cups water
¼–⅓ cup sea salt
1 large onion, sliced in ¼-inch thick wedges
1 cup carrots, sliced on a thin diagonal
½ red onion, sliced in ¼-inch thick wedges
1 lb pickling cucumber, washed and quartered
1 cup cauliflower flowerettes, sliced in half
1 cup broccoli flowerettes, sliced in half

Combine the water and salt. Stir until the salt dissolves completely. Place the raw vegetables in a large gallon jar, and pour the salt water over them until the vegetables are completely covered. Cover the mouth of the jar with a thin layer of cotton cheesecloth, and let sit for 2 to 3 days (in warm weather), or 3 to 4 days (in cool weather). Cover the jar and refrigerate. Keep pickles in the refrigerator for another 2 to 3 days. To serve, simply rinse under cold water. These will keep about 1 month in the refrigerator.

For variety: Add ½ cup sauerkraut or a little brown rice vinegar to the salt brine for a different flavor.

Quick Daikon Pickles

> **4 cups daikon, sliced in very thin rounds**
> **¼ tsp sea salt**

Place the daikon and sea salt in a pickle press, mix thoroughly, cover, and apply pressure. Let sit for 2 to 3 hours. Remove, rinse, and serve. To store, remove from press, place in a glass jar, seal, and refrigerate.

Desserts ─────────────────────────────────

Sugar-free natural desserts are preferred for optimal health and beauty. Below are several easy to make recipes.

Fruit Kanten

This natural, sugar-free gelatin is made from agar-agar, a variety of sea vegetable. It has natural laxative properties.

> **3 medium apples, pears, peaches or nectarines, sliced thin**
> **1 quart apple juice**
> **pinch of sea salt**
> **5–6 Tbsp agar-agar flakes (read directions on package)**

Place the sliced fruit, juice, sea salt, and agar-agar flakes in a pot, stir, and bring to a boil. Reduce the flame to medium-low and simmer for about 2 to 3 minutes. Pour the hot mixture into a glass baking or casserole dish, individual fruit cups, or mold. Refrigerate until jelled (about 45 minutes to 1 hour), or place in a cool place until jelled (1 to 2 hours).

Baked Apples

Wash several baking apples and place in a baking dish with a small amount of water or apple juice. Cover the dish and bake approximately 20 minutes or so at 350° F or until tender. For variety, core the apples and stuff them with chopped walnuts and raisins.

Applesauce

Wash and peel several apples. Slice the apples thinly, place in a pot with a pinch of sea salt and enough water or apple juice to half-cover. Bring to a boil, reduce the flame to medium-low, and simmer until the apples are soft (about 10 minutes or so). Pour the apples and the liquid into a hand food mill set on top of a bowl. Purée the apples into the bowl. Eat hot or allow to cool before serving.

Amazaké Pudding

Amazaké, a naturally sweet drink made from fermented brown rice, is available ready-made in many natural food stores. It adds a wonderfully sweet flavor to desserts and can be eaten as is with whole grain porridges and other natural breakfast cereals.

> 1 quart amazaké
> 4 tsp kuzu, diluted in 4–5 tsp water
> ¼ cup walnuts, chopped and roasted
> ⅛ cup raisins

Place the amazaké in a pot. Dilute the kuzu and pour into the pot. Stir in well. Bring to a boil, stirring constantly to prevent lumping. Reduce the flame to low and simmer for about 1 minute. Remove and place pudding in individual dessert cups or in a bowl. Garnish with roasted walnuts and raisins. Allow to cool or serve at room temperature.

Stewed Fruit

> 1 quart apple juice
> ¼ cup raisins
> pinch of sea salt
> 2 cups apples, sliced thin
> 1 cup pears, sliced thin
> 2 Tbsp kuzu, diluted in 3 Tbsp water

Place the apple juice, raisins, and sea salt in a pot, cover, and bring to a boil. Reduce the flame to low and simmer for 10 minutes. Add the apples and pears, cover, bring to a boil again, and reduce the flame to low. Simmer until the fruit is soft, about 10 minutes. Dilute the kuzu and stir thoroughly into the fruit mixture. Simmer until the kuzu causes the juice to thicken, stirring constantly to prevent lumping. When thick and translucent, remove from the flame and place in a serving bowl or individual dessert cups. Serve warm or slightly chilled.

Fish and Seafood

Low-fat white-meat fish is a healthful alternative to other varieties of animal food that are high in saturated fat and cholesterol.

Broiled Sole

> 4 sole fillets, washed
> tamari soy sauce
> 1 lemon
> chopped parsley for garnish

Place the sole on a cookie sheet. Sprinkle with several drops of tamari soy sauce. Slice a lemon in half and squeeze several drops of juice on top of each fillet. Broil 5 to 7 minutes until the sole is tender. Remove, place on a serving platter, and sprinkle a little chopped parsley on each fillet for garnish. A tablespoon of grated daikon may be served with each piece of sole.

For variety: Other types of white-meat fish, such as scrod or cod, may be prepared in the same manner.

Sautéed Vegetables and Steamed Scrod

> 1½ lb fresh scrod (or other white-meat fish)
> 1 cup onions, sliced in thin half-moons
> ½ cup carrots, sliced in matchsticks
> ¼ cup celery, sliced on a thin diagonal
> ½ cup green string beans, sliced on a thin diagonal
> dark sesame oil
> ½ cup water
> fresh gingerroot
> 1–2 tsp tamari soy sauce
> chopped parsley for garnish

Place a small amount of dark sesame oil in a skillet and heat up. Add the onions and sauté 1 to 2 minutes.

Wash the scrod, place in a bowl, and soak for about 5 minutes.

Set the carrots, celery, and green string beans on top of the onions, but do not stir. Next, place the scrod on top of the vegetables. Add the water to the skillet. Grate fresh gingerroot, and squeeze the juice over each piece of scrod. Sprinkle a few drops of tamari soy sauce over each piece of scrod. Bring the water to a boil, cover, and reduce the flame to medium-low. Simmer until the vegetables are tender and the fish is done. Serve in the skillet or place in a serving dish. Garnish with a small amount of chopped parsley.

Trout Soup

This soup is especially good for restoring vitality and reducing fatigue.

> 1 whole trout, insides removed
> dark sesame oil
> 1½ cups burdock, shaved
> 1½ cup carrots, sliced in matchsticks
> 4–5 cups water
> 2–2½ tsp puréed barley miso
> ½ tsp fresh ginger juice
> chopped scallions for garnish

Wash the trout and leave the head, tail, fins, and bones intact. Slice the fish into 2-inch chunks.

Brush a small amount of dark sesame oil in the bottom of a pressure cooker and heat up. Add the burdock, and sauté for 2 to 3 minutes. Set the carrots and trout on top of the burdock but do not mix. Add the water, cover the cooker, place on a high flame, and bring up to pressure. Reduce the flame to medium-low and cook for 50 minutes. Remove from flame and allow the pressure to come down. Remove the cover and place the cooker on a low flame. Add the puréed miso and ginger juice. Simmer, uncovered, for 2 to 3 minutes. Place in individual serving bowls and garnish with a small amount of chopped scallions.

Fish Stew

> 1–1½ lb fresh cod, scrod, or other white-meat fish
> 1 strip kombu, 3–4 inches long, soaked and cubed
> 4–5 shiitake mushrooms, soaked 10–15 minutes, de-stemmed, and quartered
> ½ cup daikon, ¼-inch thick half-moons
> ½ cup celery, sliced on a thick diagonal
> 1 cup onions, sliced in thick wedges
> 1 cup carrots, cut in bite-sized chunks
> ¼ cup burdock, sliced in ¼-inch thick diagonals
> 5 cups water
> pinch of sea salt
> 2–2½ Tbsp tamari soy sauce
> ½ tsp fresh ginger juice
> chopped scallions or parsley for garnish

Place the kombu, shiitake mushrooms, daikon, celery, onions, carrots, and burdock in a heavy pot. Add the water and a small pinch of sea salt. Cover and bring to a boil. Reduce the flame to medium-low and simmer until the vegetables are tender. Wash and slice the scrod and place in the pot with the vegetables. Cover and simmer until the fish is tender. Add the tamari soy sauce and ginger juice, mix, and cover. Simmer for another 4 to 5 minutes. Remove, place in serving bowls, garnish with chopped scallions or parsley, and serve.

Beverages

A variety of caffeine-free, nonstimulant beverages are recommended for optimal health and beauty. Below are several examples.

Bancha Tea

> 2 Tbsp bancha twigs
> 1½ quarts water

Place the bancha twigs and water in a teapot, cover, and bring to a boil. For a mild tea, reduce the flame to low and simmer for 3 to 5 minutes. For a stronger tea, reduce the flame to low and simmer for 10 to 15 minutes. Pour the tea through a bamboo tea strainer into individual cups. Serve hot.

Roasted Barley Tea

> 2 Tbsp roasted barley
> 1½ quarts water

Place the roasted barley and water in a teapot, cover, and bring to a boil. Reduce the flame to low and simmer for 5 minutes for a mild tea, or 10 to 15 minutes for a stronger tea. Pour tea through a bamboo tea strainer into individual cups and serve hot. In hot weather serve slightly chilled or with a slice of fresh organic lemon.

Roasted Brown Rice Tea

$\frac{1}{4}$ cup short grain brown rice
1$\frac{1}{2}$ cups water

Wash and drain the rice. Place a stainless steel skillet over a medium flame and heat up. Place the drained brown rice in the hot skillet, and dry-roast, stirring constantly to evenly roast, until the rice becomes a golden color.

Place the roasted rice and water in a teapot. Cover, bring to a boil, reduce the flame to medium-low, and simmer 15 to 20 minutes. Serve as above.

Grain Coffee

There are many prepackaged grain coffees available in natural food stores. Choose one that does not contain figs, dates, molasses, or honey. To prepare, simply place a teaspoonful of grain coffee in a cup and pour boiling water over it. Stir and drink.

Hot Apple Juice or Cider

Simply place 1 cup of juice or cider in a saucepan with 1 or 2 grains of sea salt and heat up. Drink hot.

Sweet Vegetable Drink

This drink is especially helpful in relieving the craving for sweets that results from hypoglycemia. It is wonderfully relaxing and refreshing.

$\frac{1}{4}$ cup onion, finely diced
$\frac{1}{4}$ cup carrot, finely diced
$\frac{1}{4}$ cup butternut or buttercup squash, finely diced
$\frac{1}{4}$ cup green cabbage, finely diced
4 cups spring water

Place the ingredients in a pot and bring to a boil. Reduce the flame to medium-low and simmer for 15 to 20 minutes. Strain the vegetables from the juice. The vegetables may be reserved and used in miso soup or other dishes. Drink the juice hot, or to store, place in a glass jar, seal, and refrigerate until ready to drink. Heat up before drinking.

Spring or Well Water

The best quality water for cooking or for drinking is fresh deep well water or natural spring water. Sparkling mineral waters is not recommended for daily use, but for those in generally good health, it can be enjoyed on occasion.

PART III

Natural Beauty Care

External Beauty Care

Beauty begins with the simple affirmation "I am beautiful." Never underestimate or dismiss this most important statement. Beauty continues by taking charge of our actions, however small they may be. Beauty is understanding that "I am what I project" and observing it. Beauty is taking the time to nurture the self. The care we provide to our body is only a result of this affirmation.

No beauty-care products can beautify unless we ourselves know that we are a thing of beauty. This knowledge generates the respect for our body as a sacred gift to be observed and cared for.

The importance of being beautiful is as old as the beginning of time. The ancient Hindu body of knowledge known as the *Vedas*,[1] expounded innumerably the origin of beauty. The Upanishads[2] and the Gita referred to beauty as divine in essence. The Sanskrit term *Alankara* which translates as "perfected creation" refers to beauty as the subtle combination of the magical and the aesthetic. From the verses of the Bhagavad Gita,[3] it is said "Whatever object in the Universe is outstanding, beautiful or spirited, take it to be a product of my own brilliant aspect." (X-41)

The great Hindu sages, before the ages of Western philosophers, and poets celebrated the Goddess of Beauty with numerous hymns. *Sri* or *Lakshmi* is the Sanscrit name for beauty. It is said that the beauty of the Goddess Lakshmi is beyond the imagination of mortals and eludes even the creator, Lord Brahma. Srivatsanka Misra wrote "Whatever glory the Lord enjoys, whatever beauty, grace and goodness are manifest in the universe, all that is dependent upon you. It is that they are identified with you and referred to as graced with *Sri* or Beauty."

Beauty, according to the Vedas, is composed of three dimensions. The first is known as *Alankara* or that which connotes the external beauty. It is what is seen visually; the contour and shape of the face; the texture of the skin; length and body of the hair; strength of the individual and so on. These qualities are what we know of as beauty. Rarely do we look beyond the external. The maddening rush to the hairdresser, the cosmetic surgeon, the boutiques . . . the frenzy of external pursuits for visual perfection is a spiral with no end and no resolve. The mere activity of constantly beautifying the external depletes the inner springs of fortitude and strength. Eventually the body ages and all signs of youth and firmness fade and fall. There remains an emptiness devoid of any substance. No collective wisdom to

---

[1] *Vedas:* The scriptures of the ancient sages of India, handed down orally from teacher to student throughout the generations until today.

[2] *Upanishads:* The end portion of the Vedas that deals with the knowledge of self as the ultimate non-dual reality and our identity with that reality.

[3] *Bhagavad Gita:* The song of the Lord, sometimes referred to as the "Crescent Jewel" of the great epic of the Mahabharata. The eighteen chapters of the Gita was taken out of this much larger epic. Lord Krishna shares the vision of the Upanishads with Arjuna.

brace the twilight time. No experience gathered through the springtime for the mean and cruel winter. All the juice and ripeness of the summer years sapped up in the constant frenzy for external beautification.

Cleansing the body internally as well as externally is important. The external must be clean and brilliant. A daily ritual of cleansing, toning, and simple makeup accent are recommended for maintaining the simple beauty.

The second aspect of beauty is called the *guna* or the character of the individual person. This dimension is considered to be much more important than the first. *Gunas* are determined from birth by *samskaras* or collective qualities from *karma* of the previous births or what we know of as genetic traits. There are certain distinct qualities of grace, movement, spirited emotions, and so on, in every human being. The *guna* of a person materializes through being nurtured and disciplined as a child on through maturity. As we grow our parents and teachers are meant to guide, teach, and nurture these special qualities to their fruition. Qualities such as compassion is considered the greatest quality of the human spirit as it holds all elements of understanding, patience, love, sharing, and nurturing in harmony. Learning how to use the mind is considered a *tapas*[4] or discipline. The training of the mind to become focused and attentive are the external factors of the learning process. The more important consideration is the caring and blossoming of the inner qualities of the child. In our early adulthood, we begin to apply our attentions to career training, sports training, physical training, and so on. Hence, it is necessary to balance these activities with contemplation, prayers, and rest.

The three aspects of the total beauty is like a scale, one side holds the *Alankaras* or the external ingredients, the other holds the *gunas* or internal ingredients. And the act of balancing itself is the third aspect or *Rasa*. *Rasa* is the cumulative experience or aesthetic emotions of the individual. *Rasa* deals with time as its essential factor; for only through time can experiences be accumulated and only through the knowledge of experience can the individual refine the basic emotions. In essence, when the emotion has passed through all five stages of growth, the seed, sprout, plant, flower, and fruit, it then becomes *Rasa*. The emotion or spirit that is fully lived. This is magic. This is maturity. And this is beauty in its fullness. External beauty alone is like a coconut shell painted in beautiful colors with no life inside.

It is important to maintain a vibrant and alive exterior. However the real glow shines through only from the disciplines applied to the internal self. In addition to the recommended diet regimen, the chapter on *tapas* or self-discipline explores many practices for self-improvement and fortitude. Beauty is on a continuous motion. We can only achieve the enhancement of external beauty during our youth. It is only toward the prime years of our lives that we have the opportunity to fully accomplish beauty to be our own. True beauty is that of understanding the process of beauty. It is a fickle and dangerous game to be caught up in the fancies

---

[4]*Tapas* is any discipline or disciplines chosen for your self by yourself. It is the consistent practice of any chosen activity that nurtures you and allows you to gain health, strength, beauty, and knowledge. At the beginning of any such practice, you may concentrate on any one of the above ends. In time each accomplishment naturally qualifies you to seek the other.

of youthful, external beauty. We are taught to set ourselves up in this manner only to watch everything crumble one by one as the years tick away. Through contemplation or quiet time, we can relearn the motions of growing older. We can begin to appreciate that aging gives us the only opportunity for maturing, and that maturing is *Rasa*—the golden gift that holds the key to what is real. It unlocks the essence of beauty, beauty that you alone can spend. The external concept of beauty is spent for you. It is spent by time. You have no control over it. The pure external approach leads you down the garden path and off the precipice. Internal character gives you strength and the ability to play, work, and nurture the spirit and the external to its full fruition. This fullness is *Rasa*. This is the beauty of the universe. This is your beauty reflecting the universe.

The *Alankara, guna*, and *Rasa* are the trident of the Earth's beauty. One is inseparable from the other. It is the inside, the outside, and the spiritual fortitude with which we work to refine our emotions to its most honest and clear point. It is not that we have to slave for this. We are born with this intact. It is not an achievement that is outside of us. It is an achievement in recognizing that "I am made up of all three aspects," "I recognize all three aspects to be myself." All that is necessary to do, is to live accordingly, giving time and attention to the healthy blossoming of all three aspects of natural growth.

In the beautiful story of the love between two deities of the Hindu scripture, it is told of the goddess Parvati's love for Lord Shiva. Parvati, escorted by the God of Love himself, Manmatha proudly displayed her charms before Lord Shiva. But the Lord was not moved. He did not respond to her love. Parvati recognizing the futility of her beauty yet to mature, took to *tapas* to win the Lord's love. In the end she triumphed by cleansing her emotions, and by dwelling with her inner beauty. Afterward she shone like the brilliant light of a thousand moons over the vast oceans. Goddess Parvati then won the love of Lord Shiva.

The Ayurvedic and macrobiotic approaches to beauty consider the total assemblage of the body, mind, and senses as well as the spirited emotion that is responsible for our self-image. Thus the steps given to determine your individual needs will require deliberate time and offer in your part to fully understand and use these guides for your lifelong benefits. These recommendations are for those who find that it is not sufficient to think of beauty as skin deep.

A handle on your life comes with the understanding of how the body, mind, and senses work for you; a handle to hold onto in order that you may assume the responsibilities and rewards for who you are. In being aware of your specific constitutional type you become alert to your bodily indications. You know what the results are from what you eat, why you eat what you eat, what your mind is doing or not doing. You become aware of your activities as they happen. You are able to observe yourself being angry, or being happy as opposed to being angry or happy without your observation. You are able to trace your actions and activities to their results and observe their effects in your internal and thus external self-image.

Self-image is a combination of the opinion of yourself and how this impression is projected. The external self lacks confidence and masks real beauty when the internal self is neglected. Beauty, according to principles of the Ayurvedas and macrobiotics, is presenting who we are at every stage of change, exactly as we are. The self that lacks confidence when presented for what it is holds its own beauty. That beauty is honesty. It is a self that is not fearfull of showing what it is while it is aspiring to what it would like to be. Beauty is not skin deep. It is layers and layers and layers deep. It is every cell and breath of ourselves.

As we cleanse and grow internally beauty is what we project. As change is the only certainty of life we can ascertain that beauty is always intertwined with our changes. To allow these changes to be what they are gives consistency to our lives. Fears and uncertainties come from the need for everything to remain the same. They come from resisting change. In accepting that changes are the only certain part of life we avoid setting ourselves in a rut where fears really exist and where they are very real. We project who we are at every stage and this projection changes from stage to stage. If at every stage we form an opinion of who we are, then we must allow for that opinion to change by the next stage. If we get stuck with opinions of ourselves we obstruct our progress. And thus self-opinions are unnecessary and obstructive to our natural changes and growth.

An opinion is a perception. It is what a given thing seems to be at a certain time. And even though the perception is real when it occurs, it is not necessarily what it is. We perceive everything within the limitations of what we know, and therefore as we grow, what we know changes. Thus our perceptions change. It is impossible to assume any conclusions about ourselves or others. We may observe what it is we perceive about ourselves and others and watch that perception changes as we change. This observation and reserve from arriving at conclusions about ourselves and others is our essential nature. It is from this observation that a true self-image is projected. This image is one of confidence, one that shows the distance between where we are and where we aspire to be, not in terms of our material success but in terms of our continuous self-growth. The only reason to demonstrate where we aspire to be is to reinforce our focus and personal initiative. And in the process it is encouraging to allow others to see us for who we are. When we assume the image of what we aspire to be before we arrive there we set ourselves up for many disasters. We incur expectations in others and we try and live up to them. Because we are far from equipped to deal with these expectations, we inevitably disappoint ourselves and invariably blame those whose expectations were fostered by our own premature projections.

We can accommodate our eagerness to show our individual grandeur by always knowing and showing where we are at all times with some indication of where we are going. This enthusiasm is inspirational and does not demand that which we cannot pay. We learn to give only what we are capable of giving and take only what we need. This is beauty. This is the universal beauty.

Your Skin and Hair According to Your Constitutional Type

Modern cosmetology, like Western medicine, approaches the caring processes of beauty symptomatically and superficially. The Ayurvedic and macrobiotic principles consider the life-force and the body, mind, and senses of the total person.

According to the Ayurvedas (the ancient Indian system of medicine), the human *prakriti* or constitution (first creation) is made up of the five basic elements of nature. The human constitution as determined by genetics remain constant throughout the lifetime. Only the physiological and pathological aspects of the constitution are affected by social, environmental, and cultural changes. There are three basic principles or humors born out of the five basic elements that govern the constitutional type of each individual. Each of these principles is responsible for the type of skin, hair, body, energy, and so on of each person. These three principles are responsible for the body's interaction with the internal and external elements. These three principles are known as *Vata, Pitta*, and *Kapha*. They work together in harmony to make up the entire body.

Vata is formed from ether and air and is known as the air principle of the body. It governs the nervous system and the biological movement of the body. Pitta is made up of fire and water and is known as the body fire or *agni*. It maintains the body energy or metabolic process and controls the endocrine glands and the enzymatic activities of the body. Kapha is made up of water and earth and is referred to as the body's water. Kapha maintains the body's resistance, provides the matter of the physical structure, lubricates the joints, provides moisture to the skin, and helps to heal wounds. Kapha gives biological strength and verve to the body. Pitta controls the balance between the kinetic energy of Vata and the potential energy of Kapha. Total health depends upon the harmonious coexistance of the two elements within each principle (i.e., the ether and air components within the Vata principle), and finally the overall balance of Vata-Pitta-Kapha in the body. From these three basic principles or *Tridosha* are derived the seven different types of constitution which govern our skin and hair types: (1) Vata, (2) Pitta, (3) Kapha, (4) Vata-Pitta, (5) Vata-Kapha, (6) Pitta-Kapha, (7) Vata-Pitta-Kapha. Generally most people are a combination of two of the three principles, however there are a small number of people who are purely Vata, Pitta, or Kapha and some who are a combination of all three principles.

The Ayurvedic principle of health is vast and elaborate. Chart 1 is simplified for easy assimilation and to give a general understanding of your specific differences. Modern cosmetology refers to the various skin types as dry, oily, normal, sensitive, and so on. Whereas the Vata type skin and hair are naturally dry, the Kapha type naturally oily, and the Pitta type naturally balanced, it is necessary to know that our skin and hair reflect our very nature. When the natural constitution is off balance, a Kapha type skin can be unusually dry, a Pitta type skin abnormally oily, and a Vata type skin enormously sensitive. The elements of each of our constitution determine our sensitivities to hot and cold, dryness and wetness, and our likes and dislikes.

Since the Ayurvedic principle is new to you, a brief review of how we currently

Chart 1   Analyzing Your Constitutional Type

CONSTITU-TIONAL TYPE	SKIN TYPE	SKIN COLOR	HAIR	NAILS	EYES	TEETH
VATA Ether/Air	Dry, cold, chapped Leathery Tans easily Rarely burns	Dark brown Very dark Light[1]	Brown, black Dry, tight Wavy, thin Frizzy Body hair very fine or very coarse	Brittle, dry, Ridged Tendency to bit nails	Steel blue Gray, violet Dark brown Dull, narrow Small, dry Itchy	Big Protruded
PITTA Fire/Water	Moderately oily Soft, freckled Warm, red-dish Rashes, pim-ples Tans moder-ately Burns easily	Reddish Yellowish Fair, pink Freckled Coppery	Red, auburn Reddish blonde Silver Premature gray Moderately oily Straight Premature baldness	Clear, pink Well formed Pliable	Sharp, alert Green, hazel Gray, very light Light brown Light blue Vibrant blue Gleaming	Moderate size Yellowish Nicely shaped
KAPHA Water/Earth	Very oily Dense, soft Smooth, silky Cool Tans evenly Burns when overexposed	Pale white Fair Gleaming complexion	Jet black Dark brown Very brown Moderately wavy	Strong, pale Evenly shaped Square	Bright, big Clear, blue Black, sensual Very white Thick lashes Sometimes itchy	Strong white Moderate size

---

[1] Coloring is relative to the racial background, as a causation who is Vata will tend to a light complexion with a sallow tone. A dark skinned person who is Kapha will tend to have gleaming light tone.

[2] Birth control pills and devices mask the natural menstruation symptoms.

[3] A Vata type can be overweight if the diet is poor and Kapha producing. Excess weight of a Vata type will be carried in the midriff. Infrequently, a Kapha type can also be underweight due to poor diet and excess activities.

approach beauty is necessary. The skin is the largest organ of the body. It is porous and thus absorbs matter that is placed on it. It is a strong and yet delicate system. There are three layers that work to replenish the constantly flaking dead skin cells of the epidermis or outer layer. The dermis or second layer provides food to the outer skin. It houses the nerves, blood vessels, hair follicles, oil and sweat glands and the collagen. The oil and sweat glands form an emulsion that protects the outer skin. This emulsion is known as *collagen* and its depletion is responsible for aging, sagging, and wrinkling of the skin. Underneath both layers of skin is the

BODY FRAME	NATURAL CRAVINGS	ELIMINATION	PHYSICAL ACTIVITY	EMOTIONAL TEMPERAMENT	INDICATE TYPE
Thin[3], tall Angular, lanky Narrow frame Very short Flat chested Nose—bent/sharp Strong bodies Minor physical 　abnormalities	Salty/sour taste Appetite ex- 　tremes	Feces—dry/hard Urine—scant Sweat—minimal Mensus— 　scant,[2] irreg- 　ular, blood 　clots, dark, 　severe cramps	Extremely 　active Extreme 　variability Sleeps poorly Sun lovers	Low tolerance of 　pain, noise, and 　bright lights A "raw" nervous 　system Uneasy, Erratic Introspective Inclined to spiritual 　disciplines	
Medium height Medium weight Medium chest Generally slim, 　well-shaped Chiseled nose Muscular tendency	Sweet, bitter, Astringent taste Healthy appetite	Feces—soft 　yellowish, 　large quantity Urine—large 　quantity Sweat—profuse Mensus[2]—heavy, 　long, bright 　red, moderate 　cramps	Intense, hot Sleeps well Prefers cooler 　temperatures	Adaptable Irritable Alert Very intelligent Successful Self-centered	
Heavy[3] Sometimes obese Symmetrical Well-developed Soft, not 　muscular Well-lubricated 　joints Wide framed	Pungent, bitter Astringent taste Appetite con- 　sistent, 　moderate	Feces—slow/ 　thick oily, 　moderate 　quantity Urine—moder- 　ate, golden 　brown Sweat—moderate Mensus[2]— 　regular, 　moderate, pale, 　mild discomfort	Sluggish Great stability Oversleeps Sun lovers	Very stable Very calm Attached Narrow-minded 　tendency Forgiving Contemplative	

fatty layer or subcutaneous tissue which buffers the outer skin from shock as well as maintains the body heat.

Normally the skin types are referred to as dry, oily, normal, sensitive, or combination skin. Generally the Vata type skin would be considered the dry skin type, the Pitta type skin normal, and the Kapha type skin oily. The sensitive type skin would be either Pitta or Vata types. And the combination skin would be one of the following: Vata-Pitta, Vata-Kapha, Pitta-Kapha, or Vata-Pitta-Kapha.

A Guide to Analyze Your Chart and Determine Your Specific Regimen

Since the chart and determinations are new to you take some time with your self-analysis in Chart 1. Make a few copies of the chart. Indicate categorically the answers that represent you. Add up your answers by category.

EXAMPLE

	Vata	Pitta	Kapha
Category Distribution	24 points	12 points	4 points
Ratio	60%	30%	10%
Deduction	Thus the constitution of this example for the purpose of determining the body, skin, and hair type regimens is Vata-Pitta, with a predominance of Vata.		
Instructions	Refer to following section on How to Choose Your Category When You Are a Combination of Two or More Constitutional Types. Make a copy of the paragraph pertaining to your skin type. The type deduction for this example is 65% Vata/35% Pitta. Refer to chapter 4 for formula recommendations.		

The categories of natural body, skin, and hair treatments recommended in the following chapters offers a precise and comprehensive program for your specific body and skin quality.

Chart 1 provides only a general guide to determine your constitutional type. It will serve as a guide to assist in understanding your body and skin types as non-separate from the elements of nature. This chart is provided specifically for determining your predominant constitution and for the purpose of choosing your external health formulas.

Very rarely is anyone a purely Vata, purely Pitta, or purely Kapha type. Generally we are a combination of two types as Vata-Pitta, Vata-Kapha, or Pitta-Kapha. Use your predominant type to guide you through the category you are to choose from. Analyze the chart by indicating the descriptions most appropriate for you. It can be that your skin is Vata type, your hair is Pitta or Kapha type and so on. Simply add up how many points are in each group. For example, if 3 points in Vata, 2 points in Kapha, your general type for the purposes of this book will then be 60% Vata/40% Kapha. Your choice of regimen and formulas will be more from the Vata category and less from the Kapha category. If you are more than 75% of one principle (e.g., 75% Vata/25% Kapha), then you may choose exclusively from your predominant category. When choosing formulas from your less predominant category, be careful to select the formulas that are more suitable to your needs. Your needs will change from time to time but your basic constitutional type will not change. Very often our impressions of how we see ourselves will change considerably after we begin to understand our body, mind, and spirit. After you have been participating in your internal and external health and beauty regimen for approximately six months, redo your analysis of your constitutional type. You will find that certain traits have shifted either to your more predominant type or to your less predominant type. You may adjust your regimen accordingly. After a few years of consistent commitment to your health and beauty care, you will find your analysis of your constitutional chart will remain more and more constant.

Generally, you assume the qualities of a principle other than your predominant constitutional principle due to your lifestyles, for example, the food you eat may be more Kapha producing foods and if you are constitutionally a 60% Vata/40% Kapha, you may appear to be 80% Kapha/20% Vata after years of living in disharmony with your true nature.

It is important that when you analyze the chart to determine your constitutional type that you are honest with yourself. Remember that for the true purposes of your health and beauty care this analysis is between you and yourself.

How to Choose Your Category When You Are a Combination of Two or More Constitutional Types

The categories of Vata, Pitta, and Kapha formulas are geared to the predominance of Vata, the predominance of Pitta, and the predominance of Kapha.

For instance, if you are 100% Vata, 100% Pitta, or 100% Kapha, you will choose completely from your appropriate category. However since the chances of someone being 100% of any one of the three humors are rare, the categories were formulated to accommodate the predominant factor of your constitutional combinations. For instance if you are 70% Kapha/30% Vata, you will choose from the Kapha category. (Keep in mind that in the rare occasion you may have a more Vata type problem of dry skin in which case you may choose formulas from the Vata category.) The same holds true for 70% Vata/30% Kapha, and all other combinations. It is important to understand that you need to use your own discrimination as to whether your skin is oilier than normal, or drier than normal; whether it is warmer or it is cooler, and so on.

If you are approximately 75%/25% combination, choose exclusively from your predominant category.

> 75% Vata/25% Pitta—Choose from the Vata category.
> 75% Vata/25% Kapha—Choose from the Vata category.
> 75% Pitta/25% Vata—Choose from the Pitta category.
> 75% Pitta/25% Kapha—Choose from the Pitta category.
> 75% Kapha/25% Vata—Choose from Kapha category.
> 75% Kapha/25% Pitta—Choose from Kapha category.

If you are approximately 65%/35% combination choose mostly from your predominant type category and occasionally from the lesser type category.

65% Vata/35% Pitta—Choose predominantly from the Vata category and occasionally from the Pitta category. Check the qualities of both these principles on your chart and determine whether your skin needing more Vata type recommendations or Pitta type recommendations. For instance, if your skin is oilier, warmer, and redder than usual, you will need to choose more from the Pitta category. However if it is drier, cooler, and not red, you will stay within the Vata category of recommendations. Stay mostly within the predominant skin type category when your skin normalizes.

65% Vata/35% Kapha—Choose predominantly from the Vata category and occasionally from the Kapha category. Check the qualities of these two principles on your chart and determine whether your skin is needing more Kapha type treatment. For instance, if it is drier than normal, you will need to stay within Vata recommendations. If it is oilier than normal you will need to choose from the Kapha recommendations. Revert back to the Vata recommendations as soon as your skin normalizes.

65% Pitta/35% Vata—Choose predominantly from the Pitta category and occasionally from the Vata category. Check the qualities of both these principles on your chart and determine whether your skin is needing more Pitta type recommendations or Vata type recommendations. For instance, if your skin is drier, cooler and your hair is drier, coarser, and more frizzy than usual, you will need to choose more from the Vata category. However if the skin is warm and oilier and your hair is moderately oily, you will stay within the Pitta category of recommendations. Stay mostly within the predominant category of recommendations when your skin normalizes.

65% Pitta/35% Kapha—Choose predominantly from the Pitta category and occasionally from the Kapha category. Check the qualities of these two principles on your chart and determine whether your skin is needing more Kapha type recommendations or Pitta type recommendations. For instance, if your skin is oilier and cooler than normal and you are sweating less than usual, then you will need to choose more from the Kapha category of recommendations. However if your skin is less oily, warmer, and you are sweating more profusely, you will stay within the Pitta category of recommendations. Stay mostly within the predominant category of recommendations when your skin normalizes.

65% Kapha 35% Vata—Choose predominantly from the Kapha category and occasionally from the Vata category. Check the qualities of these two principles on your chart and determine whether your skin is needing more Kapha type recommendations or more Vata type recommendations. For instance, if your skin is oilier and cooler than normal, you will definitely stay in the Kapha recommendations. If it is drier than normal, you will need to choose from the Vata recommendations. Revert back to mostly Kapha recommendations as soon as your skin normalizes. Both Vata and Kapha types tend to have cold skin.

65% Kapha/35% Pitta—Choose predominantly from the Kapha category and occasionally from the Pitta category. Check the qualities of both these principles on your chart and determine whether your skin is needing more Kapha type recommendations or Pitta type recommendations. For instance, if your skin is less oily and warmer than normal and you are sweating more than usual, you will then need to choose from the Pitta category of recommendations. However if the skin is oilier and cooler and sweats less, then you will stay within the Kapha category of recommendations. Stay mostly within the predominant category of recommendations when your skin normalizes.

If you are approximately 45–55%/45–55% combination which is almost half-and-half, choose from both categories with the following modifications. Even if a person is half-and-half, there are still factors that make it necessary to choose one category over the other.

45–55% Kapha/45–55% Vata—Choose from both Kapha and Vata categories with the following modifications.
1. Establish whether your normal skin is of medium temperature, moderately oily, and moderately dry (in essence a nicely balanced skin type). If this is so, choose the more emollient formulas from the Kapha category (i.e., formulas from fall and the winter recommendations of the Kapha category) and the less emollient formulas from the Vata category (i.e., formulas from spring and summer recommendations of the Vata category).
2. If your skin is drier and colder than normal, choose more from the Vata category of recommendations and less from the Kapha category. If your skin is oilier and warmer than normal, choose more from the Kapha category and less from the Vata category.
One very certain fact is that you will be choosing at all times from both categories and you will begin to ascertain which formulas work the best for you through all of your changes.
3. In the fall and winter months, you will need the lubrication of the Vata formulas, as your skin and hair will naturally tend to be drier. Since winter is Kapha time, it will also increase the natural tendencies of your Kapha counterpart which are coldness and inertia. At this time the warming formulas of the Vata category will be best suited for you. Even though the fall is Vata time, you are still able to choose from the Vata category during this time.

45–55% Vata/45–55% Pitta—Choose from both Vata and Pitta categories with the following modifications.
1. Establish whether your normal skin is of medium temperature (lukewarm) and whether it is delicately moistened (very slightly dry). In essence, when it is a bit drier and warmer than the perfectly balanced skin, choose the least emollient formulas of the Vata category (formulas from the spring, summer, and fall recommendations of the Vata category and the more emollient formulas from the fall and winter recommendations of the Pitta category).

2.   If your skin is drier than just a bit dry and colder than just a bit cool, choose more from the Vata category and less from the Pitta category. If your skin is oilier than just a bit oily and warmer than just a bit warm, choose more from the Pitta category and less from the Vata category.

3.   In the winter months you will need to choose from the Vata category, as your skin tends to become drier and colder during this time. In the spring and fall you may continue to choose accordingly from both categories. In the summer months which is Pitta time, you will want to choose more from the cooling invitations of the Pitta category of recommendations.

45–55% Kapha/45–55% Pitta—Choose from both Kapha and Pitta categories with the following modifications.

1.   Establish whether your normal skin is medium temperature (lukewarm) and whether it is moderately moist (slightly oily). In essence, when it is a bit oilier and warmer than usual, choose from the formulas of the fall and winter recommendations of the Kapha category and from the least emollient formulas of the Pitta category (formulas from the spring and fall recommendations of the Pitta category).

2.   If your skin is oilier than just a bit oily and cooler than just a bit cool, then choose more from the Kapha category and less from the Pitta category. If your skin is drier than just a bit oily and warmer than just a bit warm, then choose more from the Pitta category and less from the Kapha category.

3.   In the winter months, you will need to choose slightly more from the fall and winter recommendations of Pitta category. *However, apply these treatments warm rather than recommended cooler applications of predominantly Pitta types.* You may also choose from the fall and winter recommendations of the Kapha category.

Similarly, in the summer, which is Pitta time, you will choose slightly more from the spring and summer recommendations of the Kapha category and also from the spring and summer recommendations of the Pitta category. Be sensitive to the recommendations of the Pitta category and to your Kapha counterpart and not overdo the "coolness" of your treatments.

The Vata-Pitta-Kapha Type—This is as rare a type as the purely Vata, purely Pitta, or the purely Kapha type.

Should you be in all these categories, choose the two predominant categories to be your constitutional type for the purposes of external recommendations. For instance, should your analysis be 40% Vata, 40% Kapha, and 20% Pitta, abide by the Vata-Kapha type according to the 45–55% Vata/45–55% Kapha category.

Should you have the difficult task of your type being 35% Vata, 30% Kapha, and 35% Pitta which is almost evenly distributed. Redo your chart analysis and redefine your least percentage principle (the least being the Kapha principle for this example) in order that you may decrease the Kapha percentage and increase either Vata or Pitta percentages. If this is not possible, simply abide by the Pitta (for this example) principle, since together they combine your highest percentage.

The Transient-sensitive Skin and Hair Type ────────────

There is one other skin activity which is classified as the *transient-sensitive skin and hair type*. This can be any one of the seven types. It is called *transient* since it is generally a condition of the skin that is affected by change of diet, exercise, climate, and so on and is not necessarily true to the symptoms of any of the seven categories of skin types. After a severe change of diet or living circumstances, one's skin type tends to indicate erratic symptoms such as spots, rashes or extreme sensitiveness to sunlight and cold. The body takes three to five years to adjust to new eating habits or new climate, even when the changes are for the better. In cleansing out fatty deposits, hard calcium deposits, and toxicity, the body is generally adjusting to a new life form. Often times these rashes and sensitivities take months to disappear and reoccur during the summer months year after year. Sometimes the pigmentation is affected and the area becomes lighter. The recommendation in the category listed as "transient-sensitive skin" will assist in decreasing the symptoms of these erratic occurrences. Since the cleansing process is a continuous one, patience is necessary in the eventual achievement of exquisite skin.

Whereas the Asian and African skin types can be found amongst the seven categories of skin types, there are some noteworthy differences. Asians and Africans are much more sensitive to alcohol and menthol (peppermint, camphor, oil of wintergreen or salicylic acid used in skin peeling creams and ointments). These skins have fewer pores and are generally smooth and silky with more prominent bone structure. The skin is usually much more firm and age much less because of its oilier nature. There is much more melanin granules which are responsible for the deeper pigmentation akin to Asian and African skin. Whereas this adds more protection from harmful ultraviolet rays of the sun, it also causes more sun reactions. It is a misconception that darker skins are insensitive to the sun. In some cases, darker skins are extremely sensitive to ultraviolet rays. A natural sunscreen such as recommended in the Sun and Wind Protection Formula section is necessary. These skins are more prone to hyperpigmentation, or dark spots on the face, neck, and arms. It is the deeper melanin in the skin that causes cuts and bruises to heal much darker than the normal skin color.

Naturally darker skins must be very careful when contemplating facial or body cosmetic surgery, skin peeling, electrolysis, and so on. These skins scar very easily and heal with excess scar tissues or keloids. The products and treatments in chapter 4 which oxygenize and feed skin cells while retaining the moisture content of the skin are recommended. All skin types will benefit substantially from these treatments.

Nurturing Season for Each Constitutional Type ────────────

The dominant season and time of day of your constitutional type is generally your least harmonious time (see Chart 2). These times are best spent in nurturing activities such as yoga, meditation, walks, massage, calmly working, and so on. The best times to have your meals are not during your dominant times of day. During your dominant season, be especially careful of your diet and activities.

Chart 2 Time and Energy Chart for Each Constitutional Type

CONSTITU-TIONAL TYPE	DOMINANT SEASON	DOMINANT TIME OF DAY	DOMINANT ENERGY,* EMOTIONS, AND ACTIVITY	VULNERABLE ORGANS AND AREAS OF BODY	POSITIVE MEAL TIMES	POSITIVE AND PRIMARY COLORS	POSITIVE, PRE-CIOUS STONES AND METALS
VATA Ether/Air	Fall	2:00–6:00 PM 2:00–6:00 AM	Cold, dry, light, dispressing, mobile Anxiety, fearfullness Aches, pains Controls: prana, freshness	Large intestine Pelvic, thighs, skin, bones ears	Breakfast: 7:00–8:00 AM Lunch: 0:00–1:00 PM Snack: 4:00–4:30 PM Dinner: 6:00–7:00 PM	Red, orange, yellow, green, and all combinations thereof	Amethyst, ruby, sapphire, red and yellow garnet, white moonstone, red and yellow opal, silver, and gold
PITTA Fire/Water	Summer	10:00 AM–2:00 PM 10:00 PM–2:00 AM	Fluid, hot, mercurial, light, penetrating Anger, hatred Intuition, intelligence Controls: hunger and thirst, metabolism, body fat, skin color	Small intestine Stomach, sweat glands, blood condition, eye and skin disorder	Breakfast: 7:00–8:00 AM Snack: 0:00–1:00 PM Lunch: 3:00–4:00 PM Dinner (light) 6:00–7:00 PM	Purple, blue, green, white, mauve, lilac, lavender, and all shades and combinations thereof	Amethyst, blue diamond, clear diamond, red coral, white and green garnet, white moonstone, pearl, silver, and platinum
KAPHA Water/Earth	Winter	6:00–10:00 AM 6:00–10:00 PM	Heavy, cold, dense, unclear, soft, slow, liquid, firmness Greed, attachment, calmness, forgiveness Prayerful, love Controls: body structure, liquid lubrication, energy, plasma	Head, chest, throat, nose, mouth, stomach	Breakfast (full): 10:30–11:30 AM Lunch (light) 2:00–2:30 PM Snack: 4:00–4:30 PM Dinner (light) 6:00–7:00 PM	Red, orange, yellow, green, purple All shades and combinations thereof	Agate, red diamond, red and yellow garnet, red and yellow opal, ruby, topaz, copper, and gold

* Dominant energy and emotions controlled by the elements of each type.

During your dominant period—Vata time is fall, Pitta time summer, and Kapha time winter—a Vata type will be affected negatively within Vata time, as the elements of the external is like the elements of the internal (e.g., the dryness of weather of fall affects the already dry Vata skin and hair). During the Pitta season a Vata type person will fare better because of the moisture and lubrications that summer brings as a balm to dryness. It is the basic premise of opposite attractions. Thus a Vata type will have a more watery, oilier diet than a Kapha type who will need a drier and lighter diet. In essence a Vata type will fare better within Kapha time, or a Pitta type will fare better within a somewhat Kapha time, and so on.

The end of your dominant season usually brings the dreaded emotion and physical chaos, such as disharmony with your spouse, colds, flu, changing jobs, and so on. In being aware of the negative aspects of your dominant season, you are able to plan your diet, activity, and emotional schedule carefully to avoid the end of season crash. The energy and time chart helps you to conduct yourself through your dominant time and season as well as your positive time for meals, activities, and so on. In essence it helps you to balance your time, energy, and activity.

How the Five Basic Elements Influence the Taste

Sweet taste—Combination of water and earth elements (pure Kapha principle)
Sour taste—Combination of earth and fire elements (Kapha-Pitta principle)
Salty taste—Combination of fire and water elements (pure Pitta principle)
Pungent taste—Combination of fire and air elements (Pitta-Vata principle)
Bitter taste—Combination of air and ether elements (pure Vata principle)
Astringent taste—Combination of air and earth elements (Vata-Kapha principle)

The energy that nourishes each of the constitutional types is also the energy other than that which is inherent within your type. Maintain these considerations within all of your regimens and endeavors.

Nurturing Energy for Each Different Constitutional Type

Purely Kapha type—Fire, air, and ether
     Heat, lightness/delicacy
     Space/distance
Purely Vata type— Fire, water, and earth
     Heat, fluidity/flexibility
     Consistency/stability
Purely Pitta type— Earth, air, and ether
     Space/distance
     Lightness/coolness
     Consistency/even-temperedness
     Reflection

Chapter 2 *Facial Cleansing Routines, Massage, and Baths for Each Constitutional Type*

The science of massaging the body from the bounty of nature is as old as time itself. In India a hot oil massage is used to balance the three humors of Vata, Pitta, and Kapha in the body. Comparable treatments were used in China, Egypt, Rome, Greece, and in the Nordic countries, as the primary art of therapeutic comfort and good health. More recently aromatherapy, the science of using various herbs, roots, barks combined with natural alcohols, keystones, acids, phenols, ethers, and sulfur compounds, and so on, has been adopted as an excellent external treatment to the body. For every cell in the body we are provided with millions of cells surrounding us within Mother Nature. From the food that nourishes our body to the wind that brushes our face every speck of nature corresponds with our spiritual, emotional, and physical process. Wisdom in living is choosing the corresponding elements of our selves from the external gardens. The plant and human skin are alike in structure and in function. Both are composed of 90 percent water. The surface of plant leaves are covered with a wax coating as our skin is covered with an oily substance. The plant breathes through its pores as does the body.

The plant has an outer layer of skin called the *cuticle* which is comparable to the body's epidermis, an inner layer called the *cutin* which is similar to the dermis of the skin that provides food to the outer layers and houses the nerves, blood vessels, hair follicles, oil and sweat glands, collagen and collagenic fibers. The function of the dermis is similar to that of the underlaying pectin and cellulose cell wall of the plant. The cuticle, like the epidermis, controls the exchange of moisture between the organism and its environment. It is thus understandable that the essential fluids of the plants will readily be absorbed into the skin, unlike the elaborate chemical substances in commercial cosmetics. The human skin, as is the human body, is traumatized when fed with chemicals. It is alien to the structure and the spirit of both the body and the mind. In essence, the external world is a replica of ourselves. To understand that there is no division between what is perceived inside of us and what we perceive outside of us, is to know that everything that appears to be separate from us is a projection of our own senses. In fact, we are indivisible with that which appears to be outside of us.

As the overwhelming analytical discoveries of science continues, the simple basic conclusions will always be the same. The infinite structure of our foods from nature, corresponds identically to the infinite structure of our body. The new century will find the human components still to be very much the same as it was originally. Whereas almost all of life can be synthesized in a laboratory, we are still the pervasive, unduplicatable human self made up of nature's substances. The ingenious chemical kingdom can only be at its very best, a poor imitation to nature. As we continue to replenish our bodies, minds, and spirit from the chemical kingdom we continue to tear down the aura of our defenses to ill-health. The harmony of body, mind, and spirit is health, and Mother Nature is the only provider.

Facial Massage and Cleansing Routines for Each Constitutional Type

The following section presents a nurturing routine for each constitutional type. The facial cleansing and massage routines are recommended for daily practice. The body massage, baths, foot soaking and body scrubbing routines are recommended for occasional use.

Facial Cleansing Routine for Vata Type

Note: Early evening is the best time to cleanse and massage Vata type face and body.

1. Apply a very clean warm towel to face for a few minutes.
2. Use a cleanser from your category of recommendation to clean dirt off the face. (Always use a clean cotton cloth or cleansing pad.)
3. Drop 3 teaspoons of sesame oil or camellia oil into a bowl of piping hot water. Put towel over head and steam the face for approximately 10 minutes (or use a facial steamer if available). Gently wipe steam off face, leaving some moisture on skin. Never towel off to completely dry.
4. Warm 3 tablespoons of any one of the following oils: olive, sesame, camellia, jojoba. Massage into face after steaming. See Figs. 1–5 for Vata massage, and refer to Vata formula section in chapter 4 for recommendations of additional oils to be used.
5. Wipe off oil with a clean warm cotton cloth or cleansing pad. Once weekly, apply one of the recommended masks from your skin type category by stroking slightly downward in a semicircular motion with the tip of your fingers and leave on for approximately 15 minutes. A horizontal resting position is excellent at this time while deeply and calmly breathing from the stomach. Apply hand in the rest motion over face (Fig. 1).
6. Remove mask with the palm of the hands, each hand simultaneously rubbing in a circular motion. Use the fingertips in an upward and downward motion for the forehead, nose, and chin. The dried mask will easily fall off.

Fig. 1

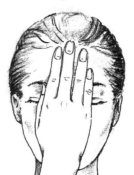

170

7. Wash skin vigorously with warm water and gently semi dry with a clean towel.

8. Apply one of the recommended astringents and moisturizers lightly in upward strokes using a cotton pad on your clean fingertips.

9. Apply a natural powder lightly to give your face a porcelain finish look. Use your eye, cheek, and lip makeup discretely.

The Rest Motion of the Hand
Use open right hand and from the top of the forehead, slowly bring it down to the bottom of face, closing the eyes along the way (Fig. 1).

Facial Massage for Vata Type

Note: Early evening is the best time for Vata type to cleanse and massage the face.

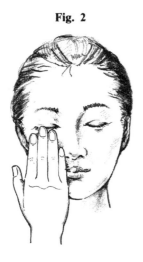

Fig. 2

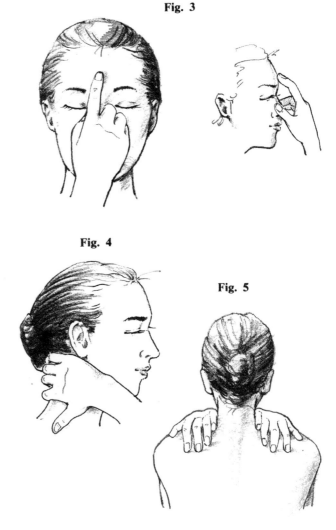

Fig. 3

Fig. 4

Fig. 5

1. Massage face with fingers in an upward motion only—in order to open pores (Fig. 2).

2. With thumb and middle finger, massage the nose (Fig. 3).

3. Massage neck with the thumbs in an upward motion (Fig. 4).

4. Using both hands facing backward, gently squeeze and release shoulders (Fig. 5).

Facial Cleansing Routine for Pitta Type

Note that early afternoon is the best time to cleanse and massage Pitta type face and body.

1. Apply a cool clean towel to the face for a few minutes.
2. Use a cleanser from your category of recommendation to clean dirt off face (always use a clean cotton cloth, or cleansing pad).
3. Drop 1 teaspoon of camellia, sunflower, or sandalwood oil into a bowl of hot water. Put towel over head and steam the face for approximately 5 minutes (or use a facial steamer if available). Gently wipe steam off face leaving moisture on the skin. Never towel off to dry.
4. Use 2 tablespoons of camellia, sunflower, or sandalwood oil at room temperature and massage face, neck, and shoulders after steaming. See Figs. 6–10 for Pitta massage.
5. Wipe off oil with a clean cool cotton cloth or cleansing pad. Once weekly, apply one of the recommended masks from your skin type category, stroking in a semicircular motion with the tip of your clean fingers and leave on for approximately 15 minutes. A horizontal resting position is excellent at this time while breathing deeply and calmly from the stomach. Place two moist cotton pads with cool water, or cool astringent (from your recommended category) over your eyes. Apply hand in the rest motion over face (see Fig. 1).
6. Remove mask with the palm of your hands in a simultaneous circular motion on the cheeks. Use the fingertips in an alternating upward and downward motion for the forehead, nose, and chin. The dried mask will easily fall off.
7. Wash skin vigorously with cool water and semi dry with a clean towel.
8. Apply one of the recommended astringents and moisturizers lightly with a gentle circular motion using a cotton pad or your clean fingertips.
9. Apply a natural powder lightly to give your face a porcelain finish look. Use your natural eye, cheek, and lip makeup discretely.

Facial Massage for Pitta Type

Fig. 6

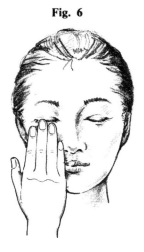

Fig. 7

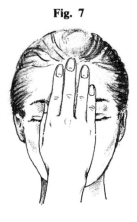

Massage face with fingers in an upward circular motion to stimulate pores.

1. Massage cheeks with fingers in an upward circular motion (Fig. 6).
2. Massage chin and forehead with fingers alternating upward and downward motion (Fig. 7).

Fig. 8   **Fig. 9**

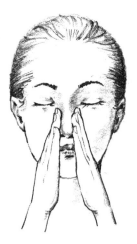

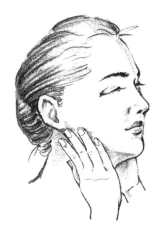

Fig. 10

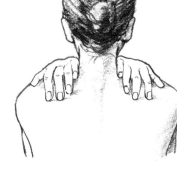

3. Using the fingers of both hands together, massage the nose with a semicircular motion (Fig. 8).

4. Using the fingers of both hands, massage the throat, neck, and shoulders in a circular motion (Fig. 9).

5. Using both hands facing backward apply moderate pressure in a squeezing motion to shoulders (Fig. 10).

Facial Cleansing Routine for Kapha Type

Note: Late morning is the best time to cleanse and massage the Kapha type face and body.

1. Apply a very warm clean towel to the face for a few minutes.

2. Use a cleanser from your category of recommendations to clean dirt off the face. Always use a clean cotton cloth, or cleansing pad.

3. Take a bowl of piping hot water, put a towel over your head and steam the face over the bowl for approximately 15 minutes (or use a facial steamer if available). Gently wipe off steam from face, leaving some moisture on the skin. Never towel off moisture completely.

4. Use 3 tablespoons of corn or sunflower oil, in a small bowl of warm water and massage deeply and slowly into face, neck, and shoulders.

5. Briskly wipe off moisture from face with a clean cotton cloth or cleansing pad. Twice weekly, apply the recommended masks from your skin type category, stroking slightly downward in a semicircular motion with the tips of your clean fingers and leave on for approximately 20 minutes. A horizontal resting position is excellent at this time while breathing deeply and calmly from the stomach. Apply hands in a rest motion over face (see Fig. 1).

6. Remove mask with the palm of your hands in a slightly downward circular motion on the cheeks. Use the fingertips in an alternating upward and downward motion for the forehead, nose, and chin. The dried mask will easily fall off.

7. Wash skin vigorously with warm to hot water and semi dry with a clean towel.

8. Apply one of the recommended astringents and moisturizers lightly with a gentle circular motion using a cotton pad or your clean fingertips.

9. Apply a natural powder to give your face a porcelain finish look. Use your natural eye, cheek, and lip makeup discretely.

Facial Massage for Kapha Type

Massage deeply and slowly in a circular, upward, and downward motion with fingers, palm of hands, and the thumb to stimulate the face.

Fig. 11

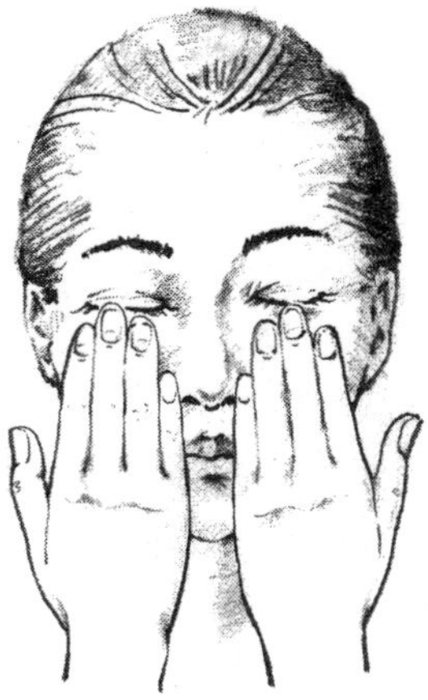

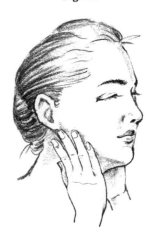

1. Massage cheeks with palm of hands with a vigorous circular and downward motion (Fig. 11).

2. Massage chin and forehead vigorously with tips of the fingers in an alternating upward and downward motion (Fig. 12).

3. Using the fingers of both hands, vigorously massage the nose with a semicircular motion (Fig. 13).

4. Using the fingers of both hands, vigorously massage the throat, neck, and shoulders in a circular motion (Fig. 14).

Fig. 12

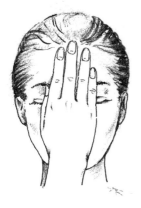

Fig. 13

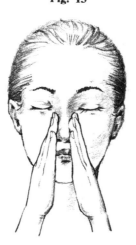

Fig. 14

Fig. 15

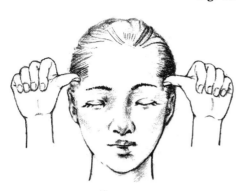

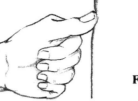

Fig. 16

5.   Using both thumbs apply acupressure to the temple working your way to the center of the forehead, down the sides of the nostril, around the cheeks to the center of the cheeks, around the top and bottom of the lips to the chin, under the ears, and down both sides of the neck (Fig. 15).

6.   Using both hands, facing backward, firmly squeeze and release the shoulders (Fig. 16).

Massage and Bath from the Bounty of Nature

Heat the oils together for the following oil massages and baths. Always add the essential oils for gels after the oils have been warmed. In an instance when water, witch hazel or glycerine is used, heat these liquids together in a separate container and then pour into the hot oil mixture. The quantity listed per formula is for one massage. Use one-third of quantity when applying to the bath water. The flour or powder is used to brush off excess oil from the skin after a massage. This procedure is optional. *Do not use the flour or powder as part of your bath formula.*

During your self-massage, concentrate on maintaining a deep and steady flow of breath. Massages and baths are synergistic. The combined effect of both is much greater than the sum total of a massage, or a bath taken independently of each other. However one is still complete without the other. Brush the body first (see Body Scrubbing for Beautiful Skin section) and then take a bath. The massage is most effective after a bath.

Note: Vata and Kapha types benefit from warm to hot baths, whereas Pitta types are best suited to a cool to lukewarm baths.

Vata Massage and Bath Oils

Note: Massage and bath oils should be very warm in temperature.

1. 0.5 oz dark sesame oil
    0.1 oz wheat germ oil
    (0.5 oz finely grounded rice flour and rice starch)

2. 0.5 carrot oil
    0.2 oz olive oil
    4 drops essential oil of neroli

3. 0.5 oz jojoba oil
    0.2 oz jojoba butter
    4 drops esential oil of hyssop

4. 0.5 oz avocado oil
    0.2 oz almond oil
    0.1 oz aloe vera gel

5. 0.5 oz almond oil
    0.1 oz borage (or evening primrose oil)
    3 drops vitamin E oil
    (0.5 oz silk powder)

6. 0.5 oz dark sesame oil
    0.2 oz very dark bancha twig tea
    3 drops essential oil of ambrette seeds (musk)
    5 drops vegetable glycerine

7. 0.5 oz soybean oil
    0.1 oz camellia oil
    4 drops essential oil of camellia

Pitta Massage and Bath Oils

Note: Massage and bath oils should be cool to lukewarm in temperature.

1. 0.5 oz sunflower oil
    0.2 oz almond oil
    (0.5 oz cinnamon powder)

2. 0.5 oz jojoba oil
    0.2 oz coconut oil
    4 drops essential oil of sandalwood
    (0.5 oz sandalwood powder)

3. 0.5 oz almond oil
    0.1 oz calamus root oil
    6 drops essential oil of peach

4. 0.2 oz evening primrose oil (or black currant oil)
    0.2 oz peanut oil
    6 drops essential oil of patchouli
    (0.5 oz rice flour and rice starch powder)

5. 0.5 oz avocado oil
   0.1 oz eucalyptus oil
   0.2 oz vegetable glycerine
   0.2 oz peppermint and pine astringent (p. 241)

6. 0.5 oz sunflower oil
   6 drops essential oil of jasmine
   (0.5 oz silk powder)

7. 0.5 oz soybean oil
   0.1 oz camellia oil
   4 drops essential oil of camellia

Kapha Massage and Bath Oils

Note: Massage and bath oils should be warm to hot in temperature.

1. 0.2 oz peanut oil
   0.2 oz witch hazel

2. 0.2 oz almond oil
   0.1 oz birch astringent (p. 259)
   6 drops essential oil of orange blossoms

3. 0.2 oz oil of lemon
   0.2 oz vegetable glycerine
   0.2 oz natural spring water
   (0.5 oz rice flour and rice starch flour)

4. 0.1 oz strawberry oil
   0.2 oz corn oil
   6 drops essential oil of juniper berries

5. 0.4 oz jojoba oil
   0.2 oz coconut oil
   (0.5 oz silk powder)

6. 0.2 oz black currant oil
   0.2 oz peanut oil
   0.1 oz camellia oil
   (0.5 oz sandalwood powder)

7. 0.4 oz corn oil
   2 drops essential oil of cloves

Essential oils for baths
The 0.5 ounce of any of the oils recommended per your constitutional type in the emollient section can be used in your bath water.

Herbal Baths from Land and Sea

Depending on the time allowance, any one of the following procedures can be done in order to have an effective bath.

1. The herbs can be grounded into a semi-powder form and mixed into the oil. This paste is diluted in one eighth of very hot water. When the water cools, draw the rest of the bath water to a suitable temperature.
2. The herbs (contained in a drawstring muslin bag) can be steeped for an hour in very hot bath water. Oil can be added to bath water if it is recommended in the formula.
3. The herbs (contained in a drawstring bag) can be left to steep overnight in one eighth filled tub of boiling water. Simply draw your bath into herbal water to a suitable temperature.

I prefer to have the herbs and leaves loose and surrounding me in my bath water. I use a sieve to remove the herbs before draining the water. I recommend using the seaweeds without an enclosure, as you will benefit from its maximum extract. I also use the soaked pieces of seaweed to rub into my body and hair; although you may prefer to shampoo the hair after your bath, you may use the herbal oil bath to wash hair as well.

There are innumerable plant extracts from the earth used for health therapy, but the sea has also been a vital source of man's good health. In Europe, West Germany, Yugoslavia, and along the Soviet Black Sea, spas apply the use of sea plants and seawater for therapeutic healing (thalassotherapy). The use of sea resources for man's health is as old as time itself. Man is connected to the ocean in a very primal way. Water is inseparable from man and is necessary to the nurturing and embracing of the body, mind, and spirit. The vegetation on the bed of the ocean is as vast as the ocean itself and these plants contain all the nutritional elements of the sea. The trace elements in seaweed are ten times more powerful than the trace elements of the earth's herbs. Sea therapy is associated with the rekindling, regeneration, and rejuvenation of the spirit, mind, and body of man. It is the external and eternal second to the primal fluids of the mother's womb.

Vata Herbal Baths from Land and Sea

1. 0.5 oz camomile
   0.5 oz marigold
   0.1 oz blue green algae powder
   0.2 oz sesame oil

2. 0.5 oz hops
   0.5 oz camomile
   6 drops essential oil of hops

3. 0.5 oz St. John's wort
    0.5 oz coneflower
    0.2 oz St. John's wort oil
    6 drops essential oil of *Laminaria digitata* (seaweed)

4. 0.1 oz glycolic extract of rosemary
    0.5 oz dried kombu
    0.1 oz olive oil
    6 drops essential oil of lavender

5. 0.1 oz glycolic extract of elecampane
    0.1 oz crude extract of licorice root
    0.1 oz glycolic extract of bladder wrack (seaweed)
    0.2 oz jojoba oil

6. 0.5 oz elderflower
    0.5 oz coneflower
    0.5 oz marigold
    0.5 oz camellia oil

7. 0.2 oz rosa mosqueta oil (rose-hip seed oil)
    0.1 oz sea salt
    0.1 oz sea kelp powder

Pitta Herbal Baths from Land and Sea

1. 0.5 oz butcher's broom
    0.5 oz marigold
    0.5 oz camomile
    0.1 oz sunflower oil

2. 0.5 oz ginseng
    0.5 oz horse chestnut
    0.1 oz glycolic extract of bladder wrack
    0.1 oz sea salt
    0.1 oz almond oil

3. 0.5 oz hops
    0.5 oz camomile
    6 drops essential oil of hops

4. 0.5 oz fennel
    0.1 oz fennel oil

5. 0.1 oz sea kelp powder
    0.1 oz sea salt
    0.1 oz coconut oil
    0.1 oz almond oil

6. 0.5 oz dried kombu
   0.1 oz peppermint oil

7. 0.1 oz blue green algae powder
   0.1 oz glycolic extract of mallow
   0.1 oz fresh parsley
   0.1 oz almond oil

Kapha Herbal Baths from Land and Sea

1. 0.5 oz glycolic extract of bladder wrack (seaweed)
   0.1 oz citrus oil

2. 0.5 oz camomile
   0.5 oz sage
   0.5 oz marigold
   6 drops essential oil of jasmine

3. 0.1 oz St. John's wort oil
   0.5 oz dried kombu

4. 0.2 oz sea kelp powder
   0.2 oz sea salt
   0.2 oz coconut oil

5. 0.5 oz glycolic extract of birch
   0.2 oz fennel
   0.1 oz fennel oil

6. 0.5 oz elderflower
   0.5 oz elecampane
   0.5 oz hops
   6 drops essential oil of hops

7. 0.2 oz glycolic extract of bladder wrack
   0.2 oz glycolic extract of mallow
   0.1 oz glycolic extract of ivy

8. 0.2 oz sea salt
   0.2 oz almond oil
   0.1 oz blue green algae powder
   6 drops essential oil

Note: In the above formulas the recommended powders and extracts are to be diluted in the bath water at the beginning of drawing your bath. The oils are to be poured into the bath directly before getting in.

Body Scrubbing for Beautiful Skin for All Constitutional Types

Scrubbing your body with a moist hot* towel is a wonderful way to activate circulation, increase the transit time of skin cells, dissolve and soften cross-linked collagen, open the pores, and melt away deposits of hard fat in the blood vessels. It energizes and refreshes the entire body and allows the skin to breathe. It is also a quick and simple way to dissolve stress and tension, both of which interfere with a fresh, healthy appearance.

Fig. 17

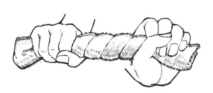

Body scrubbing can be done before or after a bath or shower, or at any time. It takes only about ten minutes and all that is needed is a sink with hot water and a medium-sized cotton towel. Turn on the hot water. Hold the towel at either end and place the center part under the stream of hot water. Wring out the towel (Fig. 17), and while it is still hot and steamy, begin to scrub with it. Do a section of the body at a time, beginning with the hands and fingers and working your way up the arms to the shoulders, neck, and face, and then downward to the chest, upper back, abdomen, lower back, buttocks, legs, feet, and toes. Scrub until the skin turns slightly red or until each part becomes warm. Reheat the towel by running it under the hot water after scrubbing each section or as soon as it starts to cool.

A Special Ginger Scrub (for Vata and Kapha types, and occasional Pitta use) ━━━

A special body scrub, prepared with ginger water, is especially refreshing. It is nice to treat yourself to this special beauty-care practice on occasion. To prepare a ginger body scrub, you will need a piece of fresh gingerroot (available at most natural or Oriental food markets), a flat metal grater, a cheesecloth, a medium-sized cotton towel, and a medium to large pot with a lid.

Grate the gingerroot on a metal grater and place a clump the size of a golf ball in a double layer of cheesecloth. Tie the cheesecloth at the top to form a sack. Then place a galloon of water in the pot and bring it up to but not over the boiling point. Just before the water starts to boil, turn the flame down to low.

Next, hold the sack over the pot and squeeze as much of the ginger juice as you can into the water. Then drop the sack into the pot. Make sure the water does not boil, as this would weaken the effect of the ginger scrub. Place the lid on the pot and let the ginger sack simmer in the water for about five minutes. Then fold your towel lengthwise several times so that it becomes long and thin. Hold it from both ends and dip the center into the hot ginger water. Wring it out tightly, and if it is too hot to place on the skin, shake it slightly. Then begin scrubbing your body as described above. Many people find plain hot water body scrubbing more convenient during the week and use the ginger scrub on the weekends. One pot of hot

*Use lukewarm water for Pitta type.

ginger water can be used for two days of body scrubs. Reheat (but do not boil) the water before using.

Dry Brush Scrubbing (for Pitta and Kapha types, and occasional Vata use) ——————

Use a natural bristle brush of medium-firm bristles. Upon rising in the early morning, sit in the *vajras* (diamond) position. Dry brush your entire body firmly but gently, beginning with the hands and working your way up the arms and shoulders, neck, face, and then downward to the chest, upper back, abdomen, lower back, buttocks, legs, feet, and toes (Fig. 18). Take your bath and wash off the dead skin. Once every week, wash your brush and dry it in the sun.

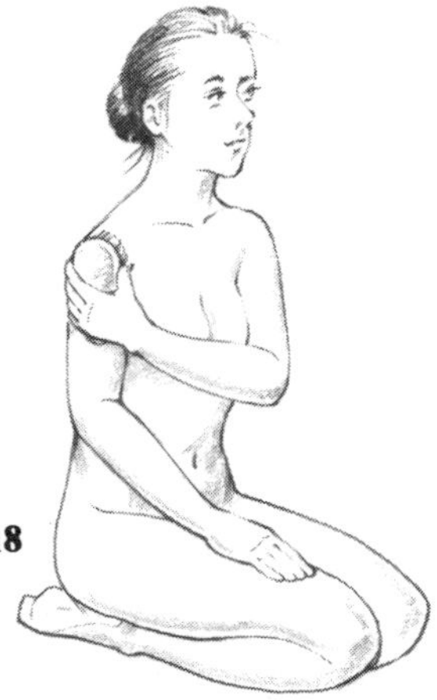

Fig. 18

Nuka Skin Wash (for all constitutional types) ————————————

Many natural beauty products can be made at home from daily foods. In Oriental countries, for example, rice bran, or nuka, was traditionally used to wash the skin and to treat various skin conditions. Nuka contains squalene, a compound found in sebum that is highly valued for its moisturizing properties. Nuka can be used to prepare a special skin wash to moisturize healthy skin, or as a part of home care for problem skin. You can purchase nuka in most natural food stores, as it is used in many macrobiotic households to prepare pickled vegetables. To prepare a nuka skin wash:

1. Put about 3 to 5 tablespoons of nuka into a white cotton sack or a sack made of thin cloth or cheesecloth. Tie the sack so that the nuka does not fall out.
2. Fill the bathtub with hot water. Place the sack into the water and squeeze it until a milky liquid comes out.
3. Mix the milky liquid into the water and use it to wash the skin, including areas where skin problems are present. After finishing your bath, dry yourself with a cotton towel.

Rice bran can also be used to make a quick skin wash. Wrap the nuka in cotton cloth or cheesecloth, as described above. Place in warm water, squeeze, and shake. The nuka will dissolve and the water will turn yellowish. A white foam may form on the surface. Lightly wash the face or other area of the body with a towel or face cloth that has been dipped into the nuka water. Pat dry with a cotton towel.

Daikon Hip Bath and Douche (for Pitta and Kapha types, and occasional Vata use) ━━━━━━━━━━━━━━━━━━━━━━━━━━━━━━━━━━━

Pimples and other blemishes frequently correlate with menstrual disorders and related problems in the female reproductive tract. Menstruation helps the body discharge excess every month, and if it is not smooth, excess that would normally be discharged may begin to gather in other parts of the body. For example, sugars and fats, which are more yin, often move upward toward the breasts, where they accumulate, or toward the face, where they are discharged in the form of pimples. In order to keep the skin healthy and beautiful, it is important to keep the reproductive tract clean and clear and to dissolve stagnation that interferes with smooth menstruation. This bath should be taken a few before or after menstruation.

The daikon hip bath has been used for this purpose for centuries. Ideally, the bath water should contain dried daikon leaves (you can use turnip greens or arame if you cannot find daikon greens). To prepare a daikon hip bath:

1. Hang fresh leaves in the shade until they turn brown and brittle.
2. Place about 4 or 5 bunches of dried leaves or a double handful of arame into a large pot. Add about 4 to 5 quarts of water and bring to a boil. Reduce the flame to medium and boil until the water turns brown. Add a handful of sea salt and stir well to dissolve.
3. Run hot water into the bathtub and add the mixture, together with another large handful of sea salt. Add only enough water to cover the body from the waist down. Sit in the tub and cover your upper body with a thick cotton towel to prevent chills and absorb perspiration (Fig. 19). If the water begins to cool, add more hot water. Stay in the bath for 10 to 12 minutes.

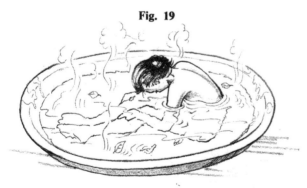

Fig. 19

The hot bath will cause your lower body to become very red as a result of an increase in circulation. This, along with the heat, will loosen fat and mucus deposits in the pelvic region.

Then, following the hot hip bath, douche with a special solution. To prepare:

1. Squeeze the juice from half a lemon into warm bancha tea, or add 1 to 2 teaspoons of brown rice vinegar to warm bancha tea. Add a 3-finger pinch of sea salt.
2. Stir and use as a douche.

The douching solution helps dissolve deposits of mucus and fat that have been loosened during the bath. The hip bath and douche can be repeated every day for up to 10 days (for a more intensive routine) or twice a day for 6 weeks (for a more moderate routine). During this time, it is important to eat well and avoid foods that contribute to the buildup of excess in the reproductive tract and throughout the body.

You can prepare a simpler version of the hip bath by dissolving a double handful of sea salt into hot bath water and sitting in it as described above. Follow the hip bath with the special douching solution as indicated.

Dried daikon (or turnip) greens are also helpful in relieving skin conditions such as eczema, acne, and psoriasis. Prepare the dried leaves as indicated above. However, rather than pouring the mixture into the bathtub, dip a cotton towel into the pot, and squeeze it lightly. Apply it to the affected area, making repeated applications until the skin turns red. Dry with a cotton towel.

Foot Soaking (for all constitutional types)

Fig. 20

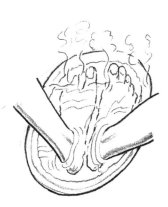

Soaking the feet in hot water helps soften callouses and hard skin, activate circulation, and refresh the entire body. Fill the tub with enough hot water to cover the feet. Place both feet into the hot water and soak for about 5 minutes (Fig. 20). Dry with a cotton towel. The feet can be soaked regularly in this manner, especially if hard callouses are present.

A ginger foot soak is also nice on occasion. Prepare a pot of hot ginger water as described above. Scrub your body as described in the section on Body Scrubbing for Beautiful Skin, and when you are finished, place both feet into the hot water. Soak for about 5 minutes and dry with a towel.

Massage for Beautiful Nails

The health and appearance of the nails depends on good circulation and a smooth, active flow of energy along each of the meridians. Daily body scrubbing activates these functions and is an excellent natural method of nail care. Simple self-massage, or Dō-In as it is known in macrobiotics, also activates energy flow and circulation, and helps restore normal color and texture to the nails. This very simple routine can be done any time.

1. Grasp the thumb of one hand between the thumb and index finger of the other. Begin to rub with a circular or back-and-forth motion. Start at the base of the thumb and work your way out to the tip. Do the outside, both sides, and inside of the thumb. Repeat several times, until the thumb feels energized and stimulated.

2. Use your thumb to press the point located at the base of the nail (Fig. 21). Apply pressure, hold for several sec-

Fig. 21

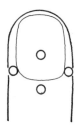

onds, and quickly release. Repeat several times to stimulate the nail bed.

3. Apply pressure to the points on either side of the nail in the above manner. Then proceed to the center of the nail itself. Repeat several times before proceeding to the next point.

Repeat the above steps for each of the fingers.

Fig. 22

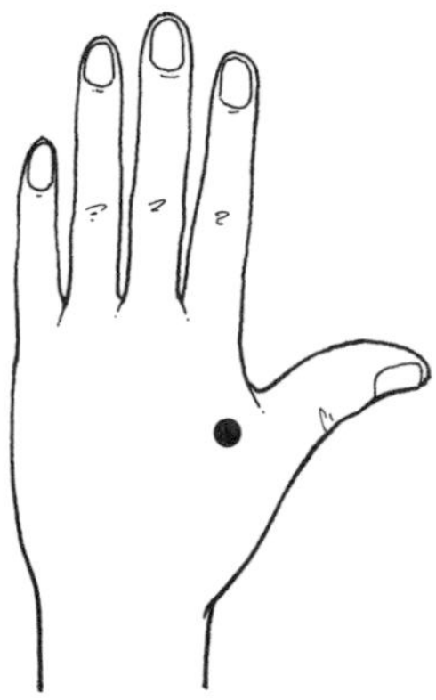

4. Then, use your thumb to rub and massage the large instestine point (Fig. 22). This releases any remaining stagnation in the meridians flowing along the thumb (lung) and index finger (large intestine). Use a deep but gentle circular motion and massage for a minute or two.

Repeat above steps on the opposite hand.

5. Conclude by relaxing both hands completely and then shaking and vibrating them for about half a minute. Allow any remaining excessive energy to flow out through the fingertips.

This massage stimulates the organs and meridians that correspond to each of the fingers. After doing it, you should feel energized, relaxed, and refreshed. It can be done daily or often as a part of your natural beauty program. If you have enough time, you can also do the toenails. Sit in a cross-legged position with one foot resting on your thigh. Massage the large toe using the steps outlined above, and then proceed to each of the other toes. Then massage the kidney point located at the bottom of the foot with a deep circular motion before changing positions and repeating the procedure on the opposite foot (see the figure of the foot on p. 66). To conclude, sit with both legs extended and slightly elevated. Allow your feet and ankles to relax completely and then shake both feet vigorously for 30 seconds, allowing excess energy to flow out through the toes.

Chapter 3 *Sadhanas—Daily Self-discipline Practices*

Introduction to Pranayama and Yoga Asanas

The ancient Vedic seers of India developed an elaborate system of practices to discipline the activity of breathing. This system is known as *Pranayama*. *Prana* is the life-force that holds body, mind, and spirit together. We obtain *prana* from the atmosphere and our food. Where as the lungs play the major role in the respiratory process, *prana* is carried throughout by every cell in the body. The colon is said to produce certain volatile fatty acids which like oxygen, food and water are carriers of *prana*. The good health of the nervous system, lungs, and colon determine how much *prana* we can absorb into the body.

Pranayama is the most essential factor to well-being as it controls breath and respiration which is life. In the practice of *Pranayama*, you will quickly feel the many changes of attitudes and feelings. A deep inner calm and control over the events of your life will be felt. It is necessary to remember not to approach your meditation and yoga *asanas* mechanically. Practice breathing from the stomach by lying on your back with one hand on the stomach. At the beginning exaggerate the inhalation by deliberately pushing out your stomach. Always lengthen your exhalation time to two or three times longer than your inhalation. Too often when we begin to practice breathing meditation, there is a tendency to take a high chest breath and push our shoulders upward. The shoulders and upper chest have nothing to do with the act of breathing. Inhalation also has nothing to do with sniffing something into the nostrils. In essence, ignore the nostrils completely. As you practice *Pranayama* draw your attention to your stomach. Begin to feel your stomach push outward even before you hear the sound of your breathing. Concentrate on the sound of the breath, not on the breathing. You may feel that you are only making the noise of breathing, without breathing. The sound will pull the breath along. Remember to pay attention to the sound of the breath, while you fill your stomach with fresh, clean air. Then exhale by concentrating on the sound of the exhalation leaving the stomach and traveling slowly, very slowly upward, outward, holding the sound like a tenor holds a note, releasing it in a crescendo, from loud to soft to very soft to loud again. After practicing for a short time you will find that the breath flows naturally without any effort.

Asanas, often incorrectly referred to as yoga, are the various postures we practice for the discipline of the body. It is a gentle and powerful practice of the ancient sages of India, in order to keep harmony with body and universe. The movements are smooth and flowing. It is like warm oil pouring out of a bottle. There are no staccato or rash moves in yoga *asanas*, no jarring effects. We learn to release the body limb by limb as we enter the postures. Practice deep breathing while doing your yoga *asanas*. Never hold your breath and remember, breath is life. Choose the same sequence and time of morning and evening every day to practice your meditation and yoga *asanas*.

Morning *Pranayama* and *Asanas* for Predominantly Vata Type

Fig. 23

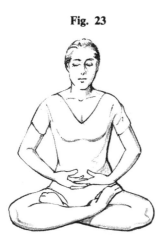

Pranayama: Approximately 15 minutes
1.   Sit in the upright yoga *mudra* position, the lotus position (Fig. 23), or a position closest to this and comfortable. Inhale through the left nostril and exhale through the right nostril. Continue by inhaling through the left nostril and exhaling through the right nostril. Alternate and repeat for approximately 5 minutes.

Fig. 24

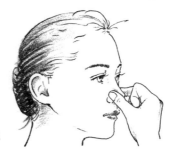
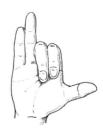

2.   Continue to sit in the position. Assume the right hand position (Fig. 24). Inhale through the right nostril, then do a swallowing motion, and then bring chin to the nape of neck. Hold breath for the same length of time as inhalation. Lift and exhale through the left nostril. Exhalation should be twice as long as inhalation. Continue by inhaling through the left nostril, swallow, put chin to nape of neck, hold the breath, and then exhale through the right nostril. Alternate 10 times.

Fig. 25

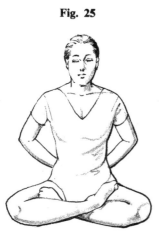

3.   From the upright yoga *mudra* position, clasp both hands in back (Fig. 25) and lower the upper body until forehead touches the floor, or as far forward as is comfortable (Fig. 26). Hold for 60 seconds, or longer if desired.

Fig. 26

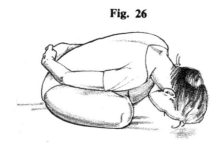

(Yoga *Asanas:* Approximately 30 minutes)

First Asana

Plough and Shoulder Stand (*Halasana* and *Sarvangasana*): Five stages; 2 stages for plough and 3 stages for shoulder stand

The plough position strengthens the upper body, aids circulation, and calms the body's energy. The shoulder stand strengthens the lower body.

Caution: Hold the position for no more than 30 minutes. Do not force any of the movements. Vata types need to be very careful of the lower back, as they are prone to spinal shifting and lower back problems. *Do not do this position if there is an existing back problem.*

Plough
1. Lie flat on back, lift leg up to 30 degrees, then to 60 degrees, and then to 90 degrees (Figs. 27 and 28).
2. Take the extended legs to the back of the head, or as far back as you can (Fig. 29). Hold for 30 seconds. This is the plough position.

Fig. 27

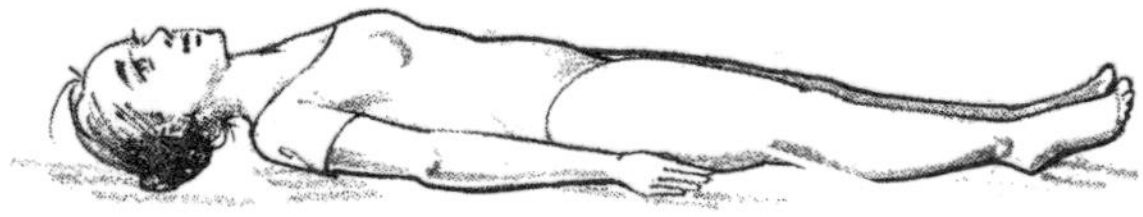

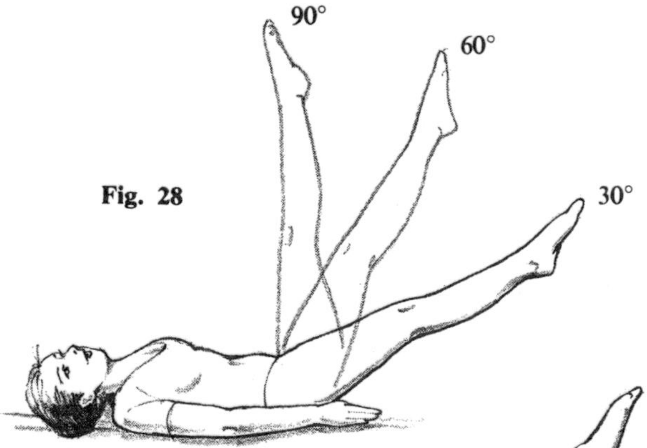

Fig. 28

Fig. 29

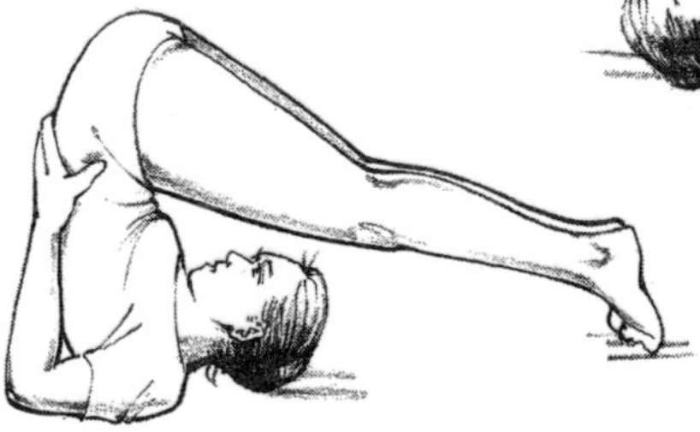

Fig. 30

Shoulder Stand
1. Bring legs forward up to shoulder stand, always controlling the movement from the lower abdomen (Fig. 30). Hold for 30 seconds.
2. Take legs back to plough position.
3. From the plough position, bring legs up to 90 degrees, then begin lowering to 60 degrees, 30 degrees, and then to

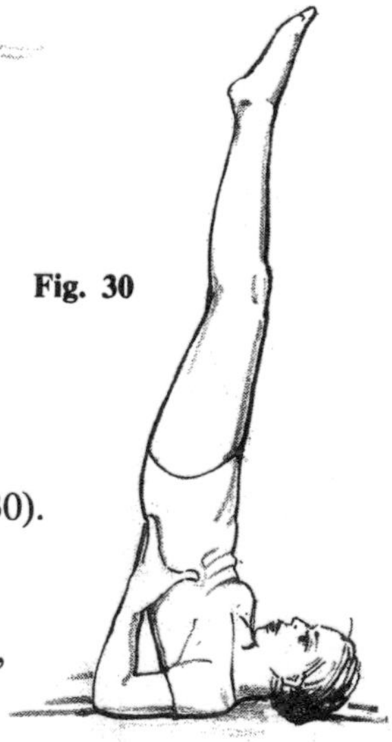

the floor. Be careful to release the back from the upper back vertebra by vertebra until the back is flat to the floor. Always release back slowly and smoothly.

SECOND ASANA

Cobra (*Bhujangasana*)
This position strengthens the lower body, relieves intestinal disorders, PMS (premenstrual) symptoms, and so on.

1.   While flat on back, extend left arm, then turn over to the stomach (turn in direction of extended arm).
2.   Lay arms alongside body in a relaxed position.
3.   Lay hand flat alongside the chest, with elbows pointing upward.
4.   Lift upper chest and head up to ceiling (Fig. 31). Be careful not to put any of the body weight on the hands. Lift up only to the point where there is no pressure on the hands. You should be able to lift hands off floor and still maintain upright chest position. Stay up for 30 seconds and slowly bring chest back to floor and extend arms alongside the body.

Fig. 31

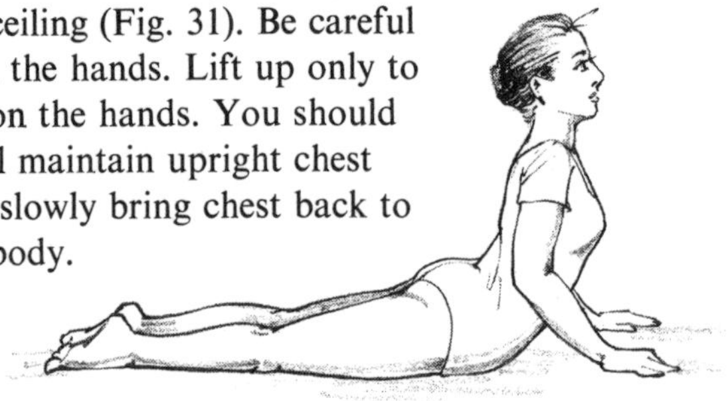

THIRD ASANA

Child's Pose, Easy Backbend, and Hard Backbend (*Vajrasana, Virasana*)

These positions strengthen the back, chest, blood circulation, and relieve tension and stiffness of muscles.

Child's Pose
1.   Sit in *seiza* position with hands on the lap (Fig. 32).
2.   Cuff both hands and place snugly against stomach (Figs. 33 and 34).
3.   Feel the bend forward, from the lower back through the vertebra to the top of the head. Bring head down to the floor (Fig. 35).

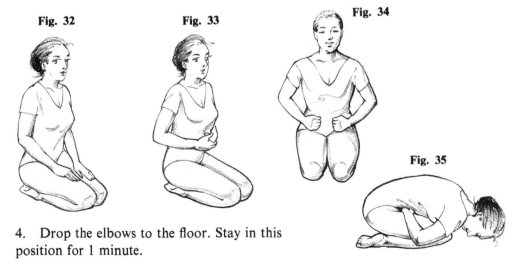

Fig. 32   **Fig. 33**   **Fig. 34**

Fig. 35

4.   Drop the elbows to the floor. Stay in this position for 1 minute.

Easy Backbend

1.   From the *seiza* position, spread the knees apart approximately 12 inches and lower your seat to the floor (Figs. 36 and 37).
2.   Lean backward and support self with elbows, bringing hands forward to touch the toes (Fig. 38). Head is in an upright position, hold for 30 seconds.

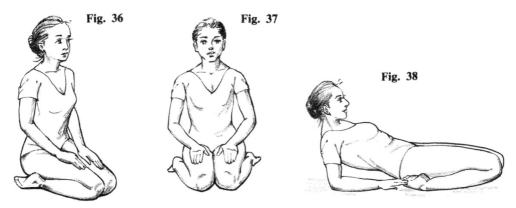

Fig. 36   Fig. 37

Fig. 38

Hard Backbend (optional)

1.   From the *seiza* position, spread the knees apart approximately 12 inches, and lower your seat to the floor.
2.   Lean backward and support self with elbows, bringing hands forward to touch the toes. Head is in an upright position, hold for 30 seconds.
3.   Follow the steps of easy backbend and lay the back and head on the floor (Fig. 39).
4.   Extend arm over head, flat on the floor. Hold the position for 30 seconds.
5.   Gently lift yourself up from either the easy or the hard backbend position and release legs by extending them forward one at a time.

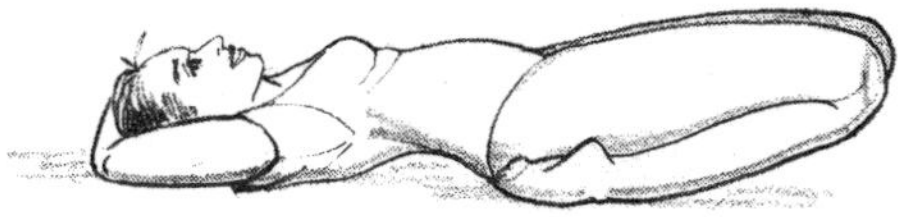

Fig. 39

FOURTH ASANAS

Difficult Head to Knee (*Paschimottanasana*)

This position strengthens the upper body, neck, and head while adding flexibility to the hamstrings.

1.   Sit with legs extended and arms to the side (Fig. 40).
2.   Slowly, from the lower back, begin to release the body forward, until the body is parallel to the extended legs, resting the face between the calves (Fig. 41).

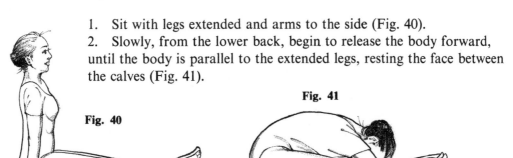

Fig. 41

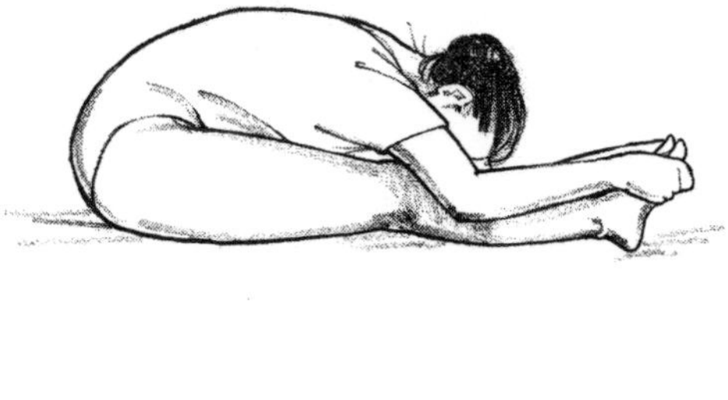

Fig. 40

Note: Do not force the body forward. If you cannot bring the body all the way down, try the easy head to knee position.

Easy Head to Knee (*Paschimottanasana*)

1. Sit with legs extended. With the help of a scarf or towel, place towel behind the feet and hold ends in each hand (Fig. 42). (The towel is an extension of your hands.)
2. Gently pull yourself forward, lowering from the bottom of the back while maintaining a straight back at all times (Fig. 43). Hold position for 60 seconds.

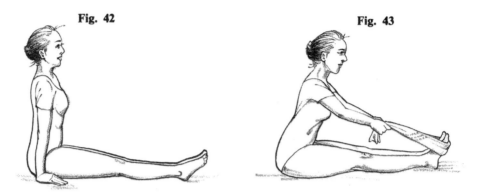

Fig. 42   **Fig. 43**

FIFTH ASANA

Half Wheel (*Ardha Cakrasana*)

This *asana* strengthens the lower body including intestines and lower back, aids circulation, and relieves PMS symptoms. This is an excellent one for Vata types.

1. Lay flat on the back, arms along the side (Fig. 44).
2. Bend the knees and bring the feet closer to the seat of the body (Fig. 45).
3. Place hands above the waist and gently begin to lift the hips and lower chest off the floor (Fig. 46). Feel a good extension of the back. Hold for 30 seconds.
4. Release the back gently to the floor. Be careful not to arch the back.
5. Extend the legs and release arms to the side.

Fig. 44

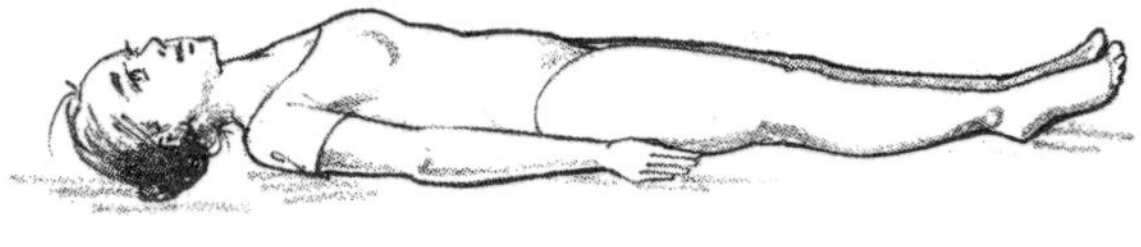

Fig. 45

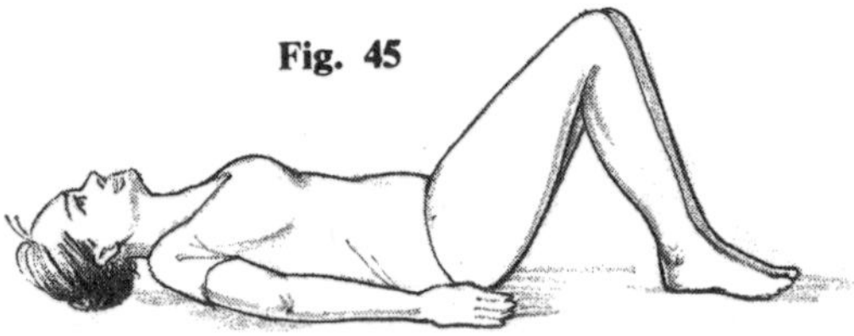

Fig. 46

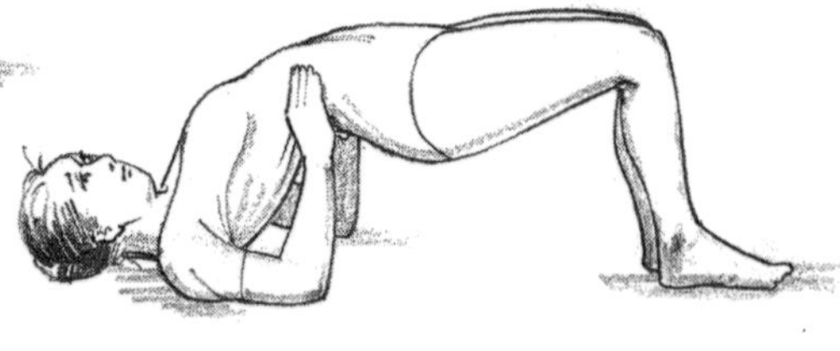

Fig. 47

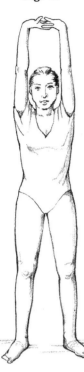

6.   Stay on the back with eyes closed, feet relaxed, arms and hands released, gently breathing. Stay for 1 to 3 minutes.

SIXTH ASANA

Palm Tree
This position strengthens and lifts the spirit and revitalizes the body.

1.   Stand up in an upright position with legs naturally apart.
2.   Intertwine fingers in front of you and lift arms to ceiling, with palms facing ceiling (Fig. 47).

Evening *Pranayama* and *Asanas* for Vata Type

Yoga *Mudra*
1.   Sit in yoga *mudra* position. Alternate breathing for 5 minutes.
2.   While sitting in yoga *mudra* position, clasp your hands behind your back and bring head to the floor. Always begin bending movement from lower back. Stay in position for a few minutes, while breathing deeply but gently.

Fig. 48

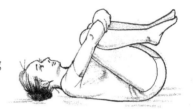

Knees to Chest
Release position and lay on the back with arms loosely on the side. Bend the knees and gently bring forward to rest on the chest. Embrace knees with arms (Fig. 48). Stay in position for a few minutes.

Corpse (*Savasana*)
Release knees and continue to be flat on back. Keep legs comfortably apart, arms loosely on the sides (Fig. 49). Gently close your eyes. Be conscious of releasing all strain and stress from the body. Remain as if lifeless and calm. Invite your attention to your *hara* (belly). Visualize your own fire kindling from the deep recesses of your being. Watch the fire blaze into flame of yellow, red to orange. Feel the heat permeate through your entire being. Allow the fire to dissolve into a translucent luminous vivid green light. Feel the warmth of this light and allow it to pervade every cell in your body. Mentally picture your body lubricated inside by

Fig. 49

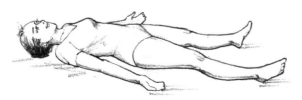

this light. Picture yourself limb by limb, beginning with your toes and invite yourself to surrender to the universal light of the self.

I let go of my toes . . .
I let go of my feet . . .
I let go of my ankles . . .
I let go of my calves . . .
I let go of my knees . . .
I let go of my thighs . . .
I let go of my groin . . .
I let go of my belly . . .
I let go of my waist . . .
I let go of my chest . . .
I let go of my breasts . . .
I let go of my neck . . .
I let go of my throat . . .
I let go of my chin . . .
I let go of my lips . . .
I let go of my nose . . .
I let go of my eyes . . .
I let go of my forehead . . .
I let go of my face . . .
I let go of my hair . . .
I let go of my head . . .
I let go of my shoulders . . .
I let go of my arms . . .
I let go of my elbows . . .
I let go of my hands
I let go . . . I let go . . . I let go. . . . I am one with the universe, I am pure consciousness. . . . I am silence.

Say your evening prayers and go to bed with a clear, silent mind.

Morning *Pranayama* and *Asanas* for Predominantly Pitta Type ————

Pranayama: Approximately 15 minutes
1.   Sit in the lotus, semi-lotus, *seiza* (diamond position), or a position closest to it with back upright and slightly forward (see Fig. 23).
2.   With right fingers in breathing position (see Fig. 24), begin to inhale through the left nostril and exhale through the right nostril, continue by breathing in through left and out of right. Concentrate on the sound of your breathing, let the thoughts flow in and flow out. Always get back to sound of the breath. Repeat left nostril inhalation for 5 minutes.
3.   With hands in lap, inhale and exhale deeply, slowly and calmly, sustaining both inhalation and exhalation as long as possible. Practice for 5 minutes.

(Yoga *Asanas*: Approximately 30 minutes)

FIRST ASANA

Plough Position and Shoulder Stand (*Halasana and Sarvangasana*): See p. 187 for instructions.

SECOND ASANAS

Cobra (*Bhujangasana*): See p. 188 for instructions.

THIRD ASANA

Half Bow (*Ardha Dhanurasana*)
This position strengthens the nervous system and aids with anger and tension.

Lie flat on the stomach and extend arms forward. Lift both legs together and raise approximately 14 inches from the floor (Fig. 50). Balance on the stomach and hold position for 30 seconds.

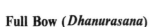

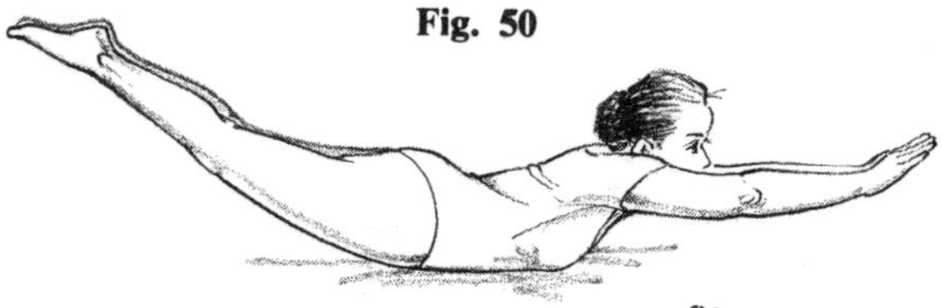

Fig. 50

Full Bow (*Dhanurasana*)
From the holding position above, bend the knees and hold the ankles. Begin gently pulling the legs in an upward position, creating a cradle effect of the body, balancing silently on the stomach (Fig. 51). Hold position for 15 minutes.

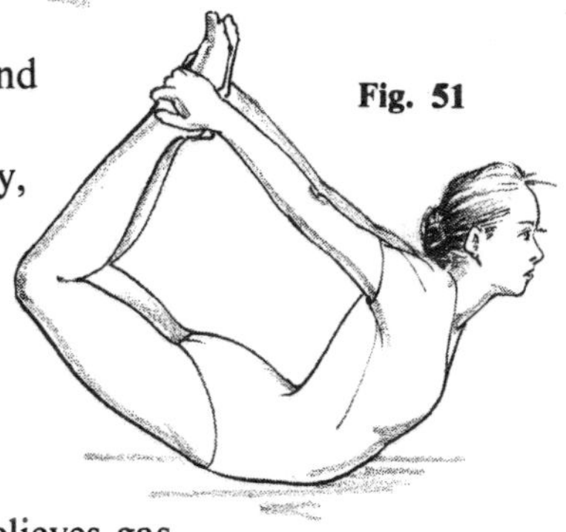

Fig. 51

FOURTH ASANA

The Locust (*Shalabhasana*)
This position strengthens the lower intestines and relieves gas.

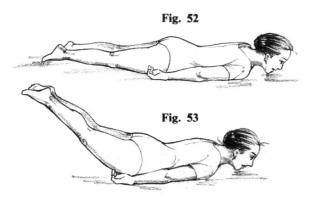

Fig. 52

Fig. 53

1. Lie on the stomach, chin squarely on the floor. Cuff the hands and place them, finger up, under the hips closer to the outside (Fig. 52).
2. Begin to lift both legs to 30 degrees, 40 degrees, and 60 degrees upward (Fig. 53). Hold the position for 30 seconds.

Fifth Asana

The Fish (*Matsyasana*)
This position strengthens the liver and digestive system and relieves headaches and stress.

1.   Lie flat on the back and place both hands underneath closer to the outside of your seat.
2.   Lift the chest and head and place tops of head on the floor with chin pointing to the ceiling (Fig. 54). Hold the position for 60 seconds.

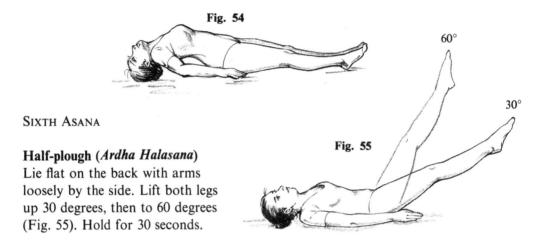

Fig. 54

Sixth Asana

Half-plough (*Ardha Halasana*)
Lie flat on the back with arms loosely by the side. Lift both legs up 30 degrees, then to 60 degrees (Fig. 55). Hold for 30 seconds.

Fig. 55

Seventh Asana

The Boat (*Naukasana*)
This position strengthens the upper body, chest, and lungs.

1.   Sit upright (90 degrees) with legs extended (Fig. 56).
2.   Lean back to approximately 60 degrees, extend arms and hands with palms facing downward. Lift both legs together to 60 degrees off the floor with arm position parallel to legs (Fig. 57). Hold the position for 20 seconds.

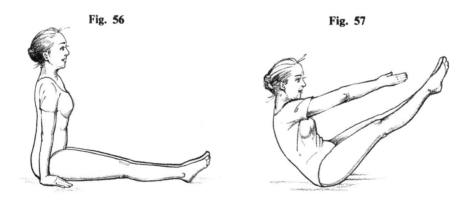

Fig. 56

Fig. 57

195

EIGHTH ASANA

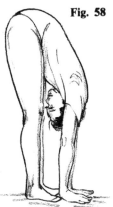
Fig. 58

Forward Bend—Standing Position (*Padahasasana*)
This position gives stability and excellent posture.

1. Stand upright, feet only a few inches apart.
2. Lift the arms to the ceiling and then bend slightly backward arching the back ever so slightly.
3. From the lower back, begin moving extended arms slowly over the head, then directly in front of you. Then move extended arms to the feet or the floor in front of your feet (Fig. 58). Hold for 30 seconds. Slowly lift up to standing position.

Evening *Pranayama* and *Asanas* for Pitta Type

Pranayama: Approximately 15 minutes
1. Sit in lotus position, semi-lotus position, or *seiza* (diamond position).
2. Assume breathing position with right hand (see Fig. 24). Inhale through the left nostril and exhale through the right nostril slowly, calmly for a few minutes.

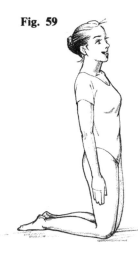
Fig. 59

Kneeling Forward Bend
Stand upright on the knees from your lower back (Fig. 59). Bring gently the head and ears down slightly between your knees (or as close to the knees as possible). Have both arms hanging loosely, fingers pointing backward alongside your body (Fig. 60). Seat position is pointing to the ceiling. Retain position for 60 seconds. Release position. Lift and straighten out.

Fig. 60

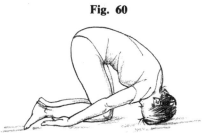

Knees to Chest: See p. 191 for instructions.

Corpse (*Savasana*)
Lie flat on your back, feet comfortably apart, arms alongside the body, palms resting comfortably upward and away from the body (see Fig. 49). Close your eyes gently. Be conscious of relieving all strain and stress from the body. Remain as if lifeless and calm. Invite your attention to your *hara* (belly). Visualize your own innate fire kindling from the deep recesses of your being. Watch this fire ignite your entire center and then allow the flames to become cool. Trace the changes of

color of the flame from deep purple through the blue to a translucent, milky pearl light. Allow this cool light to permeate your entire being. Mentally picture your body limb by limb beginning with your toes and invite it to surrender to the universal light of the self.

I let go of my toes . . .
I let go of my feet . . .
I let go of my ankles . . .
I let go of my calves . . .
I let go of my knees . . .
I let go of my thighs . . .
I let go of my groin . . .
I let go of my belly . . .
I let go of my waist . . .
I let go of my chest . . .
I let go of my breasts . . .
I let go of my neck . . .
I let go of my throat
I let go of my chin . . .
I let go of my lips . . .
I let go of my nose . . .
I let go of my eyes . . .
I let go of my forehead . . .
I let go of my face . . .
I let go of my hair . . .
I let go of my head . . .
I let go of my shoulders . . .
I let go of my arms . . .
I let go of my elbows . . .
I let go of my hands . . .
I let go . . . I let go . . . I let go. . . . I am one with the universe, I am pure consciousness. . . . I am silence.

Say your evening prayers and go to bed with a clear, silent mind.

Morning *Pranayama* and *Asanas* for Predominantly Kapha Type —————

Pranayama: Approximately 25 minutes
The *bhariska* breath is excellent for "emptying" the body of stale air. It revitalizes the body and stimulates the metabolism. All types may perform this breathing techniques, but it is especially powerful for Kapha types.

1. Bhariska—The Yogi's Breath of Fire
Sit in lotus, semi-lotus, or in a position close to this. Begin firmly and forcefully exhaling. Your breath will make a clean sharp sound. Do not concentrate on the

inhalation. This will occur naturally. Simply breathe out loudly and briskly from the stomach on counts of 3 for 30 seconds. Rest for 30 seconds and then repeat the fire breath. Practice for 3 minutes every morning.

2. *Right Nostril Inhalation*

Continue sitting and assume the breathing position with right hand (see Fig. 24). Inhale through the right nostril and exhale through the left nostril. Remember to inhale deeply through the stomach and to exhale 2 or 3 times longer than inhalation. Keep the breathing deep, calm, and slow. Repeat 20 times by inhaling through the right nostril and exhaling through the left. Repeat approximately 10 minutes.

Repeat 20 times by inhaling through the right nostril and exhaling through the left for approximately 10 minutes.

(Yoga *Asanas*: Approximately 45 to 60 minutes)

FIRST ASANA

Plough and Shoulder Stand (*Halasana and Sarvangasana*): See p. 187 for instructions.

SECOND ASANA

Cobra (*Bhujangasana*): See p. 188 for instructions.

THIRD ASANA

Half Bow (*Ardha Dhanurasna*): See p. 193 for instructions.
This position strengthens the chest and helps congestion and sinuses.

FOURTH ASANA

Full Bow (*Dhanurasana*): See p. 193 for instructions.

FIFTH ASANA

Child's Pose, Easy Backbend, and Hard Backbend (*Yajrasana, Virasana*)

Child's Pose: See p. 188 for instructions.

Easy Backbend: See p. 189 for instructions.

Hard Backbend: See p. 189 for instructions.
In steps 2 and 4 hold the position for 60 seconds.

SIXTH ASANA

Difficult Head to Knee and Easy Head to Knee (*Paschimottanasana*): See pp. 189 and 190 for instructions. In step 3 of easy head to knee, hold the position for 30 seconds.

SEVENTH ASANA

The Boat (*Naukasana*): See p. 194 for instructions.

EIGHTH ASANA

The Locust (*Shalabhasana*): See p. 193 for instructions.

NINTH ASANA

The Fish (*Matsyasana*): See p. 194 for instructions.
This position is an excellent one for Kapha type. It strengthens intestines, lungs, throat, and blood.

TENTH ASANA

Half Wheel (*Ardha Cakrasana*): See p. 190 for instructions.
This position is another excellent *asana* for Kapha type. It guards against lung, chest, and blood disorders.

ELEVENTH ASANA

Palm Tree: See p. 191 for instructions.
This position generates a lift in spirit and strengthens lungs.

TWELFTH ASANA

Forward Bend—Standing Position (*Padahasasana*): See p. 195 for instructions.
Go directly from the palm tree *asana*. In step 2 hold the position for 60 seconds.

THIRTEENTH ASANA

Wheel—Side Bending (*Chakrasana*)
This position strengthens the upper body, lungs, throat, and is excellent for upper body flexibility.

1. Extend and raise right arm 90 degrees to the body, turn the palm upward (Fig. 61).
2. Slowly move the extended arm to touch the ear.
3. Keeping arms extended by the ear, lean the body and arm toward the left

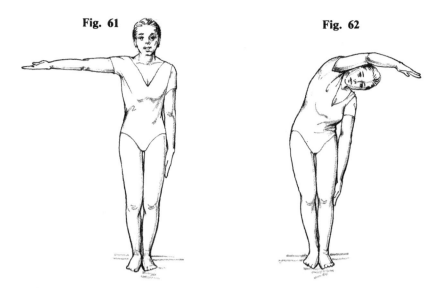

Fig. 61

Fig. 62

side, giving maximum stretch to the right side of the body (Fig. 62). Hold position for 30 seconds. Slowly straighten the body with arm still extended. Release arm to 90 degrees. Turn palms down and take arms down to the side.

4.   Repeat exercise with left arm and side. Hold position for 30 seconds.

FOURTEENTH ASANA

Triangle (*Trikonasana*)
This position gives a stretch to the entire body and strengthens all organs of upper and lower body.

1.   Assume the standing position. Spread both legs wide apart. Extend both arms horizontally (Fig. 63).
2.   Begin turning only the upper body to the left, arms still extended. Drop the right arm to touch the left toe and bring the extended left arm pointing straight up

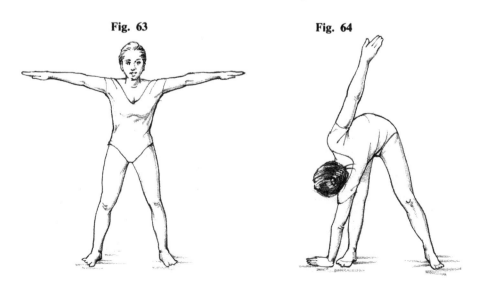

Fig. 63

Fig. 64

to the ceiling (Fig. 64). Turn your head looking in the direction of the left hand above. Head is parallel to the extended left arm. Hold for 30 seconds.

3.   Slowly bring extended left arm and head down as the extended right arm moves upward to the side. Keeping both arms extended, bring the body and head directly to the center. Bring the body to the standing position and release arms down to the side. Repeat exercise with right arm extended to the ceiling. Hold position for 30 seconds.

Evening *Pranayama* and *Asanas* for Kapha Type

Pranayama: Approximately 15 minutes

Fig. 65

1.   Repeat the *bhariska* breath (fire breath) for 60 seconds.
2.   Repeat the right nostril inhalation for 60 seconds.

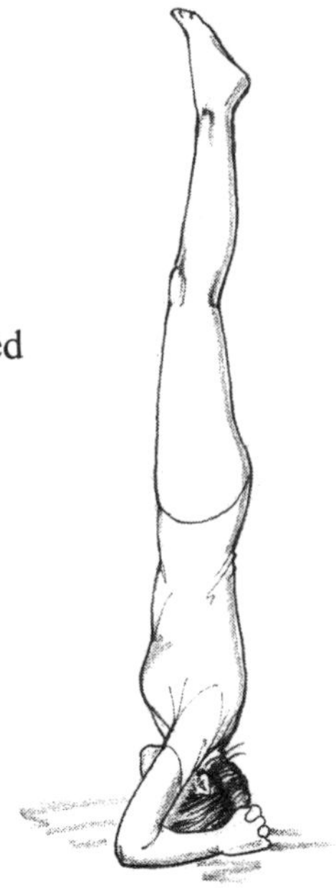

Head Stand (*Sirsasana*)

1.   Place a small pillow on the floor where the head will be placed. Use a supporting wall for those who need assistance. Kneel on hands and knees on the floor. Arms are close to the head, with backs of hands facing the wall. Fingers are intertwined and placed snugly against the back of head. Allow the head to be 2 feet away from the wall.

2.   Tighten the lower abdomen and from the point of strength push the feet and lower body off the floor upward. Simultaneously, secure hands and head position firmly while slowly extending lower body and feet upward to the ceiling (Fig. 65). Weight will be directly on top of head. Tips of feet may lean against the wall, until body is strong enough to support the weight without leaning.

3.   Hold the position for 30 seconds and slowly begin to release position by bending and bringing knees close to the body.

4.   Release the upper, then lower back and slowly bring it down to the floor vertebra by vertebra so as to unfold the body.

Release knees and continue to be flat on back. Have legs comfortably apart, arms loose, a little way from side. Lay flat on the back, arms along the side.

Corpse (*Sarasana*)

Lie flat on your back, feet comfortable apart, arms alongside the body, palms resting comfortably upward and away from the body (see Fig. 49). Gently close your eyes. Be conscious of releasing all strains and stress from the body. Remain as if lifeless and calm. Invite your attention to your *hara* (belly). Visualize your own fire kindling from the deep recesses of your being. Watch the fire blaze into flames of orange and red. Feel the heat permeate through your entire being. Allow the fire to dissolve in a translucent vibrant green light. Feel the warmth of this light and allow it to pervade every cell in your body. Mentally picture your body firm and crisp inside. Picture yourself limb by limb, beginning with your toes, and invite yourself to surrender to the universal light of the self.

I let go of my toes . . .
I let go of my feet . . .
I let go of my ankles . . .
I let go of my calves . . .
I let go of my knees . . .
I let go of my thighs
I let go of my groin . . .
I let go of my belly . . .
I let go of my waist . . .
I let go of my chest . . .
I let go of my breasts . . .
I let go of my neck . . .
I let go of my throat . . .
I let go of my chin . . .
I let go of my lips . . .
I let go of my nose . . .
I let go of my eyes . . .
I let go of my forehead . . .
I let go of my face . . .
I let go of my hair . . .
I let go of my head . . .
I let go of my shoulders . . .
I let go of my arms . . .
I let go of my elbows . . .
I let go of my hands . . .
I let go . . . I let go . . . I let go. . . . I am one with the universe, I am pure consciousness. . . . I am silence.

Say your evening prayers and go to bed with a clear, silent mind.

Yoga Exercises for the Face

These exercises are beneficial to everyone. All the various constitutional types can practice the same facial yogic exercises.

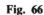

Fig. 66

Lion (*Simhasana*)
Extend tongue as far out as possible (Fig. 66). Hold for 5 seconds and then quickly withdraw tongue. Repeat 5 times.

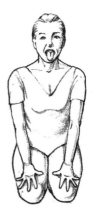

Eye Exercise
1. Eye movements side to side.
2. Eye movements up to down and then down to up.
   Extend eye movements to the very extreme.

Fig. 67

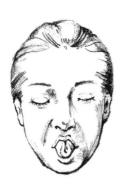

Open and Close Mouth Rotation
1. Pull the upper lip over top of front teeth and shape the mouth to an open O.
2. Widen lips to an extremely exaggerated smile, and rhythmically rotate the opening and closing of the mouth in a circular motion. Repeat the movement 10 times.

The Curved Tongue
1. Stick the tongue out halfway in a tight curve forming a canal (Fig. 67).
2. Inhale and exhale quickly through curved tongue. Repeat the movement 10 times.

Dō-In Facelift and Beauty Meditation

Daily self-massage, or Dō-In, is an excellent way to refresh and revitalize the face by activating energy and circulation. You can use the simple routine below—adapted from *The Book of Dō-In* by Michio Kushi—to tone the skin and relax tension in the face and throughout the body. It takes only several minutes to do.

1. Sit in a quiet place, relax your breathing, and apply both palms to your cheeks—the right palm to right cheek, the left palm to the left cheek (Fig. 68). Keep your hands in this position and breathe deeply at least 3 times.
2. Rub your cheeks up and down until they become warm (Fig. 69).
3. Close your eyes and place both palms over them (Fig. 70). Hold this position while you breathe in and out several times. This energizes the regions around the eyes and helps relax tension and stress.

Fig. 68   **Fig. 69**   **Fig. 70**

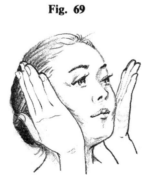
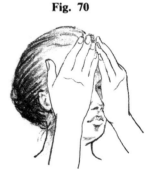

4. Keep your eyes closed and use the index, middle, and ring fingers to press firmly but gently on the bony edge of the upper eye socket, moving from the inside to the outside, and then press the bone underneath the eye (Figs. 71 and 72). Do both eyes at once and repeat several times.
5. With your eyes still closed, use the tips of the same three fingers to slowly

and gently press the front of the eyeballs (Fig. 73). Press and then quickly detach your fingers. Repeat 10 times to release stress and tension in the eyes.

Fig. 71   **Fig. 72**   **Fig. 73**

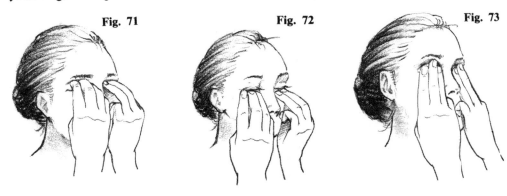

6.   Use your thumb and index finger to pinch the bridge of the nose and the corners of the eyes (Fig. 74). Push deeply for about 10 seconds and then quickly detach by pulling your fingers away from your face (Fig. 75). Repeat 3 to 5 times. This exercise is especially helpful for relieving strain and fatigue in the eyes.

Fig. 74

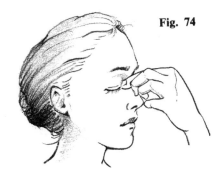

7.   Rub the sides of the nose up and down with the same fingers until it becomes warm (Fig. 76). This exercise activates the stomach and pancreas and helps make breathing more smooth and steady.

8.   Massage the area between the nose and mouth with the four fingers of both hands (Fig. 77). Use a circular motion and begin from the center and work your way to the periphery. Repeat 7 to 10 times. Then do the same thing below the mouth (Fig. 78).

Fig. 75

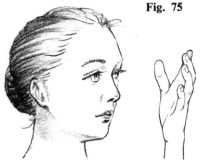

Fig. 76   **Fig. 77**   **Fig. 78**

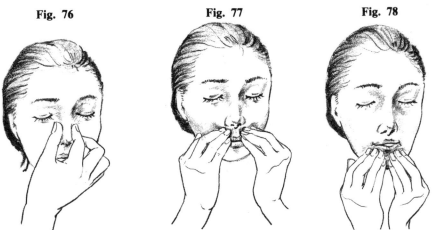

Fig. 79   **Fig. 80**

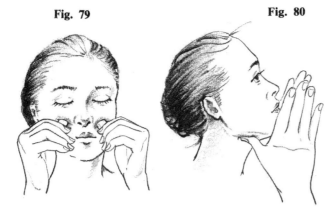

9. Place your thumbs underneath your cheekbone about a fingerwidth away from the sides of the nose (Fig. 79). Use a circular motion to rub and massage these points for about a minute. This helps relieve tension in the face caused by sinus congestion.

10. Use your thumbs to press deeply under the lower jaw, as if you are making deep indentations, from underneath the ear to below the chin (Fig. 80). Repeat 3 to 5 times. This exercise helps tone the skin and muscles of the jaw.

11. Use the index, middle, and ring fingers to press around the ear several times (Fig. 81). This increases circulation in the ear and helps improve the sense of balance.

12. Use the thumbs and index finger to pull the ears upward from the top, outward from the middle, and downward from the lobe (Figs. 82–84). Pull twice in each direction by placing your fingers in the inner region of the ear and sliding them outward, and then proceed to the next section. Repeat the entire procedure 5 times. Massaging the ears stimulates the flow of energy to the kidneys and releases stagnation in the body as a whole.

13. Use the palms to briskly strike the ears

Fig. 81

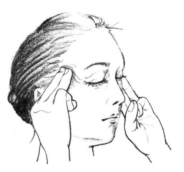

Fig. 82

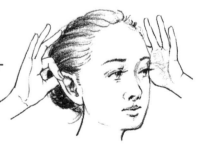

Fig. 83   **Fig. 84**

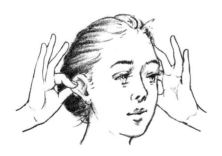
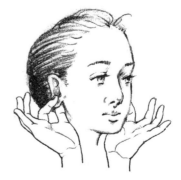

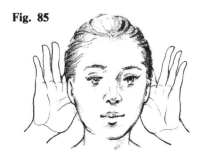

Fig. 85

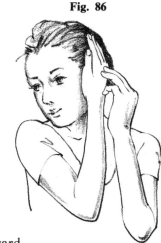

Fig. 86

with a repeating back-to-front motion (Fig. 85). Repeat about 10 to 20 times.

14. Cover the left ear with the right hand and with the first three fingers of the left hand, tap briskly on the back of the right hand, sensing sharp vibrations toward the inner ear. Tap in pairs and do about 10 pairs of taps. Reverse hands and repeat this procedure on the right ear (Fig. 86).

15. Use the index, middle, and ring fingers of both hands to gently massage the temples (Fig. 87). Rub in a circular motion for a minute or two to release tension and stagnation.

16. Make a loose fist with both hands and lightly pound the entire head (as if your hands are bouncing all over the head) covering the top, sides, front and back (Fig. 88). This stimulates circulation in the scalp and the growth of healthy new hair.

Fig. 87

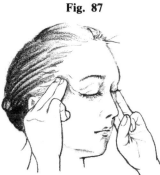

17. Use all of your fingers to vigorously massage the entire scalp with a rapid back-and-forth motion as if you were shampooing the hair (Fig. 89). Continue for about half a minute.

18. Tilt your head to the left and bang the right side of the neck with the right fist (Fig. 90). Then tilt the head in the opposite direction and bang the

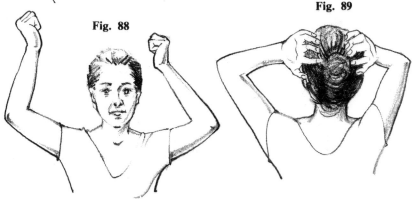

Fig. 88

Fig. 89

Fig. 90

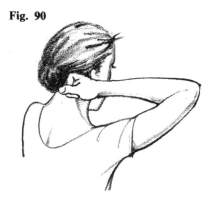

Fig. 91

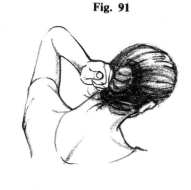

left side of the neck with the left fist (Fig. 91). Tilt the head forward and bang the back of the neck. Then allow the head to relax and fall fully forward and back several times (Figs. 92 and 93), and then side to side several times (Fig. 94). Finally, rotate the neck counterclockwise about 5 times, and then clockwise about 5 times (Fig. 95). This exercise helps release stagnation in the head and accelerates the flow of energy to the face.

Fig. 92   Fig. 93

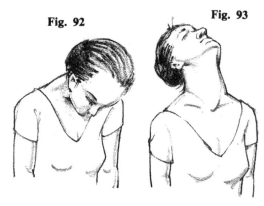

Fig. 94   Fig. 95

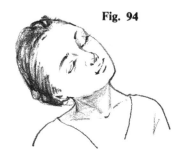

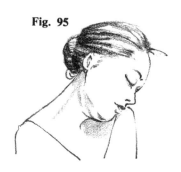

Fig. 96

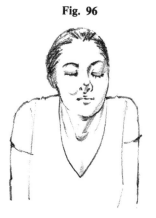

19.   Raise your shoulders, contracting your shoulder muscles as much as possible (Fig. 96). Then quickly release the contraction, completely relaxing these muscles as much as possible. Repeat 5 times. This exercise helps release tension in the neck and shoulders and activates the smooth functioning of the intestines.

20.   Use the fingers of one hand to press down and massage the opposite shoulder, tilting your head to the opposite side (Fig. 97). Repeat on the other shoulder. Use a circular massage to loosen any tension or stiffness.

Fig. 97   Fig. 98

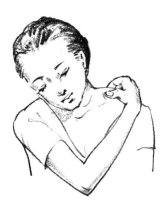

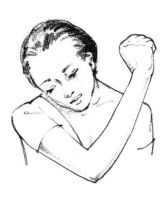

Fig. 99

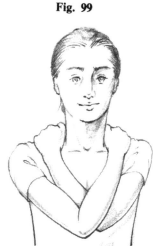

21.   Make a fist with one hand and pound the opposite shoulder about 10 to 20 times (Fig. 98). Repeat
on the other shoulder. Then pound the top of the spine
as well as the back of the neck about 10 to 20 times.

22.   Apply the palms to the opposite shoulders
and breathe in and out 3 times, slowly but deeply, to harmonize the flow of energy
throughout the body (Fig. 99).

23.   Sit comfortably, close your eyes, and let your mind and body relax (Fig.
100). Breathe naturally for about a minute, and allow energy to flow freely to every
part of your body, enlivening each cell. Then see yourself as healthy and beautiful
and hold that image for a while. Slowly open your eyes and return to normal. See
your daily life—including your diet, activity, and thoughts—as the means to
actualize this self-image.

Fig. 100

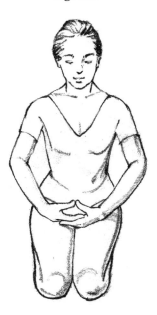

The Practice of Japa for a Silent Mind

Japa is beneficial to everyone. All the various constitutional types can practice *Japa*. It is especially helpful to Vata and Pitta types. *Japa* represents that which puts an end to the cycle of births and deaths or attaining oneness with pure consciousness through silence. *Japa* is that which destroys all impurities of the mind.

Japa is an old Vedic practice for attaining a quiet mind. Our minds are generally preoccupied and busy. We think of our dreams and our disappointments, fears, and commitments, what to eat, what to wear, where to go, how much we have, how much more we need, we think, think, and think. The mind becomes thick with sticky thoughts. Thoughts we cannot separate ourselves from.

We ask for peace and calm but do not understand that peace is silence. Silence of the mind. Peace is being able to quietly thin the mind of its erratic thoughts.

Japa provides a physical action that draws the mind to a single point. In using a rosary or *japa mala* (which are usually 54 or 108 beads), you are able to turn a bead one at a time while repeating a specific *mantra* (which is a short grouping of words that has a sound; repetition of this sound generates a deep vibration in accord with the heart and eventually achieves a silencing of unwanted, extraneous thoughts; Figs. 101 and 102).

In practicing *Japa*, the *mantra* should be repeated audibly and with the same time intervals. One very excellent *mantra* that is practiced by the students of the Vedas is *Om Namo Shivaya*. The Sanscrit words meaning "the eternal sound of the Lord's name." You may use any meaningful *mantra* of your choice. It is important that it has some deep meaning to you, for only then will sincerity and perseverance be present.

Using the *mala*, each bead representing the completion of *Om Namo Shivaya* is then turned, then on to the next bead, repeating *Om Namo Shivaya* and continue on until you have reached the beginning of the *mala*. There is usually an extra bead to indicate that you have finished one rotation of the *mala*. You may also use an "Om" sign, a "Cross," the "Star of David," a crystal of your choice or any important symbols as a pendant to indicate the beginning of your *mala*.

The beginning and end of each *mantra* denotes the beginning and end of each thought. *Japa* is not a series of continuous thoughts. It is the crisp beginning and end of each singular *mantra*. Thus the same *mantra* is repeated, each with its own separate beginning and end. In-between each *mantra* is the silence. The repetition of the *mantra* allows us the silence in-between the *mantras*. This silence is pure consciousness. This silence is you, before thoughts and activities are superimposed upon you. This silence is peace. This silence is meditation. Maintaining this silence is meditation. At the beginning and for some time other thoughts will come while practicing the *mantra*. Always go back to the sound of the *mantra*. Do not worry about the thoughts. Allow them to flow in and flow out, by going back to the sound of the *mantra*. The thoughts will resolve themselves into the silence. It is important that you do not concentrate on the thoughts that enter your mind, or else you will become obsessed with these thoughts and they will build into monumental thoughts. Let them be. If the mind continuously goes back to the thoughts, keep repeating your *mantra* and concentrate on the sound of your voice. Eventually the thoughts will dissolve. *Japa* teaches us to recognize silence and to become comfortable with a silent mind.

Fig. 101

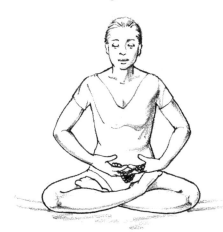

Fig. 102

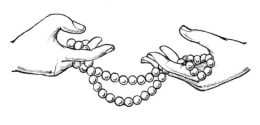

Chapter 4 *Natural Beauty Formulas*

Healthy, wholesome skin is on the balance between lucidity and opacity. A skin that has lustre and brilliance is the best sign of good health. The foods we eat, the exercise or yoga *asanas* and meditation we practice, the conscious effort we make to maintain strength, fortitude, and honesty in our attitudes in our daily lives makes the glow from within. This translucent glow is good health. Perfect skin is balanced by a porcelain-like appearance or opacity of the outer skin. This is also a result of vital cell activity programmed by the above mentioned *sadhanas* or daily disciplines. Daily *sadhanas* maximize the benefits in the training of the mind and the body. For instance, choose the same times every day for your meals, meditation, exercises, body cleansing, work hours, and so on. This builds a continuous motion of harmony and consistency in your life. Do not become fanatical about any routine. There will be times when circumstances invade your daily practice. Allow the circumstances to flow in and to flow out of your life. Get back to your regular schedule as soon as possible. The beauty of life is that it is ever changing, it can never be the same thing day after day. Every day has its own mood, trials, and joys. Take it as it comes, accept it, and flow with it. You know not where it will go, nor is it important to know where it goes. Simply know that it goes. The few consistent *sadhanas* that we set up to do daily are all a conscious effort of self-discipline. Life's tide has a tendency to pull us out to sea on a big adventure and then deposit us back on its banks at the end of its daily excitement. Know before the tide comes in that it is coming and stay back away from its forces, unless you choose to go on the adventure. When you can watch her go and greet her back from shore, you are beginning to get somewhere. Always be considerate to your mistakes. Do not try to get perfect scores because there is no such thing as a perfect score. Beauty has only to do with learning the lessons as they come, even if it takes us several times to learn the same lesson. Eventually we learn from our mistakes and that is what matters. If we learn one out of every thousand lessons, that is truly a good score.

As your health improves, so will the texture and glow of the skin. When the skin begins to express her own aliveness you will find it more and more unnecessary to apply heavy makeup to the face after cleansing. By using your makeup lightly, discretely, and occasionally you will find that you are not naked at all without great amounts of it. Allow the skin to breathe and inhale fresh air. By all means, put on the perfectly adorned face should the venue call for it.

> No birds are seen flying about
> No clouds lined with rainbow
> Yet the sky is most beautiful
> Natural beauty needs no adornment
> (*Bharvari Kirataryniya* IV.23)

The Value of Nature's Formula

In choosing a good natural cosmetic it is important to understand how beneficial the product is to the skin. A good product must have both natural healing ability as well as being absorptive. It is essential to use products that will not harm the normal functions of the skin as the skin absorbs indiscriminately. Products made from petrochemical ingredients and mineral oils are unhealthy and dangerous to the skin. They encourage phytotoxicity and photosensitivity and inhibit the skin's normal moisture producing capacity.

A good natural product must also have a good absorption base, before the skin can reap the full benefit of the product. In ancient Indian and Chinese cosmetic applications, various sulfur compounds and acids were used effectively. Today the natural essential oils have a wide variety of organic compounds which serve as a good absorptive base. Nature has provided the best ingredient for cosmetics from the beginning of time. Skin absorption occurs through the hair follicles and oil glands, as certain substances penetrate the outer and second layers of the skin and are absorbed into the circulatory system.

While it is important not to be caught up with complex terminology, it is beneficial to know certain terms, listed in the end of this chapter, that are frequently used in both commercial and natural cosmetic markets. The basic chemistry of healthy cosmetics is as old as the earth itself. The simple beauty applications of the ancient cultures contain similar ingredients to any clean, natural cosmetic product today. We use a mere fraction of the wealth of good natural ingredients available to us today for beautification. Healthy, wholesome skin does not need the unconscious chemical compounds and slick marketing techniques used in commercial cosmetic products today.

As the awareness and consciousness begin to enhance that which is given from nature, the senses become more subtle and are able to distinguish the grosser characteristics of perfumed chemicals. Once the senses are attuned to the freshness of nature's herbs, oils and minerals, they will be your best guide to detecting an unclean product. It is prudent to prepare yourself for the powerful subtleties of nature's beauty. The chemical kingdom has mimicked nature's beauty by exaggerating all of her delicacies of scent and aura and as a result our senses are trained to the grosser pursuits. Beauty, as in a scent, is a very subtle thing. We depend on nature for our existence. Our body is the microcosm of the entire creation. We are indivisible with that which appears to be outside of us. For every cell in our body, we are provided with millions of cells by Mother Nature, surrounding us. From the food that nourishes us to the wind that brushes our face, every speck of nature corresponds with our spiritual, mental, and physical process. Wisdom in living is choosing the corresponding of our internal self from the external gardens. To understand that there is no division between what is perceived as inside and what is perceived as outside of the body, is to know that everything that appears to be separate from us is a projeccton of the mind and senses.

As the overwhelming analytical discoveries of science continues, the simple basic conclusion will always be the same. The infinite structure of our foods correspond identically to the infinite structure of the body. The new century will find the human components to be very much the same as it always was. Whereas almost all of life can be synthesized in a laboratory, we are still the pervasive, unduplicatable human self made up of nature's substances.

Our ingenious chemical kingdom, can only be at its very best, a poor imitation to nature. If we continue to replenish our body and minds from the chemical kingdom we continue to tear down the aura of our defenses against ill-health. Absolute beauty is absolute health. The harmony of body, mind, and spirit is health. And Mother Nature is still our only source of food, food for the spirit and food for the body and food for the skin.

Vata Type Nature's Formula

Vata Astringents

Musk Astringent

> 10 drops ambrette seed essential oil (musk)
> 10 oz natural spring water
> 8 oz vegetable glycerine
> 1 Tbsp each of the following herbs: fennel, elderflower, camomile, blue mallow, marigold, nettle, coltsfoot
> 1 Tbsp styrax benzoin gum
> 2 tsp grapefruit peel oil
> 1 Tbsp pure gord juice

Bring water and glycerine to a boil. Add herbs and benzoin gum as soon as water begins to boil. Remove from heat until lukewarm. Strain through a clean muslin cloth by twisting each end of cloth in the opposite direction (mixture of herbs is in the center of cloth which is securely folded over to contain herbs).

Add the grapefruit peel oil, ambrette seed essential oil, and the gord juice to mixture. Pour into a clean glass jar. Cover and shake to mix. Keep in a cool place or refrigerate.

Peppermint-Licorice Astringent

> 6 drops peppermint oil
> ½ tsp licorice root powder
> 10 oz natural spring water
> 10 oz vegetable glycerine
> 1 oz each of the following herbs: horse chestnut, peppermint, hops
> 2 tsp natural ascorbic acid (powdered)
> 6 drops camellia oil

Bring water and glycerine to a boil. Add herbs, ascorbic acid, and licorice root powder to water. As soon as water begins to boil remove from heat until lukewarm. Strain herbs through clean muslin cloth (follow previous instructions).

Add the peppermint and camellia oils to this mixture. Pour into a clean glass jar. Cover and shake to mix. Keep in a cool place or refrigerate.

Evening Primrose Gel Astringent (*winter*)

> 6 drops evening primrose oil
> 1 tsp carrageen powder extract
> 5 oz natural spring water
> 5 oz vegetable glycerine
> 1 Tbsp sweet almond seed oil
> 6 drops lemon peel oil

Dissolve carrageen powder extract in 2 tablespoons of cold water. Bring water and glycerine to a boil. Remove from heat. Stir in cold carrageen mixture to water mixture until slightly consistent gelling occurs. Add the almond seed oil, evening primrose oil, and the lemon peel oil to mixture. Stir and pour into a clean glass jar. Keep in a cool place or refrigerate.

Lavender-Almond Astringent—Gentle Astringent (*all year*)

> 6 drops lavender essential oil
> 2 oz almond seed oil
> 10 oz elderflower water

Steep 4 ounces of dried elderflowers in 14 ounces of water until it boils. Remove herbs when water is lukewarm. Add almond seed and lavender essential oils to elderflower water.

Goldenseal and Apricot Astringent (*summer*)

> 1 Tbsp goldenseal powder (tumeric)
> 6 drops apricot essential oil
> 6 drops tincture of styrax benzoin gum
> 10 oz natural spring water
> 2 Tbsp aloe vera gel

Add benzoin gum and goldenseal powder to water and bring to a boil. Remove water from heat until lukewarm. Add aloe vera gel and apricot essential oil to mixture. Pour into a cool jar. Cover and shake to mix. Keep in a cool place or refrigerate.

Honey Astringent (*all year*)

> 4 Tbsp honey
> 10 oz water
> 2 tsp lemon peel oil

Bring water to a boil. Remove from heat until lukewarm. Dilute honey and lemon peel oil. Pour into a clean glass container and shake until an even consistency is reached. Keep in a cool place or refrigerate.

Winter Musk Astringent

> 10 oz musk astringent (p. 212)
> 8 oz vegetable glycerine
> 2 Tbsp camomile
> 1 Tbsp marigold
> 1 Tbsp sage
> 1 Tbsp rosemary
> 1 Tbsp ascorbic acid (natural vitamin C powder)
> 1 tsp St. John's wort oil
> 6 drops rosewood bark oil

Bring musk astringent and glycerine to a boil. Add camomile, marigold, sage, and rosemary, and ascorbic acid. Remove from heat until lukewarm using straining method of musk astringent. Add St. John's wort oil and rosewood bark oil to mixture. Pour into a clean glass jar. Cover and shake to mix. Store in a cool place or refrigerate.

Orange Blossoms Astringent (*spring*)

> 10 oz rose water (see recipe below)
> 6 oz vegetable glycerine
> 1 tsp neroli oil
> 6 drops grapefruit peel oil

Warm the rose water with glycerine. Do not boil. Add the neroli and grapefruit peel oils to mixture. Pour into a clean glass jar. Cover and shake to mix. Keep in a cool place or refrigerate.

Rose Water

> 4 oz fresh rose petals
> 4 oz natural spring water
> 4 oz vegetable glycerine

Combine water and glycerine and heat to 155°F. Add rose petals to boiling water. Allow to steep until water cools. Remove petals and use remaining rose water for all formulas requiring rose water.

Blue Honeysuckle Astringent (*spring*)

> 10 drops honeysuckle essential oil
> 4 Tbsp elecampane leaves
> 2 Tbsp hops
> 10 oz natural spring water
> 2 oz witch hazel

Infuse the elecampane leaves and hops in boiling water. The elecampane leaves will turn the water blue. Add the witch hazel to boiling water. Remove from heat until lukewarm. Remove the leaves from water and add the honeysuckle essential oil to mixture. Pour into a clean glass jar. Cover and shake to mix. Keep in a cool place or refrigerate.

Pure Gold Astringent (*fall*)

Gold water: Put 1 ounce of pure gold piece in 20 ounces of spring water and boil until 10 ounces of spring water remains. Remove gold piece and use the remaining water for all formulas requiring gold water. Gold piece can be used an infinite number of times.

> 10 oz pure gold water (or a piece of pure plain gold jewelry)
> 1 Tbsp goldenseal powder (tumeric)
> 10 oz natural spring water
> 6 oz glycerine
> 1 Tbsp jojoba oil

Bring spring water, glycerine, and goldenseal powder to a boil. Remove from heat until lukewarm. Add gold water to solution. Add warm jojoba oil. Pour into a clean glass jar. Cover and shake to mix. Keep in a cool place or refrigerate.

Sweet Fennel Astringent (*all year*)

Steep 4 ounces of sweet fennel leaves and roots in 14 ounces of boiling natural spring water. Remove roots and leaves after water cools. Use 10 ounces of this water for following formula.

> 10 oz sweet fennel water
> 2 oz vegetable glycerine
> 1 Tbsp styrax benzoin gum
> 2 oz light sesame oil
> 6 drops vitamin E oil

Bring the sweet fennel water and glycerine to a boil. Add the styrax benzoin gum to water mixture. Heat the sesame and vitamin E oils in a separate container. Pour oil mixture into water mixture. Pour into a clean glass jar. Cover and shake to mix. Keep in a cool place or refrigerate.

Vata Tonics

Bedtime Tonic (*for fatigue*)

> 1 Tbsp jojoba butter
> 1 oz wheat germ oil
> 2 Tbsp plain yogurt

Heat jojoba butter and wheat germ oil together. Stir butter-oil mixture into cool yogurt. Apply to a clean face and leave on for 15 minutes. Wash off with warm water and moisturize before bed.

Skin Tonic for Very Dry Skin

> 1 Tbsp olive oil
> 1 tsp glycerine
> ¼ oz avocado pulp

Warm olive oil with glycerine. Blend into avocado pulp until a creamy consistency is reached. Apply to a clean face and leave on for 20 minutes. Wash off with warm water and moisturize before bed.

Skin Tonic for Red, Irritated Skin

1/2 cup fresh milk
1 tsp kuzu or arrowroot starch
1 tsp honey
6 drops vitamin E oil

Boil milk until it begins to cream. Dilute kuzu or arrowroot starch in a few table-spoons of cold water. Add starch mixture to hot milk, after the cream of milk has been removed. Mix honey into mixture and stir until it gels. Mix the vitamin E oil into the cream separately. Apply the milk-starch-honey gel to a clean face. Leave on for 15 minutes. Wash off with warm water. Semi dry the face with a clean towel. Then massage the skimmed cream and vitamin E oil mixture into the skin and leave on overnight.

Occasional Day Skin Tonic

1 tsp ghee (purified sweet butter)
1/2 tsp sesame oil
1/2 tsp glycerine
2 drops evening primrose oil
1 Tbsp aloe vera gel

Warm the ghee and sesame oil, add glycerine, evening primrose oil, and aloe vera gel, and blend mixture together. Apply tonic to a clean face and leave on for 20 minutes. Wash off with warm water. Semi dry face with clean towel. Moisturize or apply makeup.

Tonic for Nervous Skin

6 very ripe strawberries
1/4 tsp orris powder
1 Tbsp olive oil
2 drops hops essential oil

Pulp strawberries in suribachi or blender, add orris powder and olive oil and mix in thoroughly. Apply tonic to a clean face. Leave on for 15 minutes. Wash off with warm water. Semi dry with towel. Massage the hops essential oil into face and leave on overnight.

Vata Masks

Clay Masks

Clay was used for skin treatments in India and China even before the time of Buddha. Clays are the best insulation for the skin, as it is composed largely of silica. Clay is absorbent and cleans the skin without itching. It is a tonic for the complexion and stimulates the flow of blood under the skin. In India a yellow clay called *gachni* was smeared on the body to relieve the heat of the sun.

The purest of all known clay is called *kaolin*, or China clay, from Mt. Kaolin in China. It has been used for medicinal purposes for centuries in China and by the aristocrates of Europe as a face powder. It is a pure white clay mineral composed of a mixture of rain and aluminum silicate. The most well-known clay in the United States is the fuller's earth. This was formed millions of years ago from huge deposits of diatoms, single-celled algae, on land that was once the ocean floor, where the sea had receded. Many millions of tons are mined yearly as diatomaceous earth, or fuller's earth.

In recent years many new clays have entered the market, amongst which is a very fine crystal clay mined in Arizona by American Indians. Clays are our direct healing connection to our earth. Choose your clay carefully from the variety available.

Clay masks are beneficial to a predominantly Kapha skin type which are oily and excessively moist. Predominantly Vata skin type which is dry and taut should moisturize the skin before use and lessen the time of application of a clay mask.

All types of skin will gain beneficial results from the clay. A clay mask should be applied occasionally to the entire body.

Kaolin Mask (*spring and summer*)

> 0.5 oz kaolin clay
> 0.2 oz vegetable glycerine
> 0.3 oz aloe vera gel
> 0.1 oz olive oil

Warm glycerine, aloe vera gel, and olive oil together. Blend in the kaolin clay to mixture. Use a few drops of olive oil to lightly moisturize face and then apply the clay mask. Leave on for 15 minutes. Rub off the mask from face. Wash face with warm water.

Fuller's Earth Mask (*all year*)

> 0.4 oz fuller's earth
> 0.3 oz elderflower water (p. 213)
> 0.1 oz sesame oil

Warm elderflower water and sesame oil together and add the fuller's earth. Apply a thin application of sesame oil to face before applying the mask. Apply mask and leave on for 15 minutes. Rub off the mask from face. Wash face with warm water.

Avocado Clay Mask (*all year*)

> 0.3 oz avocado oil
> 4 drops avocado essential oil
> 0.4 oz clay of your choice
> 0.1 oz spring water

0.1 oz brown algae extract

Warm the spring water and avocado oil mixture and dilute the brown algae extract. Brown algae extract causes a film to form on mask. Blend the clay into mixture. Apply a thin film of avocado oil on the face before applying mask. Leave on for 10 to 15 minutes. Peel off the mask. Wash face with warm water. Apply the drops of avocado essential oil to face afterward.

Clay and Gel Mask (*all year*)

> **0.3 oz clay of your choice**
> **0.1 oz natural amino acid gel**
> **0.1 oz vegetable glycerine**
> **0.1 oz gord extract**
> **0.1 oz powdered extract of oats**
> **0.2 oz jojoba oil**

Warm the glycerine, gord extract, and amino acid gel together. Dissolve the powdered extract of oats in mixture and allow to gel. Mix clay and jojoba oil into the gel mixture. Apply to clean face. Leave on for 10 to 15 minutes. Wash off with warm water. Use a few drops of jojoba oil to moisturize the face afterward.

Cucumber and Clay Mask (*summer*)

> **0.3 oz cucumber slices**
> **0.3 oz fuller's earth**
> **0.2 oz vegetable glycerine**

Boil cucumber slices and glycerine on slow heat. Purée cucumber in glycerine mixture with a fork. Add the fuller's earth to mixture. Apply the mask to a clean face. Leave on for 15 minutes. Wash off with warm water. Moisturize face afterward.

Cucumber Mask (*summer*)

> **12 slices unpeeled cucumber**
> **2 oz vegetable glycerine**
> **1 oz rice bran**
> **4 drops jojoba oil**

Warm the glycerine and cucumber slices together. Strain and squeeze moisture through a clean muslin bag into a clean bowl. Add the rice bran to mixture to make a paste and blend jojoba oil into paste. Apply paste to a clean face. Leave on for 15 minutes. Wash off face with warm water.

Gentle Milk Mask (*all year*)

> **1 oz fresh milk**
> **1 oz elderflower water (p. 213)**
> **2 oz rice flour**
> **few drops jojoba oil**

Warm elderflower water and milk together, add rice flour and make a paste. Apply to a clean face. Leave on for 20 minutes. Wash off with warm water. Moisturize with a few drops of jojoba oil and water.

Clear Peel-off Mask (*all year*)

> 0.2 oz sea kelp powder
> 0.1 oz acacia gum
> 0.5 oz vegetable glycerine
> 1 oz sesame oil
> 4 drops corn acid

Dissolve sea kelp powder and acacia gum in warm glycerine. Heat the sesame oil in a separate container. Add the corn acid to sea kelp, gum, and glycerine mixture and simultaneously combine the mixture with the hot oil. Stir briskly, as mixture gels. Apply to a clean face while mixture is warm. Leave on for 15 to 20 minutes. Mask will dry to a semi-taut feeling. Peel off mask and wash face with warm water. In the winter, add a few drops of evening primrose oil to rinse water.

Honey and Yogurt Mask (*summer*)

> 1 oz honey
> 1 oz plain yogurt
> 0.5 oz sesame oil
> 0.5 oz sorbitol

Warm sesame oil, honey, and sorbitol together. Blend in a yogurt to a cream consistency. Apply warm mixture to a clean face for 20 minutes. Wash off with warm water.

Slippery Elm Gel Mask (*all year*)

> 0.2 oz slippery elm powder
> 0.2 oz aloe vera gel
> 0.8 oz natural spring water

Dissolve slippery elm powder in hot water until it gels. Blend in aloe vera gel. Apply warm mixture to a clean face for 15 minutes. Wash off with warm water.

Camomile Mask (*spring and fall*)

> 3 drops essential oil of camomile
> 0.5 oz almond milk
> 0.5 oz oatmeal flour

Warm the almond milk. Blend in oatmeal flour. Add the essential oil of camomile. Apply warm mixture to a clean face. Leave on for 20 minutes. Rub off mask with clean fingers. Wash off with warm water.

Apricot and Peach Mask (*spring and fall*)

> 0.2 oz unpeeled apricot pieces

0.2 oz unpeeled peach pieces
0.1 oz fruit pectin extract
0.3 oz natural spring water
0.3 oz vegetable glycerine
0.02 oz neroli essential oil

Dissolve the fruit pectin extract in water. Pour glycerine into water and heat. Put the unpeeled pieces of apricot and peach into glycerine-water mixture. Bring to a boil. Purée fruits with a fork. Mixture will thicken as a result of pulp and fruit pectin extract. Allow to cool to lukewarm. Add the drops of neroli essential oil. Apply to a clean face for 20 minutes. Wash off with warm water. This mask like a jam can be kept for several applications. (The recipe lists the ingredients for one application.)

Vata Emollient Creams

Elderflower Cream (*fall*)

10 oz elderflower water (p. 213)
2 oz beeswax
1 oz olive oil
0.2 oz squalene extract (from olive oil)
1 oz almond oil
0.1 oz vitamin E oil
0.5 oz glycerine
0.1 oz borax

Melt beeswax in olive oil on slow heat (beeswax melts at approximately 148°F). Dissolve squalene extract in mixture and add almond and vitamin E oils and heat mixture to 165°F. Simultaneously, combine the elderflower water, glycerine, and borax together and heat to 165°F. Pour the water mixture into oil mixture while briskly stirring. Remove from heat and stir until mixture cools and thickens. Pour into a clean glass jar and keep in a cool place.

Camellia and Licorice Cream (*all year*)

1 oz camellia oil
0.5 oz licorice extract
1.5 oz sesame oil
1 oz carrot seed or root oil
1 oz Japan wax (from Japanese sumac or hazel tree)
1 oz vegetable glycerine
3 oz musk astringent (p. 212)
1 oz glycyrrhizic acid (from licorice root)

Combine the camellia oil, sesame oil, and carrot oil. Melt the Japan wax in oil mixture and heat slowly to approximately 155°F. Simultaneously combine glycerine, musk astringent, licorice extract, and glycyrrhizic acid in a separate container and heat to 155°F. Pour the oil-wax mixture into the astringent-acid mixture. Remove from heat and stir briskly until mixture cool and creamy. Pour into a clean glass jar. Keep in a cool place.

Lavender Cream (*spring*)

4 drops lavender essential oil
4 oz lavender-almond astringent (p. 213)
2 oz chaulmoogra seed oil
1 oz cottonseed oil
0.5 oz rice bran oil
0.5 oz karite (African) butter
1 oz vegetable glycerine
0.5 oz sea kelp powdered extract

Combine oils and melt karite butter to approximately 155°F. Simultaneously combine lavender-almond astringent and glycerine and dissolve the powdered extract into this solution. Heat and stir to approximately 155°F. Pour heated oil mixture into astringent mixture and stir briskly until cream gels. Remove from heat and continue stirring until mixture cools. Pour into a clean glass jar. Keep in a cool place.

Marigold Cream (*summer*)

½ oz fresh marigold flowers
2 oz natural rice vinegar
4 oz natural spring water
1 oz vegetable glycerine
1 oz yellow beeswax
4 oz cottonseed oil
1 oz sweet almond oil
8 drops vitamin E oil

Allow the fresh marigold flowers to sit in vinegar and water in a sealed jar in the sun for 1 week. Shake the mixture daily. Remove the flowers from the marigold water and add glycerine to it. Heat to approximately 145°F. Melt the yellow beeswax slowly in the mixture of cottonseed and almond oils and heat to approximately 145°F. Add the heated oil mixture to the marigold water mixture and stir briskly until mixture stiffens. Remove from heat, add the drops of vitamin E oil to preserve it and continue stirring until cream is cool. Pour into a clean glass container. Keep in a cool place.

Sweet Fennel Cream

Repairs irritated skin and adds a glowing golden color to the skin.

4 oz fennel water (p. 215)
1 oz jojoba wax
4 oz cocoa butter
4 drops storax oil

1 oz light sesame seed oil

Heat fennel water to approximately 155°F. Melt jojoba wax slowly in cocoa butter in a separate container and heat to approximately 155°F. Pour water mixture into wax mixture and stir briskly. Remove from heat, add storax and sesame seed oils to preserve it and continue stirring until cream cools. Pour into a clean glass jar. Keep in a cool place.

Rich Oil Blend Cream (*all year*)

2 oz almond oil
0.5 oz wheat germ oil
0.5 oz avocado oil
1 oz jojoba wax
0.1 oz lecithin powder (**Make sure it is chemical-free and derived from vegetable sources.**)
1 oz pure spring water
1 oz vegetable glycerine
4 drops cetyl alcohol
6 drops neroli essential oil

Melt the jojoba wax slowly in the mixture of oils (excluding the neroli essential oil). Heat until approximately 155°F. Dilute the lecithin powder in water and combine with glycerine in a separate container. Heat to approximately 155°F. Remove from heat and add the drops of cetyl alcohol. Pour the oil and wax mixture into the water mixture and stir briskly until mixture thickens and cools. Blend in the drops of neroli essential oil. Pour into a clean glass jar. Keep in a cool place.

Rose Cream (*all year*)

6 oz rose water (p. 214)
0.5 oz rose oil
1 oz beeswax
1 oz camellia oil
1 oz almond oil
0.5 oz ascorbyl palmitate (a natural vegetable source fat-soluble vitamin C)
0.2 oz borax

Melt beeswax in the camellia and almond oils slowly and heat to approximately 155°F. Combine rose water, ascorbyl palmitate, and borax and heat to approximately 155°F. Pour oil-wax mixture into water mixture. Add rose oil and stir briskly until cream stiffens and cools. Pour into a clean glass jar.

Pure Gold Cream

10 oz pure gold water (p. 215)
2.5 oz vegetable glycerine
0.1 oz borax
0.5 oz natural amino acid gel
1 oz jojoba butter and oil
0.1 oz vitamin E oil
0.5 oz evening primrose oil

Heat the gold water, glycerine, borax, and natural amino acid gel until mixture begins to thicken. Combine jojoba butter and oil, vitamin E oil, and evening primrose oil in a separate container and heat. Pour oil-butter mixture into gold water solution. Stir briskly until cream cools. Pour into a clean glass jar. Keep in a cool place.

Evening Primrose Cream

> **0.5 oz evening primrose oil**
> **10 oz karite butter**
> **0.1 oz Japan wax**
> **1 oz glycerine**
> **0.02 oz borax**

Heat the karite butter and evening primrose oil together and melt Japan wax slowly in oil mixture. In a separate container, heat glycerine and borax mixture. Add the oil mixture to glycerine-borax mixture. Stir briskly until mixture cools. Pour into a clean glass jar. Keep in a cool place.

Vata Oils

Recommendations of oils from plants, flowers, seeds, roots, herbs, nuts, fruits, and barks for body and facial use.

The following are some of the oils most suitable to the dryness and tautness of predominantly Vata type skin. Depending on the degree of moisture requirement of skin, the following oils may be used for a facial and body massage. A thin application of your evening cream on your face before bedtime will also be necessary. For example, if the skin is very dry, a few drops of rosa mosqueta oil may be massaged into the face and neck before using your rosa mosqueta cream. The oils are listed in order of their highest emollience and heating factors.

Common Oils
Olive oil
Avocado oil
Carrot oil
Chaulmoogra oil
Almond oil
Soybean oil
Cottonseed oil
Rapeseed oil
Poppyseed oil
Hops oil

Expensive Oils
Borage oil
Evening primrose oil
Rosa mosqueta oil
Jojoba oil
St. John's wort oil
Camellia oil
Wheat germ oil
Vitamin E oil
Rice bran oil
Fennel oil
Ginger oil (3 to 5 percent mix with water)
Rosewood bark oil (5 percent mix with water)

Natural Butter
Karite butter
Jojoba butter
Ghee (clarified butter, a dairy product)

Expensive Oils

White pine bark oil
  (2 percent mix with
  water)

Hyssop herbs oil (5 to 10
  percent mix with
   water)

Balm oil of lavender
  (5 to 10 percent mix
  with water)

Essential Oils (In no specific order, use very little—approximately a few drops.)

Arnica	Lavender	Ambrette seed (musk)
Camomile	Rose	Honeysuckle
Echinacea	Lotus	Elecampane
Magnolia	Hops	Cananga
Almond	Elderflower	Cassie
Neroli	Ylang-ylang	Sweet basil (tulsi)
Jasmine	Geranium (test for	Cade oil
Apricot	allergy before using)	Cajeput oil

Vata Moisturizing Lotions

Camomile Lotion

   2 oz camomile flowers (dried)
   12 oz natural spring water
   2 oz rosemary tops (dried)
   2 oz vegetable glycerine
   0.05 oz borax
   2 oz almond oil
   0.2 oz vitamin E oil
   1 oz beeswax

Boil spring water and steep camomile flowers and rosemary tops. Remove flowers and tops when water cools. Mix camomile and rosemary water with glycerine and borax. Heat to 145°F. In a separate container heat the almond and vitamin E oils and beeswax slowly until wax melts. Pour water-glycerine mixture into oil-wax mixture. Allow to cool and pour into a clean glass jar. Cover and shake to mix. Keep in a cool place.

Camellia and Licorice Lotion

   2 oz camellia oil
   0.5 oz licorice extract
   8 oz musk astringent (p. 212)

2 oz vegetable glycerine
0.5 oz willow bark extract
0.1 oz cetyl alcohol

Heat musk astringent and glycerine together. Dilute licorice and willow bark extracts in astringent mixture. In a separate container, heat the camellia oil. Pour oil and cetyl alcohol into warm astringent mixture. Pour into a clean glass jar. Cover and shake to mix. Keep in a cool place.

Lavender Lotion

4 drops essential oil of lavender
8 oz lavender-almond astringent (p. 213)
2 oz chaulmoogra seed oil
1 oz cottonseed oil
0.5 oz karite butter
0.5 oz sea kelp powdered extract
1 oz sorbitol
6 drops tincture of benzoin acid

Heat essential oil of lavender, chaulmoogra seed and cottonseed oils, and karite butter to 145°F. Dissolve sea kelp powdered extract in lavender-almond astringent and add sorbitol to mixture and heat in a separate container to 145°F. Pour oil mixture into astringent mixture and add benzoin acid. Stir briskly until a creamy lotion consistency is reached. Allow to cool. Pour into a clean glass jar. Cover and shake to mix. Keep in a cool place.

Marigold Lotion

8 oz marigold water (p. 221)
2 oz sesame oil
0.5 oz glycolic extract of linden tree
0.1 oz ascorbyl palmitate

Warm the marigold water and sesame oil together. Dissolve the glycolic extract of linden tree and ascorbyl palmitate in warm mixture. Allow to cool. Pour in a clean glass jar. Cover and shake to mix. Keep in a cool place.

Sweet Fennel Lotion

8 oz fennel water (p. 215)
0.1 oz fennel oil
0.1 oz ascorbyl palmitate
1 oz almond oil
2 oz cocoa butter

Heat fennel water and dissolve the ascorbyl palmitate. Combine fennel and almond oils and cocoa butter and heat in a separate container. Add the water mixture to the oil mixture. Allow to cool. Pour into a clean glass jar. Cover and shake to mix. Keep in a cool place.

Rich Oil Blend Lotion

> 2 oz almond oil
> 0.5 oz wheat germ oil
> 0.5 oz avocado oil
> 0.1 oz neroli essential oil
> 1 oz jojoba butter
> 2 oz natural spring water
> 2 oz sorbitol
> 0.1 oz lecithin powder (Make sure it is chemical-free and derived from vegetable sources.)
> 2 drops cetyl alcohol

Heat the oils and butter to 145°F. Combine water and sorbitol and heat to 145°F. Dissolve lecithin powder in water mixture. Add oil-butter mixture to water mixture. Blend in drops of cetyl alcohol. Stir briskly until a lotion consistency is reached. Allow to cool. Pour into a clean glass jar. Cover and shake to mix. Keep in a cool place.

Rosa Mosqueta Lotion

> 2 oz rosa mosqueta oil (rose-hip seed oil)
> 1 oz jojoba oil
> 6 drops essential oil of ylang-ylang
> 6 drops vitamin E oil
> 2 oz rose water (p. 214)
> 2 oz vegetable glycerine
> 4 oz natural spring water
> 6 drops stearyle alcohol (from vegetable fat sources)

Heat the oils together to 145°F. Combine rose water, glycerine, and spring water and heat to 145°F. Add stearyle alcohol to water mixture. Pour water mixture into oil mixture. Stir briskly until a lotion consistency is reached. Allow to cool. Pour into a clean glass jar. Cover and shake to mix. Keep in a cool place.

Rose Lotion

> 4 oz rose water (p. 214)
> 6 drops essential oil of rose
> 4 oz almond milk
> 0.5 oz ascorbyl palmitate
> 2 oz almond oil

Heat rose water and almond milk together. Dissolve ascorbyl palmitate in mixture. Combine essential oil of rose and almond oil and heat in a separate container. Add water mixture to oil mixture. Stir briskly until mixture cools. Pour into a clean glass jar. Cover and shake to mix. Keep in a cool place.

Pure Gold Lotion

> 8 oz pure gold water (p. 215)
> 2 oz sorbitol

0.2 oz natural amino acid gel
2 oz jojoba oil
0.1 oz vitamin E oil

Heat gold water and sorbitol together. Dissolve amino acid gel in water mixture. Heat oils together in a separate container. Pour oil mixture into water mixture. Stir briskly until a fluid golden lotion is acquired. Allow to cool. Pour into a clean glass jar. Keep in a cool place.

Vata Cleansing Creams

Mint and Almond Cleansing Cream (*all year*)

2 Tbsp peppermint leaves
2 Tbsp spearmint leaves
2 oz almond meal
6 drops almond essential oil
8 oz pure spring water
1 oz rice starch
2 oz cottonseed oil
2 oz camellia oil
2 drops storax oil

Steep the peppermint and spearmint leaves in boiling water. Remove leaves after liquid cools. Dissolve almond meal and rice starch in mint water and slowly heat to approximately 145°F. Combine the cottonseed and camellia oils in a separate container and heat to approximately 145°F. Add oil mixture to the gelling mix water. Remove from heat and add the storax oil to preserve it. Stir briskly until mixture cools. Blend in almond essential oil. Pour into a clean glass jar. Keep in a cool place.

Rice Bran Cleansing Cream (*perishable—do not keep beyond use*)

2 oz rice bran
1 oz rose water (p. 214)
1 oz vegetable glycerine
1 oz honey

Bring rose water and glycerine to a boil. Dilute honey in warm water mixture. Add rice bran. Mix well and apply to face. Scrub and leave on for 10 minutes before washing with warm water.

Milk Cleansing Cream (*winter*)

2 oz fresh milk
2 oz rice flour
2 drops essential oil of hops

Warm milk, add rice flour, and mix thoroughly. Scrub into clean face. Leave on for 30 minutes. Wash off with warm water. Semi dry the face and apply essential oil of hops to face before bed.

Gentle Cleanser I (*all year*)

> 0.5 oz cocoa butter
> 0.5 oz almond oil
> 6 drops vitamin E oil
> 0.5 oz honey
> 1 oz rose water (p. 214)
> 0.2 oz yucca leaves extract

Heat cocoa butter, oils, and honey to approximately 135°F. Combine rose water and yucca leaves extract in a separate container and heat to 135°F. As mixture begins to foam, remove from heat and pour in oil-honey mixture. Massage into clean face and leave on for 20 minutes. Rinse off with clean water.

Gentle Cleanser II (*all year*)

> 0.5 oz elderflower water (p. 213)
> 0.5 oz glycolic extract of kelp
> 0.5 oz wheat germ
> 4 drops sandalwood oil
> 4 drops wheat germ oil

Heat elderflower water and glycolic extract of kelp to approximately 135°F. Add wheat germ and drops of oils into mixture. Blend in thoroughly and scrub face with cleanser. Leave on for 15 minutes and wash off with warm water.

Apricot Cleanser (*all year*)

> 0.5 oz finely grounded apricot kernels
> 2 drops essential oil of apricot
> 0.5 oz almond oil
> 0.5 oz musk astringent (p. 212)
> 4 drops vitamin E oil

Warm the almond oil and musk astringent together, mix in the finely grounded apricot kernels. Blend in the essential oil of apricot and vitamin E oil. Scrub face, leave on for 5 minutes and wash off with warm water.

Vata Cold Creams

Almond Cold Cream (*all year*)

> 4 oz sweet almond oil
> 1 oz rice bran wax
> 0.5 oz rice bran oil
> 5 oz elderflower water (p. 213)
> 0.04 oz borax
> 2 drops tincture of benzoin

Heat the rice bran wax over very low heat (rice bran wax melts at 175°F). Remove from heat and stir in the almond and rice bran oils. In a separate container, heat the elderflower water and borax. Pour the water mixture into the oil-wax mixture and stir briskly, adding the drops of benzoin to preserve the cream. Stir until cool and pour into a clean glass jar. Keep in a cool place.

Eucalyptus Cold Cream (*all year*)

Eucalyptus water: Steep eucalyptus leaves in 0.5 ounces of boiling water. Leave to cool. Remove leaves and use water for the following formula.

> 0.5 oz eucalyptus water
> 6 drops eucalyptus oil
> 2 oz sesame oil
> 2 oz cocoa butter
> 0.5 oz glycerine
> 8 drops cetyl alcohol

Heat eucalyptus and sesame oils and cocoa butter together to 155°F. Heat eucalyptus water and glycerine to 155°F. Pour water mixture into oil-butter mixture. Add cetyl alcohol and stir briskly until cream cools. Pour into a clean glass jar. Keep in a cool place.

Jojoba Cold Cream (*all year*)

> 2 oz jojoba oil
> 1 oz jojoba butter
> 1 oz jojoba wax
> 0.5 oz vegetable glycerine
> 4 oz musk astringent (p. 212)

Combine the jojoba oil, butter, and wax and slowly heat together to 145°F. Heat the glycerine and musk astringent together to 145°F. Add the oil mixture to the astringent mixture, stirring briskly until cream cools and thickens. Pour into a clean glass jar. Keep in a cool place.

Rose Cold Cream (*all year*)

> 0.25 oz rose oil
> 0.5 oz rose water (p. 214)
> 1 oz beeswax
> 2 oz olive oil

Melt the beeswax in olive oil over very slow heat and add the rose oil. Warm the rose water and slowly pour into oil-wax mixture. Stir briskly until the cream cools. Pour into a clean glass jar. Keep in a cool place.

Apricot Cold Cream

> 2 oz apricot kernel oil
> 0.8 oz beeswax
> 0.2 oz squalene extract (from olive oil)
> 0.04 oz borax

Heat all ingredients together in slow heat until wax is melted. Remove from heat and stir briskly until mixture stiffens. Put into a clean glass jar. Keep in a cool place.

Camellia and Licorice Cold Cream

>   2 oz camellia oil
>   0.2 oz licorice extract
>   1 oz cocoa butter
>   1.2 oz beeswax
>   0.06 oz borax

Heat all ingredients together on slow heat until wax is melted. Remove from heat and stir briskly until mixture stiffens. Put into a clean glass jar. Keep in a cool place.

Vata Sun and Wind Protection Lotions

Note: The recommended sun and wind protection lotions are also applicable for men's and children's use.

Ultimate Sunscreen (*for maximum protection*)

>   5 oz natural spring water
>   0.2 oz benzyl alcohol (natural herbal alcohol)
>   2.5 oz jojoba butter
>   0.02 oz essential oil of hops
>   1 oz rosa mosqueta oil (rose-hip seed oil)
>   0.5 oz carrot oil
>   0.05 oz vitamin E oil
>   0.1 oz naringin extract from grapefruit seed
>   0.5 oz paba amino benzoic acid (PABA)
>   0.05 oz ascorbyl palmitate (fat-soluble vitamin C)
>   0.05 oz natural vitamin A powder

Heat the spring water, benzyl alcohol, and jojoba butter together to 135°F to form a base for sunscreen lotion. Add the essential oil of hops to solution. In a separate container slowly heat the rosa mosqueta oil, carrot oil, vitamin E oil, and naringin extract and dissolve the PABA powder, ascorbyl palmitate, and vitamin A powder in mixture. Pour this oil mixture into the base mixture, stirring briskly to reach a creamy consistency. Pour into a clean glass jar. Keep in a cool place. Shake well before using.

Comfrey-Aloe Sunscreen

Steep 2 ounces of comfrey leaves in 4 ounces of boiling water. Remove leaves when water cools. Use 2 ounces of water for the following formula.

>   2 oz comfrey water
>   0.5 oz aloe vera gel
>   1 oz vegetable glycerine

0.5 oz PABA powder
0.2 oz panthenol powder
2 oz balsam oil
0.5 oz vitamin E oil
0.5 oz jojoba oil

Heat the comfrey water, glycerine, aloe vera gel, and PABA and panthenol pow-deres together to 135°F. Combine the oils in a separate container and heat to 135°F. Pour hot oil into water mixture. Stir briskly until mixture is cool and con-sistent. Pour into a clean glass jar. Keep in a cool place.

Walnut-Yarrow Sunscreen

2 oz walnut oil
0.2 oz yarrow extract
2 oz comfrey water (recipe from formula above)
0.2 oz PABA powder
0.5 oz hydroglycolic extract of linden tree
0.5 oz glycolic extract of St. John's wort
1 oz carrot oil
0.1 oz benzyl alcohol

Heat water, yarrow extract, PABA powder, and extracts of linden and St. John's wort together. Combine walnut and carrot oils in a separate container and heat. Pour the oil mixture into water mixture and stir briskly. Blend in the benzyl alcohol. Allow lotion to cool. Pour into a clean glass jar. Keep in a cool place.

Sunscreen Butter

2 oz karite butter
0.5 oz carrot oil
0.1 oz vitamin E oil
0.5 oz hydroglycolic extract of marigold
0.5 oz hydroglycolic extract of camomile
0.5 oz PABA powder
0.1 oz ascorbyl palmitate

Heat the karite butter and oils to 135°F. Blend the hydroglycolic extracts of mari-gold and camomile to mixture and dissolve the PABA powder and ascorbyl palmitate in mixture. Stir until mixture is buttery. Pour into a clean glass jar and refrigerate.

Allantoin Sun Protector

0.04 oz allantoin crystals (from comfrey roots)
1 oz natural spring water
0.5 oz extract of yarrow
0.1 oz benzyl alcohol
2 oz cocoa butter
0.1 oz hyssop extract oil
0.2 oz immortelle flowers extract oil
0.5 oz PABA powder

Heat the spring water, extract of yarrow, benzyl alcohol, cocoa butter, and extracts' oils together to 135°F. Dissolve the allantoin and PABA powder in mixture. Stir briskly until lotion is cool and consistent. Pour into a clean glass jar. Keep in a cool place.

Mild Sunburn Cream

2 oz cocoa butter
2 oz jojoba wax
2 oz rose water (p. 214)
2 oz elderflower water (p. 213)

Heat cocoa butter and jojoba wax to 145°F. Heat waters to 145°F. Slowly pour wax-oil mixture into water and stir briskly until mixture becomes cool and creamy.

After Sun Rosa Mosqueta and Aloe Vera Cream

0.2 oz rosa mosqueta oil
0.5 oz aloe vera gel

Mix the two together and apply to face immediately after sun or wind exposure.

The following is a list of effective oils for the prevention of sun- and windburns.

Jojoba oil	Lavender oil	Marigold (calendula) oil
Walnut oil	Sandalwood oil	Chaumoogra (glyno-
Horse chestnut oil	Sunflower oil	cardia) oil
Butcher's broom oil	Calamus root oil	Neroli oil
Balsam oil	Elderflower oil	(Aloe vera gel)

Vata Shampoos

Rosemary and Sage Shampoo (*for dark brown and black hair*)

0.5 oz rosemary extract
0.5 oz sage oil
½ bar natural Castile (pure olive oil) soap
2 oz natural spring water

Grate soap into thin slivers. Bring water and rosemary extract to a boil. Dilute soap until water becomes sudsy. Add to sage oil. Allow to cool. Pour into a clean glass bottle. Cover and shake to mix before each use. Keep in a cool place.

Camellia Shampoo (*for dry hair*)

2 oz camellia oil
½ bar all vegetable soap
2 oz natural spring water
0.2 oz eucalyptus oil

Grate soap into slivers. Bring water to a boil. Dissolve soap until water becomes sudsy. Heat camellia and eucalyptus oils in a separate container. Add to soapy water. Allow to cool. Pour into a clean glass bottle. Cover and shake before each use. Keep in a cool place.

Seaweed Shampoo

> 1 oz sea kelp powder
> 3 oz natural spring water
> 0.1 oz natural amino acid powder
> 0.2 oz cottonseed oil
> 0.2 oz yucca leaves extract
> 0.1 oz frankincense resin (bark-gum)
> 1 oz aloe vera gel

Bring water to a boil. Dissolve sea kelp powder and amino acid powder in hot water. In a separate container, heat the cottonseed oil and add yucca leaves extract and frankincense resin. Add warm oil mixture to hot water and powder mixture. Stir briskly until all extracts have dissolved completely. Allow to cool. Add the aloe vera gel and pour into a clean glass bottle. Cover and shake before use. Keep in a cool place.

Kombu and Ivy Shampoo

> 2 oz dried kombu
> 0.5 oz ivy leaves or berry extract
> 0.1 oz quillai bark extract
> 1 oz olive oil
> 3 oz camomile water (p. 250)
> 0.2 oz benzyl alcohol

Steep the ivy leaves in boiling water. Allow to cool, and use the water.

Soak the dried kombu in a small bowl of natural spring water, barely covering it. Allow to sit for 2 hours. Remove the kombu (you may use it to cook with) and use the gel-like water and add the extracts of ivy, quillai bark, and olive oil. In a separate container, heat the camomile water and add the benzyl alcohol. Stir briskly until mixture cools. Pour into a clean glass jar. Cover and shake before use. Keep in a cool place.

Balsam Shampoo

> 1 oz balsam peru glycolic extract
> 0.3 oz dried bay leaves
> 4 oz natural spring water
> 1 oz horsetails glycolic extract
> 6 drops lemon juice
> 1 oz carrot oil
> 6 drops vitamin E oil

Steep the bay leaves in the boiling spring water, until water cools. Remove leaves and reheat the bay-leaf water, adding the balsam and horsetails glycolic extracts and lemon juice. In a separate container, heat the carrot oil and vitamin E oil. Add oils to the water mixture, stirring briskly until it cools. Pour into a clean glass jar. Cover and shake to mix before use. Keep in a cool place.

Lavender and Evening Primrose Shampoo (*for all hair colors*)

Steep 4 ounces each of lavender, coltsfoot, nettle, and horsetails in 12 ounces of boiling water. Allow to cool and use water for the following formula.

6 drops essential oil of lavender
0.5 oz evening primrose oil
10 oz herbal water
2 oz quillai bark extract
1 oz sea kelp extract
0.1 oz naringin extract
2 oz cottonseed oil
0.2 oz benzyl alcohol

Heat the herbal water and dissolve quillai bark, sea kelp, and naringin extracts. Heat the evening primrose and cottonseed oils in a separate container. Add oils to water mixture. Add benzyl alcohol and essential oil of lavender to mixture. Stir briskly until mixture cools. Pour into a clean glass jar. Cover and shake to mix before use. Keep in a cool place.

Jojoba Shampoo

Steep 2 ounces of horsetail and coltsfoot in 6 ounces of boiling water. Remove the herbs after water cools. Use herbal water for the following formula.

2 oz jojoba oil
0.5 oz jojoba butter
6 oz herbal water
0.5 oz vegetable glycerine
0.5 oz yucca leaves extract
0.1 oz benzyl alcohol

Heat the herbal water and add glycerine and yucca leaves extract. Heat the jojoba oil and butter in a separate container and add to water mixture. Add benzyl alcohol and stir briskly until mixture cools. Pour into a clean glass jar. Keep in a cool place.

Shampoo of the Sea

1 oz dried seaware
6 oz natural spring water
0.5 oz sea kelp extract
0.5 oz blown algae extract
0.2 oz sea salt
0.2 oz glycolic extract of mallow

0.2 oz glycolic extract of ginseng
0.1 oz sulfur amino acid (inorganic, but non-toxic and safe)
0.5 oz camellia oil
6 drops wheat germ oil

Boil the dried seaware in spring water. Allow to cool. Remove seaware and use the water. Reheat the slightly gel-like water and add the sea kelp and brown algae extracts, sea salt, extracts of mallow and ginseng, and sulfur amino acid. Blend mixture thoroughly and add the camellia oil and wheat germ oil. Allow to cool and pour into a clean glass jar. Cover and shake to mix before each use. Keep in a cool place.

Vata Hair Conditioners

Balsam and Wine Conditioner (*for auburn hair and redheads*)

0.5 oz glycolic extract of balsam peru
1 oz dark Burgundy wine
0.5 oz carrot oil
0.8 oz glycolic extract or horsetails

Heat the wine and carrot oil together. Add the glycolic extracts of balsam peru and horsetails to solution. Massage into wet hair and scalp. After shampooing leave on for 10 to 15 minutes. Rinse with cool water.

Sage and Walnut Conditioner (*for black hair*)

0.3 oz sage oil
0.2 oz black walnut oil
1 oz birch astringent (p. 259)
0.5 oz glycolic extract of bladder wrack

Heat the birch astringent, sage oil, and black walnut oil together. Add the glycolic extract of bladder wrack to mixture. Massage into wet hair and scalp after shampooing. Leave on for 10 to 15 minutes. Rinse with cool water.

Camellia, Cade, and Mallow Conditioner (*for dry hair*)

0.5 oz camellia oil
0.5 oz cade oil
0.5 oz glycolic extract of mallow
2 oz natural spring water
0.02 oz allantoin
0.02 oz sulfur amino acid
6 drops wheat germ oil

Heat the water and dissolve the allantoin and sulfur amino acid. Heat the camellia and cade oils in a separate container. Stir in the glycolic extract of mallow and drops of wheat germ oil. Pour oil mixture into water solution and mix well. Massage into wet hair and scalp after shampooing and leave on for 20 minutes. Wash off with warm water and then cool water.

Seaweed Conditioner (*for normal hair of all colors*)

Seaware water: Soak one piece of seaware in 0.5 ounce of boiling hot water for 30 minutes. Remove seaware and use gel-like water for the following formula.

>   0.5 oz seaware water
>   0.2 oz blue green algae powder
>   0.5 oz extract of sea kelp
>   3 drop essential oil of cassie (cassie absolute)

Warm the seaware water and dissolve blue green algae powder in it. Add the extract of sea kelp in mixture. Massage conditioner into wet hair after shampooing. Leave on for 30 minutes. Rinse off with cool water. Towel hair dry and apply with the palm of hands the drops of essential oil of cassie.

Ginseng and Walnut Conditioner (*for normal hair of all colors*)

Rosemary water: Steep a few rosemary leaves in 1 ounce of boiling water for 30 minutes. Remove leaves and use rosemary water for the following formula.

>   0.5 oz extract of ginseng
>   0.5 oz walnut oil
>   1 oz rosemary water
>   0.5 oz glycerine
>   0.5 oz vitamin B complex powder
>   0.5 oz coconut oil
>   0.2 oz aloe vera gel

Heat the rosemary water and glycerine together. Dissolve the vitamin B complex powder and extract of ginseng in rosemary water and glycerine solution. In a separate container heat the coconut and walnut oils. Add the aloe vera gel to oil mixture and blend into water-powder mixture. Massage into wet hair after shampooing. Leave on for 30 minutes. Rinse with cool water.

Vata Hair Rinses and Colors

Henna Rinse I (*for auburn hair and redheads*)

>   0.5 oz henna powder
>   1 oz dark Burgundy wine
>   6 drops carrot oil
>   6 drops lemon

Heat wine and mix in henna powder. Add drops of carrot oil and lemon, and mix into a paste. Using a fine toothbrush, apply the paste to strands of hair at a time. Leave on for 20 minutes. Wash off with lukewarm water.

Henna Rinse II (*for dark brown hair*)

>   0.5 oz henna powder
>   1 oz very dark bancha twig tea

6 drops dark sesame oil
6 drops lemon

Heat bancha twig tea and mix in henna powder. Add drops of dark sesame oil and lemon and mix into paste. Using a fine toothbrush, apply the paste to strands of hair at a time. Leave on 20 minutes. Wash off with lukewarm water.

Henna Rinse III (*for black hair*)

0.5 oz henna powder
1 oz indigo water (see recipe below)
6 drops lemon
6 drops black walnut oil

Steep indigo leaves in 1 ounce of boiling water until water becomes blue-black. Mix the henna powder into indigo water and add drops of lemon and walnut oil. Make into a paste. Using a fine toothbrush apply paste to strands of hair. Leave on for 20 minutes. Wash off with lukewarm water.

Note: Henna should *not be used* for blonde, silver, gray, bleached or damaged hair.

Camomile and Rosemary Rinse (*for blonde hair*)

1 oz camomile and rosemary
4 oz natural spring water
3 drops lemon juice
6 drops essential oil of ylang-ylang

Steep camomile and rosemary in boiling spring water until water cools. Remove herbs and add lemon juice and essential oil of ylang-ylang to herbal water. Apply to wet hair and scalp after shampooing and/or conditioning. Towel dry and leave rinse on the hair.

Goldenrod and Vervain Rinse (*for light blonde hair*)

1 oz goldenrod and vervain
4 oz natural spring water
6 drops peppermint oil
3 drops lemon juice

Steep goldenrod and vervain in boiling spring water until water cools. Remove herbs and add peppermint oil and lemon juice to herbal water. Apply to wet hair and scalp after shampooing and/or conditioning. Towel dry and leave rinse on the hair.

Mullein and Saffron Rinse (*for golden blonde hair*)

1 oz mullein
0.1 oz saffron powder
4 oz natural spring water

6 drops apple cider vinegar
6 drops cananga essential oil

Steep the mullein in boiling water until water cools. Remove the herbs and dilute the saffron powder into water. Add the drops of apple cider vinegar and cananga essential oil to rinse. Apply to wet hair and scalp after shampooing and/or conditioning. Towel dry and leave rinse on the hair.

Sage, Birch, and Walnut Rinse (*for black hair*)

1 oz sage and birch
6 drops walnut oil
4 oz natural spring water
6 drops malt vinegar

Steep the sage and birch in boiling water until water cools. Remove herbs and add the malt vinegar and walnut oil to water. Apply to wet hair and scalp after shampooing and/or conditioning. Towel dry and leave rinse on the hair.

Twig and Musk Rinse (*for auburn hair*)

1 oz bancha twigs
6 drops essential oil of ambrette seed (musk)
4 oz natural spring water
6 drops malt vinegar

Steep the bancha twigs in boiling water until water cools. Remove twigs and add malt vinegar and essential oil of ambrette seed to water. Apply to wet hair and scalp after shampooing and/or conditioning. Towel dry and leave rinse on the hair.

Thyme, Sage, and Rosemary Rinse (*for auburn and black hair; spring and summer*)

0.5 oz fresh thyme
1 oz sage and rosemary
4 oz natural spring water
6 drops lemon juice
6 drops sandalwood oil

Steep the thyme, sage, and rosemary in boiling water until water cools. Remove herbs and add the lemon juice and sandalwood oil to herbal water. Apply to wet hair and scalp after shampooing and/or conditioning. Towel dry and leave rinse on hair.

Vata Hair Oils

Camomile Oil (*for light-colored hair; all year*)

1 oz camomile tea
3 oz sunflower oil

Heat the sunflower oil and allow camomile tea to sit in hot oil until oil cools. Remove herbs and pour oil into a clean glass jar. Apply to hair occasionally.

Camellia Oil (*for all hair colors*)

Apply the pure camellia oil to hair for additional sheen occasionally. Use with a touch of water in the palm of hands.

Ylang-Ylang Oil

The pure oil of ylang-ylang is also excellent for additional hair sheen. Use with a touch of water in the palm of hands.

Evening Primrose Oil (*for all hair colors; fall and winter*)

> 6 drops evening primrose oil
> 6 drops glycerine
> 6 drops elderflower water (p. 213)

Mix the evening primrose oil, glycerine, and elderflower water in palm of hands and massage into strands of hair.

Golden Jojoba Oil (*for all hair colors; all year*)

> 6 drops jojoba oil
> 6 drops rose water (p. 214)

Mix the jojoba oil and rose water in palm of hands and massage into the strands of hair.

Thyme-Sage Oil (*for dark hair; all year*)

> 0.1 oz thyme oil
> 0.5 oz sage
> 3 oz olive oil
> 0.2 oz witch hazel

Heat the olive oil and allow the sage to sit in the hot oil until it cools. Remove the herbs and add thyme oil and witch hazel to sage oil. Mix thoroughly and pour into a clean glass bottle.

Lavender Oil (*for all hair colors; spring and summer*)

> 1 oz lavender
> 6 drops essential oil of lavender
> 4 oz water
> 6 drops sorbitol

Steep the lavender in boiling water. Remove the herbs from water and add the essential oil of lavender and sorbitol. Pour oil mixture into a clean glass bottle. Use a few drops in the palm of hands and massage into the strands of hair.

Black Oil (*for black hair; spring and summer*)

> 1 oz Jacob's ladder (Cut plant in summer while it is in bloom.)
> 3 oz walnut oil

Boil the pieces of Jacob's ladder in walnut oil under slow flames until the oil becomes black. Allow to cool and pour into a clean glass jar. Use a few drops of oil with a few drops of water in the palm of hands. Massage into the strands of hair.

Neroli-Orange Oil (*for light color hair; spring and summer*)

> 3 drops essential oil of neroli
> 6 drops orange juice
> 3 drops glycerine

Mix all ingredients together in palm of hands and massage into the strands of hair.

Gold Oil (*for blondes and black hair; all year*)

> 4 oz gold water (p. 215)
> 0.2 oz glycerine
> 0.5 oz almond oil
> 0.5 oz jojoba oil
> 6 drops wheat germ oil
> 6 drops essential oil of honeysuckle

Heat the gold water and glycerine. Add the almond, jojoba, wheat germ, and essential oils to mixture. Mix thoroughly and pour into a clean glass jar. Keep in a cool place. Use a few drops in the palm of hands. Massage into the strands of hair.

Pitta Type Nature's Formula

Pitta Astringents

Patchouli Astringent (*all year*)

> 10 drops patchouli essential oil
> 10 oz water
> 6 oz witch hazel
> 1 tsp licorice powder
> 1 Tbsp styrax benzoin gum
> 1 Tbsp coltsfoot
> 1 Tbsp nettle
> 2 Tbsp cilantro leaves
> 2 Tbsp dried pipessewa leaves
> 1 tsp calamus root oil

Bring water and witch hazel to a boil. Then add licorice powder, styrax benzoin gum, coltsfoot, nettle, cilantro and pipessewa leaves to boiling water. Remove from heat until lukewarm. Strain mixture through a clean muslin cloth by twisting each end of cloth in the opposite direction. (Mixture of herbs is in the center of cloth which is securely folded over to contain herbs.) Add patchouli essential oil and calamus root oil to water mixture. Pour into a clean glass jar. Cover and shake to mix. Keep in a cool place or refrigerate.

Camomile Astringent (*winter*)

> 6 drops camomile essential oil
> 2 Tbsp camomile glycolic extract
> 10 oz water
> 8 oz vegetable glycerine
> 2 Tbsp pure gord juice
> ½ tsp pine needle oil

Bring water and glycerine to a boil. Add camomile glycolic extract and gord juice to boiling water. Remove from heat until lukewarm. Add camomile essential oil and pine needle oil. Pour into a clean glass jar. Cover and shake to mix. Keep in a cool place or refrigerate.

Aloe Vera Gel Astringent (*winter*)

> 2 Tbsp aloe vera gel
> 16 oz water
> 8 oz vegetable glycerine
> 4 Tbsp elderflower
> 1 tsp sweet almond oil
> 1 tsp lemon peel oil

Bring water and glycerine to a boil. Add elderflower and remove mixture from heat until lukewarm. Strain mixture using the method explained in patchouli astringent. To the elderflower solution, add the aloe vera gel, almond and lemon peel oils. Pour into a clean glass container. Cover and shake to mix. Keep in a cool place or refrigerate.

Peppermint and Pine Astringent (*summer*)

> 2 Tbsp peppermint leaves
> ½ tsp white pine bark extract
> ½ tsp pine needle oil
> 10 oz water
> 4 oz vegetable glycerine
> 2 Tbsp eucalyptus leaves

Bring water and glycerine to a boil. Add peppermint and eucalyptus leaves to boiling water, remove from heat until lukewarm. Remove leaves from solution and add white pine bark extract and pine needle oil. Stir until an even consistency is reached. Pour into a clean glass jar. Cover and shake to mix. Keep in a cool place or refrigerate.

Horse Chestnut Astringent (*all year*)

> 2 Tbsp horse chestnut
> 10 oz water
> 8 oz vegetable glycerine
> 1 Tbsp rosemary
> 1 Tbsp marigold
> 2 tsp ascorbic acid
> 1 tsp blue or marsh mallow glycolic extract
> 1 tsp St. John's wort oil

Bring water and glycerine to a boil. Add rosemary, marigold, and ascorbic acid and remove from heat until lukewarm. Strain mixture using the method explained in patchouli astringent. Add the mallow glycolic extract and St. John's wort oil. Stir until an even consistency is reached. Pour into a clean glass jar. Cover and shake to mix. Keep in a cool place or refrigerate.

Magnolia Tanning Astringent (*spring and summer*)

> 10 drops magnolia essential oil
> 10 oz water
> 4 oz glycerine
> 4 Tbsp rhatany
> 2 Tbsp hops
> 1 tsp hyssop extract

Bring water and glycerine to a boil. Add rhatany and hops and remove from heat until lukewarm. Strain mixture using the method explained in patchouli astringent. Add hyssop extract and magnolia essential oil. Pour into a clean glass jar. Cover and shake to mix. Keep in a cool place or refrigerate.

Almond Astringent (*spring*)

> 2 Tbsp sweet almond oil
> 8 oz elderflower water (p. 213)
> 2 oz witch hazel
> 1 tsp myrrh extract
> 1 tsp licorice extract

Bring elderflower water and witch hazel to a boil. Add the myrrh and licorice extracts and remove mixture from heat until lukewarm. Add the almond oil to mixture. Pour into a clean glass jar. Cover and shake to mix. Keep in a cool place or refrigerate.

Mint Astringent (*summer*)

> 2 Tbsp spearmint
> 12 oz water
> 6 oz witch hazel
> 2 Tbsp pennyroyal
> 1 Tbsp glycolic extract of cinnamon
> 6 drops storax oil

6 drops clove oil

Bring water and witch hazel to a boil. Add pennyroyal and spearmint to mixture and remove from heat until lukewarm. Strain mixture using the method explained in patchouli astringent. Add the glycolic extract of cinnamon, storax oil, and clove oil to mixture. Stir until even consistency is reached. Pour into a clean glass jar. Cover and shake to mix. Keep in a cool place or refrigerate.

Blue Jasmine Astringent (*spring*)

10 drops essential oil of jasmine
4 Tbsp elecampane leaves
10 oz water
4 oz witch hazel
1 Tbsp maple syrup

Infuse the elecampane leaves into boiling water. The leaves will turn water blue. Add the witch hazel to boiling water. Remove from heat until lukewarm. Remove the leaves from water and add the maple syrup. Stir until an even consistency is reached. Add the essential oil of jasmine. Pour into a clean glass jar. Cover and shake to mix. Keep in a cool place or refrigerate.

Pure Silver Astringent (*all year*)

Silver water: Add 1 ounce of pure silver piece or new silver quarters to 20 ounces of natural spring water. Boil until 10 ounces of water remain. Remove the silver piece and use remaining water for all formulas requiring silver water. Silver piece coin can be used an infinite number of times.

10 oz silver water
6 oz glycerine
1 tsp sandalwood oil

Bring silver water and glycerine to a boil. Remove from heat until lukewarm. Add warm sandalwood oil. Pour into a clean glass jar. Cover and shake to mix. Keep in a cool place or refrigerate.

Pitta Tonics

Skin Tonic for Fatigue

8 slices cucumber (unpeeled)
2 Tbsp sunflower oil

Place cucumber slices in a small container of hot water for a few minutes. Place the soaked, mushy pieces in a clean muslin bag or cloth. Squeeze the pulp of the cucumber and sunflower oil firmly with milking of the cow motion, until all the juice has been squeezed out of the bag. Use the warm cucumber water to wash face, before applying cucumber tonic. Apply to face and leave on for 10 minutes. Wash off with cucumber water before going to bed.

Occasional Day Skin Tonic

$\frac{1}{2}$ semi-ripe banana
$\frac{1}{2}$ tsp wheat germ oil
1 Tbsp vegetable glycerine

Blend all ingredients in a suribachi or blender. Apply to face after cleaning for 10 minutes. Remove with cool water before applying moisturizer or makeup.

Bedtime Skin Tonic (*for red, irritated skin, before bed*)

$\frac{1}{2}$ cup fresh milk
1 tsp kuzu or arrowroot starch
6 drops vitamin E oil

Boil milk until it begins to cream. Dilute kuzu or arrowroot starch in a few table-spoons of cold water. Add starch mixture to hot milk, after the cream has been removed. Stir until it gels. Mix the vitamin E oil into the cream separately. Apply the milk and strach gel to a clean face. Leave on for 10 to 15 minutes. Wash off with cool water. Semi dry the face with a clean towel. Then massage the skimmed cream and vitamin mixture into skin and leave on overnight.

Radiant Skin Tonic (*for occasional morning use*)

4 Tbsp elderflower water (p. 213)
$\frac{1}{2}$ tsp jojoba butter
2 Tbsp maple syrup

Warm the elderflower water and melt the jojoba butter and maple syrup in it. Use this paste to massage into face and leave on for 15 minutes. Rinse off with cool water. Towel to semi dry and moisturize.

Tonic for Itchy Skin

$\frac{1}{2}$ tsp kelp extract
2 Tbsp water
$\frac{1}{2}$ tsp St. John's wort oil
$\frac{1}{2}$ tsp thyme oil

Mix the kelp extract in water. Warm the St. John's wort and thyme oils and pour kelp solution slowly into it. Stir until oils are well blended in. Apply thin coat of mixture to a clean face and leave on overnight.

Note: Salves for sunburnt, chapped, and irritated skin are covered under Transient-sensitive Skin formulas, in the Transient-sensitive Skin and Hair section.

Pitta Masks

Kaolin Mask (*spring and summer*)

0.5 oz kaolin clay

0.3 oz aloe vera gel
0.2 oz vegetable glycerine

Mix the kaolin clay and aloe vera gel in warm glycerine. Apply to a clean face. Leave on for 15 minutes. Rub the dry flakes of clay off face. Wash face with cool water.

Cucumber and Clay Mask (*summer*)

0.3 oz cucumber pulp
0.3 oz fuller's earth
0.2 oz vegetable glycerine

Boil glycerine on slow heat. Purée the cucumber into a pulp with a fork. Add the fuller's earth to mixture. Apply this mask to clean face. Leave on for 15 minutes. Wash off with cool water.

Fuller's Earth Clay (*all year*)

0.5 oz fuller's earth
0.4 oz patchouli astringent (p. 240)
0.1 oz sunflower seed oil

Warm the patchouli astringent and the sunflower seed oil. Add the clay to mixture. Apply to a clean face. Leave on for 15 minutes. Rub off mask from face. Wash with cool water.

Clay Mask I (*winter*)

0.4 oz clay of your choice
0.2 oz jojoba oil
0.3 oz vegetable glycerine

Mix the clay and jojoba oil in warm glycerine. Apply to a clean face. Leave on for 15 minutes. Rub the flakes of clay off face. Wash with lukewarm water and then moisturize.

Clay and Gel Mask (*all year*)

0.3 oz clay of your choice
0.1 oz natural amino acid gel
0.2 oz vegetable glycerine
0.1 oz gord extract
0.1 oz powdered extract of oats

Warm the glycerine, gord extract, and amino acid gel together. Dissolve the powdered extract of oats in mixture and allow to gel. Mix clay into mixture. Apply to a clean face and leave on for 20 minutes. Wash face off with cool water.

Cucumber Mask (*summer*)

12 unpeeled cucumber slices

2 oz vegetable glycerine
1 oz rice bran
2 drops peppermint oil

Warm the glycerine and cucumber slices together. Strain and squeeze mixture through a clean muslin bag into a clean bowl. Add the rice bran to mixture to make a paste. Blend in drops of peppermint oil into a paste. Apply paste to a clean face. Leave on for 20 minutes. Wash off face with cool water.

Gentle Milk Mask (*all year*): See p. 218 for recipe. Apply to a clean face. Leave on for 20 minutes. Wash off with cool water.

Clear Peel-off Mask (*all year*)

0.2 oz sea kelp powder
0.1 oz acacia gum
0.5 oz vegetable glycerine
1 oz coconut oil
4 drops corn acid

Dissolve sea kelp powder and acacia gum in warm glycerine. Heat the coconut oil in a separate container. Add the corn acid to sea kelp, gum, and glycerine mixture and simultaneously pour in the hot oil mixture. Stir briskly as mixture gels. Apply to a clean face while mixture is warm. Leave on for 15 to 20 minutes. Mask will dry to a semi-taut feeling. Peel mask off and wash face with warm water. In the summer add a few drops of thyme oil or St. John's wort oil in rinse water.

Sage Mask (*all year*)

0.1 oz sage oil
0.2 oz coconut oil
0.1 oz brown algae extract
0.5 oz natural spring water

Heat coconut and sage oils. Dissolve brown algae extract in water and heat until it begins to gel. Add hot oils. Allow mask to cool. Apply to a clean face. Leave on for 15 minutes. Wash off with cool water.

Apricot and Peach Mask (*fall*)

0.2 oz unpeeled apricot pieces
0.2 oz unpeeled ripe peach pieces
0.1 oz fruit pectin extract
0.3 oz natural spring water
0.3 oz vegetable glycerine

Dissolve the fruit pectin extract in water. Pour glycerine into water and heat. Put the unpeeled apricot and peach pieces into glycerine-water mixture. Bring to a boil. Purée fruits with a fork. Mixture will thicken as a result of pulp and fruit pectin extract. Allow to cool. Apply to a clean face for 20 minutes. Wash off with cool water. This mask like a jam can be kept for several applications. (The recipe lists the ingredients for one application.)

Slippery Elm Gel Mask (*all year*): See 219 for recipe. Apply to clean face for 20 minutes. Wash off with cool water.

Peppermint Mask (*spring and summer*)

> 3 drops essential oil of peppermint
> 1 oz almond milk
> 0.2 oz fuller's earth
> 0.5 oz gram (chick-pea) flour

Warm the almond milk. Blend in clay and gram flour. Add the essence of peppermint. Allow mixture to cool. Apply to a clean face for 20 minutes. Rub off mask with clean fingers. Wash off face with cool water.

Pitta Emollient Creams

Horse Chestnut Cream

> 10 oz horse chestnut astringent (p. 242)
> 2 oz sun-bleached Japan wax (from the sumac or hazel tree)
> 1 oz sunflower oil
> 0.2 oz squalene extract (from olive oil)
> 1 oz almond oil
> 0.1 oz vitamin E oil
> 0.5 oz glycerine
> 0.1 oz borax

Melt Japan wax in sunflower oil (Japan wax melts at approximately 118°F). Dissolve squalene extract in oil-wax mixture and add almond and vitamin E oils. Heat mixture to 165°F. Simultaneously combine the horse chestnut astringent, glycerine, and borax in a separate container and heat to 165°F. Pour water mixture into oil mixture, while stirring briskly. Remove from heat and stir until mixture cools and thickens. Pour into a clean glass jar. Keep in a cool place.

Camellia and Licorice Cream

> 1.5 oz camellia oil
> 0.5 oz licorice extract
> 1 oz sunflower oil
> 1 oz rice bran wax (tan-colored wax)
> 2 oz elderflower water (p. 213)
> 2 oz glycerine
> 0.1 oz glycyrrhizic acid (from licorice root)

Combine camellia oil and sunflower oil. Melt rice bran wax in oils (rice bran wax melts at 175°F) and slowly heat to 155°F. Simultaneously combine elderflower water, glycerine, licorice extract, and glycyrrhizic acid in a separate container and heat to 155°F. Pour oil-wax mixture into water-acid mixture. Remove from heat and stir briskly until mixture is cool and creamy. Pour into a clean glass jar. Keep in a cool place.

Aloe Vera Gel Cream

> 1 oz aloe vera gel
> 0.5 oz glycolic extract of buthcer's broom
> 0.5 oz glycolic extract of horse chestnut
> 0.5 oz glycolic extract of horsetails
> 0.2 oz orange peel oil
> 2 oz glycerine
> 0.5 oz locust bean gum

Warm the aloe vera gel with glycolic extracts and orange peel oil. Heat glycerine in a separate container and dissolve the locust bean gum in it. Add the warm gel mixture to glycerine-gum mixture. Stir until an even gel consistency is reached. Pour into a clean glass jar. Keep in a cool place.

Sandalwood Cream

> 1 oz sandalwood oil
> 2 oz almond oil
> 0.5 oz glycerine
> 0.5 oz myrrh extract
> 0.5 oz lecithin (natural lecithin from soybeans or avocado)
> 6 drops cetyl alcohol

Heat the sandalwood oil and almond oil to 155°F. Combine the glycerine, myrrh extract, and lecithin in a separate container and heat to 155°F. Add the cetyl alcohol to glycerine mixture. Stir briskly as the alcohol and lecithin begin to thicken the glycerine mixture. Remove from heat and add glycerine-acid mixture to the oils. Blend in mixture and stir briskly until cream cools. Pour into a clean glass jar. Keep in a cool place.

Jojoba Cream

> 1 oz jojoba butter
> 1 oz jojoba oil
> 1 oz patchouli astringent (p. 240)
> 1 oz vegetable glycerine
> 0.2 oz lecithin (natural lecithin from soybeans or avocado)
> 0.1 oz benzoic gum
> 6 drops cetyl alcohol
> 6 drops patchouli essential oil

Heat jojoba butter and oil to 155°F. Simultaneously heat the patchouli astringent, glycerine, lecithin, and benzoic gum in a separate container to 155°F. Remove from heat and pour the astringent mixture into oil mixture. Add cetyl alcohol and stir while cream begins to emulsify. Blend in the patchouli essential oil. Pour into a clean glass jar. Keep in a cool place.

Magnolia Cream

2 oz magnolia astringent (p. 242)
4 drops essential oil of magnolia
1 oz witch hazel
0.5 oz ascorbyl palmitate (fat-soluble vitamin C from vegetable sources)
2 oz sunflower oil
1 oz almond oil
1 oz kuzu starch

Heat the magnolia astringent, witch hazel, and ascorbyl palmitate to 155°F. Combine the sunflower and almond oils in a separate container and heat to 155°F. Dilute kuzu starch in 1 ounce of cold water and add to the hot astringent mixture. Stir briskly as mixture begins to gel. Add hot oil mixture to the astringent-kuzu mixture and stir briskly until cream cools. Blend in essential oil of magnolia into the cream. Pour into a clean glass jar. Keep in a cool place.

Rose Cream

6 oz rose water (see recipe below)
0.5 oz rose oil
1 oz rice bran wax
2 oz almond oil
0.2 oz borax
6 drops lemon peel oil

Melt rice bran wax in almond oil and heat to 155°F. Combine rose water and borax and heat to 155°F. Pour oil-wax mixture into water mixture. Add rose oil, drops of lemon peel oil and stir briskly until cream stiffens and cools. Pour into a clean glass jar. Keep in a cool place.

Rose Water

4 oz rose petals
4 oz natural spring water
4 oz witch hazel

Combine witch hazel and water and heat to 155°F. Add rose petals to water mixture and allow to stay until water cools. Remove petals and use the remaining rose water for all formulas requiring rose water.

Mint Cream (*for irritated, dry, red skin*)

6 drops essential oil of peppermint
2 oz peppermint and pine astringent (p. 241)
1 oz calamus root oil
1 oz sunflower oil
6 drops thyme oil
0.5 oz cinnamon powder
4 drops corn acid
4 drops cholesterol alcohol (from vegetable sources)

Heat all oils together. Mix peppermint and pine astringent and cinnamon powder and heat in a separate container. Pour astringent mixture into oil mixture. Add drops of corn acid and cholesterol alcohol and stir briskly into mixture until cream thickens. Pour into a clean glass jar. Keep in a cool place.

Camomile Cream (*summer*)

> ½ lb fresh or dried camomile flowers
> 0.5 oz glycolic extract of camomile
> 2 oz natural vinegar
> 4 oz natural spring water
> 1 oz vegetable glycerine
> 1 oz rice bran wax
> 1 oz sunflower oil
> 1 oz sweet rice oil
> 6 drops orange peel oil

Allow the camomile flowers to marinate in vinegar and water in a sealed glass jar for 1 week in the sun. Shake the mixture daily. Remove the flowers from jar and use 4 ounces of camomile water. Mix with glycerine and glycolic extract of camomile and heat to approximately 145°F. Melt the rice bran wax slowly in the mixture of sunflower and rice oils in a separate container and heat to 145°F. Add the heated oil mixture to the camomile water-camomile extract mixture and add drops of orange peel oil. Stir briskly until cream cools and thickens. Pour into a clean glass jar. Keep in a cool place.

Jasmine Oil Blend Cream (*for occasional use when skin is unusually dry and tired*)

> 6 drops essential oil of jasmine
> 0.5 oz jojoba oil
> 0.2 oz evening primrose oil
> 0.5 oz karite (African) butter
> 0.5 oz elderflower water (p. 213)
> 1.5 oz glycerine
> 0.2 oz benzoin gum
> 6 drops cetyl alcohol
> 0.2 oz lecithin (natural lecithin from soybeans and avocado)

Heat the jojoba and evening primrose oils and karite butter to 145°F. Combine the elderflower water, glycerine, and benzoin gum in a separate container and heat to 145°F. Add the cetyl alcohol and lecithin to this mixture and stir actively until mixture thickens. Pour into the oil and butter mixture. Add the essential oil of jasmine and stir mixture briskly until it cools. Pour into a clean glass jar. Keep in a cool place.

Pure Silver Cream

> 10 oz silver water (p. 243)
> 0.1 oz licorice acid (glycyrrhizic)
> 2.5 oz sorbitol

0.1 oz borax
0.5 oz natural amino acid gel
1 oz cocoa butter
0.5 oz calamus root oil
0.1 oz vitamin E oil

Heat the silver water, licorice acid, sorbitol, borax, and natural amino acid gel, until mixture begins to thicken. Combine the cocoa butter, calamus root oil, and vitamin E oil in a separate container and heat. Pour oil-butter mixture into silver water solution. Stir briskly until cream cools. Pour into a clean glass jar. Keep in a cool place.

Pitta Oils

Recommendation of oils from plants, seeds, roots, herbs, fruits, nuts, and barks for body and facial use. The following are some of the oils most suitable to the warm, reddish, medium-moisturized Pitta skin. Oils that need to be diluted with water are thus indicated. Depending on the varying degree of moisture inhibition or requirement of the skin, the following oils may be used for facial or body massages, in the winter months when predominantly Pitta type skin may require both a facial massage with oil as well as a cream application to the face. The following oils are listed in order of their highest emolliency and cooling factors.

More Common Oils	*More Expensive Oils*	*Butters*
Soybean oil	Calamus root oil	Ghee
Sunflower oil	Thyme oil (use 5 to 10	Karite butter
Rice oil	percent butter mix	Jojoba butter
Almond oil	with water)	
Coconut oil	Marjoram oil	
Safflower oil	Licorice oil	
	Peppermint oil	
	Spearmint oil	
	Pennyroyal oil	
	Corn mint oil	
	Fennel oil	
	Parsley oil	
	Sandalwood oil	
	Chaulmoogra oil	
	Cade oil	
	St. John's wort oil	
	Camellia oil	
	Olibanum oil (use 5 per-	
	cent mix with water)	
	Evening primrose oil	
	Jojoba oil	
	Borage oil	

Essential Oils (In no specific order, use only a few drops.)

Clove	Rose	Sweet basil (tulasi)
Honeysuckle	Jasmine	Marigold
Eucalyptus	Camellia	Camomile
Menthol	Magnolia	Enchinacea
Cardamom	Apricot	Elecampane
Sandalwood	Lavender	Calamus
Juniper berries	Ylang-ylang	Cade
Citronella	Hops	Cajeput
Patchouli	Elderflower	Arnica

Pitta Moisturizing Lotions

Camomile Lotion: See p. 224 for recipe.

Camellia and Licorice Lotion

> 1 oz camellia oil
> 0.5 oz licorice extract
> 8 oz elderflower water (p. 213)
> 2 oz glycerine
> 0.1 oz glycyrrhizic acid (from licorice root)

Heat elderflower water and glycerine together. Dissolve licorice extract in water-glycerine mixture and add the glycyrrhizic acid. Heat the camellia oil in a separate container and pour oil into the water mixture. Stir briskly until lotion cools. Pour into a clean glass jar. Cover and shake to mix. Keep in a cool place.

Horse Chestnut Lotion

> 8 oz horse chestnut astringent (p. 242)
> 0.5 oz glycerine
> 0.1 oz squalene extract (from olive oil)
> 0.5 oz aloe vera gel
> 1 oz almond oil
> 0.1 oz vitamin E oil

Heat horse chestnut astringent, glycerine, squalene extract, and aloe vera gel together. In a separate container heat the almond and vitamin E oils. Pour oils into astringent mixture. Stir briskly until mixture cools. Pour into a clean glass jar. Cover and shake to mix. Keep in a cool place.

Aloe Vera Gel Lotion

> 1 oz aloe vera gel
> 2 oz natural spring water
> 2 oz vegetable glycerine
> 0.5 oz glycolic extract of butcher's broom

0.2 oz orange peel oil

Heat water and glycerine together, add aloe vera gel and glycolic extract of butcher's broom. Blend into a lotion consistency. Add the orange peel oil. Allow to cool. Pour into a clean glass jar. Keep in a cool place.

Sandalwood Lotion

0.5 oz sandalwood oil
8 oz camomile astringent (p. 241)
0.2 oz myrrh extract
1 oz almond oil
6 drops cetyl alcohol

Heat the camomile astringent and add the myrrh extract to it. Heat the sandalwood and almond oils in a separate container and add to the astringent mixture. Stir brisky and add drops of cetyl alcohol. Stir until lotion is cool and flowing. Pour into a clean glass jar. Cover and shake to mix. Keep in a cool place.

Jojoba Lotion

1 oz jojoba oil
6 oz patchouli astringent (p. 240)
1 oz sorbitol
0.1 oz lecithin (natural lecithin from soybeans or avocado)
0.1 oz benzoic gum
6 drops patchouli essential oil

Heat the pathcouli astringent and sorbitol together. Dissolve the lecithin and benzoic gum in astringent mixture. Heat the jojoba and patchouli essential oils and pour into the astringent mixture. Stir briskly as lotion cools. Pour into a clean glass jar. Cover and shake to mix. Keep in a cool place.

Magnolia Lotion

8 oz magnolia astringent (p. 242)
4 drops essential oil of magnolia
1 oz almond milk
1 oz vegetable glycerine
0.5 oz ascorbyl palmitate
1 oz almond oil

Heat the magnolia astringent, almond milk, vegetable glycerine, and ascorbyl palmitate together. Heat the almond oil and essential oil of magnolia in a separate container and pour into the astringent-milk mixture. Stir briskly until lotion cools. Pour into a clean glass jar. Cover and shake to mix. Keep in a cool place.

Mint Lotion

6 oz peppermint and pine astringent (p. 241)
6 drops essential oil of peppermint
4 drops cholesterol alcohol (from vegetable sources)

    0.5 oz cinnamon powder
    1 oz calamus root oil
    6 drops thyme oil

Heat the peppermint and pine astringent and add cholesterol alcohol and cinnamon powder to it. In a separate container heat the calamus oil, thyme oil, and essential oil of peppermint. Pour oils into astringent mixture. Stir briskly until lotion cools. Pour into a clean glass jar. Cover and shake to mix. Keep in a cool place.

Jasmine Oil Blend Lotion

    6 drops essential oil of jasmine
    0.5 oz St. John's wort oil
    0.5 oz jojoba oil
    0.1 oz evening primrose oil
    6 oz elderflower water (p. 213)
    1 oz glycerine
    0.2 oz benzoic gum
    6 drops cetyl alcohol

Heat the St. John's wort, jojoba, and evening primrose oils together. In a separate container, heat the elderflower water, glycerine, and benzoic gum together. Pour the oil mixture into the water mixture and add drops of cetyl alcohol. Blend in the essential oil of jasmine. Stir briskly until lotion cools. Pour into a clean glass jar. Cover and shake to mix.

Pure Silver Lotion

    8 oz silver water (p. 243)
    2 oz sorbitol
    0.2 oz licorice acid (glycyrrhizic)
    1 oz cocoa butter
    0.5 oz calamus root oil
    6 drops vitamin E oil

Heat the silver water, sorbitol, and licorice acid together. In a separate container, heat the cocoa butter and calamus root and vitamin E oils together. Pour the butter-oil mixture into the silver water solution. Stir briskly until a silvery fluid texture is achieved. Allow lotion to cool. Pour into a clean glass jar. Cover and shake to mix. Keep in a cool place.

Pitta Cleansing Cream

Maple Syrup Cleanser (*perishable*)

    0.2 oz maple syrup
    0.5 oz vegetable glycerine
    0.5 oz coconut oil
    1 oz wheat germ

Warm the vegetable glycerine, maple syrup, and coconut oil together. Add the wheat germ to mixture. Scrub face thoroughly. Wash off with cool water.

Clay Cleanser (*perishable*)

> 0.5 oz kaolin clay
> 1 oz elderflower water (p. 213)
> 0.4 oz rice flour
> 0.1 oz cinnamon powder

Heat elderflower water and add clay, rice flour, and cinnamon powder. Scrub face thoroughly. If skin is slightly oily, leave cleanser on face for 5 minutes. Wash off with cool water.

Peppermint and Almond Cleanser (*all year*)

> 8 oz peppermint and pine astringent (p. 241)
> 2 oz almond meal
> 2 oz almond oil
> 1 oz rice starch
> 2 drops storax oil

Heat the peppermint and pine astringent. Dissolve rice starch in 1 ounce of natural spring water and add to astringent. Stir thoroughly until water begins to gel. Blend in almond meal, warm almond oil, and storax oil to mixture. Put into a clean glass jar. Store in a cool place.

Milk Cleansing Cream (*winter*): See p. 227 for recipe.

Gentle Cleanser I (*all year*)

> 1 oz cocoa butter
> 0.5 oz calamus root oil
> 6 drops vitamin E oil
> 1 oz rose water (p. 214)
> 0.2 oz yucca leaves extract

Heat cocoa butter and calamus root and vitamin E oils to 135°F. Combine rose water and yucca leaves extract in a separate container and heat to 135°F. As mixture begins to foam, remove from heat and pour into the oil-butter mixture. Stir briskly. Massage into clean face and leave on for 20 minutes. Rinse off with cool water.

Gentle Cleanser II (*all year*): See p. 228 for recipe.

Aloe Vera Cleanser (*perishable, dead cells remover; spring*)

> 0.5 oz aloe vera gel
> 1 oz arrowroot starch
> 2 oz boiling water
> 0.5 oz finely grounded azuki powder (leaving some fine grains in powder)

Dissolve arrowroot starch in 1 ounce of cold water. Stir in 2 ounces of boiling water and add grounded azuki powder. Stir briskly and pour into a clean muslin bag. Strain and squeeze mixture through bag into a bowl. Use azuki residue in the bag to scrub the face thoroughly. Wash off with cool water. Mix the aloe vera gel with starch-azuki fluid and rub into the face. Leave on for 15 minutes. Wash off with warm water.

Apricot Cleanser (*all year*)

> **0.5 oz finely grounded apricot kernels**
> **2 drops essential oil of apricot**
> **0.5 oz almond oil**
> **0.5 oz almond astringent (p. 242)**
> **4 drops vitamin E oil**

Warm the almond oil and astringent together. Mix in finely grounded apricot kernels. Blend in essential oil of apricot and vitamin E oil. Scrub face. Leave on for 5 minutes, and wash off with cool water.

Pitta Sun and Wind Protection Lotions ──────────

Note: The recommended sun and wind protection lotions are also applicable for men's and children's use.

Ultimate Sunscreen (*for maximum protection*): See p. 230 for recipe.

Comfrey-Aloe Sunscreen: See p. 230 for recipe.

Walnut-Yarrow Sunscreen: See p. 231 for recipe.

Sunscreen Butter: See p. 231 for recipe.

Allantoin Sun Protector: See p. 231 for recipe.

Mild Sunburn Cream: See p. 232 for recipe.

Fresh Cucumber Ointment

> **6 slices unpeeled cucumber**
> **2 oz warm horse chestnut or butcher's broom oil**

Warm the cucumber slices in oil and squeeze mixture thoroughly through a clean muslin cloth. Apply the pulp directly to sun or wind irritated skin. Leave on for 30 minutes. Wash off with cool water.

Cilantro Cream

> **2 oz cilantro water (p. 266)**
> **0.5 oz balsam oil**

0.5 oz walnut oil
0.5 oz rice bran wax
0.1 oz yarrow extract
3 drops cetyl alcohol

Combine balsam oil and walnut oil. Slowly melt rice bran wax in oils. Combine the cilantro water and yarrow extract and heat to approximately 145°F. Pour melted wax-oil mixture into the water mixture and add drops of cetyl alcohol. Stir until mixture is cool and thick. Pour into a clean glass jar. Keep in a cool place.

The following is a list of effective oils for the prevention of sun- and windburns.

Jojoba oil	Lavender oil	Marigold (calendula) oil
Walnut oil	Sandalwood oil	Chaulmoogra
Horse chestnut oil	Sunflower oil	(glyrocardia) oil
Butcher's broom oil	Calamus root oil	Neroli oil
Balsam oil	Elderflower oil	(Aloe vera gel)

Pitta Shampoos

Seaweed Shampoo: See p. 233 for recipe.

Kombu and Ivy Shampoo: See p. 233 for recipe.

Balsam Shampoo: See p. 233 for recipe.

Lavender and Evening Primrose Shampoo (*for all hair colors*): See p. 234 for recipe.

Shampoo of the Sea: See p. 234 for recipe.

Pitta Hair Conditioners

Balsam and Wine Conditioner (*for auburn hair and redheads*): See p. 235 for recipe.

Seaweed Conditioner (*for normal hair of all colors*): See p. 236 for recipe.

Ginseng and Walnut Conditioner (*for normal hair of all colors*): See p. 236 for recipe.

Pitta Hair Rinses and Colors

Henna Rinse I (*for auburn hair and redheads*): See p. 236 for recipe.

Henna Rinse II (*for dark brown hair*): See p. 236 for recipe.

Camomile and Rosemary Rinse (*for blonde hair*): See p. 237 for recipe.

Goldenrod and Vervain Rinse (*for light blonde hair*):   See p. 237 for recipe.

Mullein and Saffron Rinse (*for golden blonde hair*):   See p. 237 for recipe.

Sandalwood and Hibiscus Rinse (*for redheads*)

> 6 drops sandalwood oil
> 1 oz hibiscus tea
> 4 oz natural spring water
> 6 drops apple cider vinegar

Steep the hibiscus tea in boiling water until it cools. Remove the tea and add apple cider vinegar and sandalwood oil to water. Apply to wet hair and scalp after shampooing and/or conditioning. Towel dry and leave rinse on the hair.

Twig and Musk Rinse (*for auburn hair*):   See p. 238 for recipe.

Thyme, Sage, and Rosemary Rinse (*for sunburn and black hair; spring and summer*): See p. 238 for recipe.

Pitta Hair Oils

Camomile Oil (*for light color hair*):   See p. 238 for recipe.

Camellia Oil (*for all hair colors; all year*)

Apply the pure camellia oil to hair for additional sheen occasionally. Use with a touch of water in the palm of hands.

Ylang-Ylang Oil (*for all hair colors; all year*)

The pure oil of ylang-ylang is also excellent for additional hair sheen. Use with a touch of water in the palm of hands.

Evening Primrose Oil (*for all hair colors; fall and winter*):   See p. 239 for recipe.

Golden Jojoba Oil (*for all hair colors; all year*):   See p. 239 for recipe.

Apricot-Rosemary Oil (*for redheads; all year*)

> 0.1 oz apricot kernel oil
> 0.5 oz rosemary
> 2 oz sunflower oil
> 0.2 oz glycerine

Heat the sunflower oil. Allow rosemary to sit in hot oil until oil cools. Remove the rosemary and add apricot kernel oil and glycerine to rosemary oil. Mix thoroughly and pour into a clean glass bottle. Use a few drops in the palm of hands and massage into the strands of hair.

Sage and Thyme Oil (*for dark hair; all year*)

    0.5 oz sage
    0.1 oz thyme oil
    3 oz olive oil
    0.2 oz witch hazel

Heat the olive oil and allow the sage to sit in hot oil until oil cools. Remove the sage and add thyme oil and witch hazel to sage oil. Mix thoroughly and pour into a clean glass bottle.

Lavender Oil (*for all hair colors; spring and summer*): See p. 239 for recipe.

Neroli-Orange Oil (*for light color hair; spring and summer*): See p. 240 for recipe.

Silver Oil

    4 oz silver water (p. 243)
    0.2 oz glycerine
    1 oz coconut oil
    6 drops vitamin E oil
    6 drops essential oil of hyssop

Heat the silver water and glycerine together. Add the coconut oil, vitamin E oil, and essential oil of hyssop to mixture. Mix thoroughly and pour into a clean glass jar. Keep in a cool place. Use a few drops in the palm of hands. Massage into the strands of hair.

Kapha Type Nature's Formula

Kapha Astringents

Sweet Birch Astringent (*all year*)

    2 Tbsp sweet birch
    10 oz water
    8 oz witch hazel
    1 Tbsp sage
    1 Tbsp rosemary
    1 Tbsp styrax benzoin gum
    10 drops juniper tar oil

Bring water and witch hazel to a boil. Add the sweet birch, sage, rosemary, and styrax benzoin gum as soon as water begins to boil. Remove from heat until luke-warm. Strain through a clean muslin cloth by twisting each end of cloth in the opposite direction. (Mixture of herbs is in the center of cloth which is securely folded over to contain herbs.) Add juniper tar oil to mixture. Pour into a clean glass jar. Cover and shake to mix. Keep in a cool place or refrigerate.

Lily of the Valley Astringent (*all year*)

> 6 drops lily of the valey essential oil
> 10 oz water
> 8 oz witch hazel
> 2 Tbsp elderflower
> 2 Tbsp marigold
> 2 Tbsp coneflower
> 2 Tbsp butcher's broom
> ¼ tsp zinc oxide (powder)
> ¼ orris powder

Bring water and witch hazel to a boil. Add herbs and powders to boiling solution. Remove from heat until lukewarm. Strain (using the method above) and add lily of the valley essential oil. Pour into a clean glass container. Cover and shake. Keep in a cool place or refrigerate.

Summer Hibiscus Astringent

> 6 drops hibiscus oil
> 10 oz water
> 6 oz witch hazel
> 2 oz glycerine
> ½ tsp glycolic extract of rhatany
> 2 Tbsp gord juice
> 1 tsp ascorbic acid (natural vitamin C powder)
> ½ tsp pure citrus oil

Bring water, witch hazel, and glycerine to a boil. Remove from heat until lukewarm. Add glycolic extract of rhatany, gord juice, ascorbic acid powder, and hibiscus and citrus oils. Stir until an even consistency is reached. Pour into a clean glass jar. Cover and shake to mix. Keep in a cool place or refrigerate.

Peppermint Astringent (*spring*)

> 1 tsp peppermint oil
> 10 oz rose water (p. 249)
> 6 oz glycerine

Warm rose water and add glycerine and peppermint oil. Pour into a clean glass jar. Cover and shake to mix. Keep in a cool place or refrigerate.

Blue-Rose Astringent (*summer*)

> 1 oz fresh rose petals
> ¼ pint rose water (p. 249)
> 1 oz elecampane leaves
> ½ pint natural rice vinegar

Soak rose petals and elecampane leaves in rice vinegar for 1 week. Remove petals and leaves and add warm rose water to the solution (which will be bluish from the elecampane leaves). Pour into a clean glass jar and keep in a cool place. Before using, dilute 1 teaspoon to 4 tablespoons of water.

Elderflower and Aloe Vera Gel Astringent (*winter*)

6 Tbsp elderflowers
2 Tbsp aloe vera gel
16 oz water
8 oz witch hazel
2 tsp lemon peel oil

Bring water and witch hazel to a boil. Add elderflowers and remove mixture from heat until lukewarm. Strain mixture using the method explained in sweet birch astringent. To the elderflower solution, add the aloe vera gel and lemon peel oil. Pour into a clean glass jar. Cover and shake to mix. Keep in a cool place or refrigerate.

Honey-Citrus Astringent (*fall*)

4 Tbsp honey
1 tsp grapefruit peel oil
12 oz water
$\frac{1}{2}$ tsp cetyl alcohol
6 drops neroli oil

Bring water to a boil. Add cetyl alcohol. Remove from heat until lukewarm. Add the honey and grapefruit peel and neroli oils. Stir until an even consistency is reached. Pour into a clean glass jar. Cover and shake to mix. Keep in a cool place or refrigerate.

Allspice Astringent (*all year*)

10 oz water
8 oz witch hazel
1 tsp benzyl alcohol
6 oz coneflower
2 Tbsp nettle
1 Tbsp eucalyptus leaves
1 Tbsp blue or marsh mallow
$\frac{1}{4}$ tsp licorice powder
1 tsp lemon grass oil

Bring water and witch hazel to a boil. Add benzyl alcohol, herbs, and licorice powder. Remove from heat until lukewarm. Strain mixture using the method as explained in sweet birch astringent. Add lemon grass oil to mixture. Pour into a clean glass jar. Cover and shake to mix. Keep in a cool place or refrigerate.

Cinchona Bark Astringent (*summer*)

2 tsp red or yellow cinchona glycolic extract
10 oz water
8 oz witch hazel
1 Tbsp styrax benzoin gum
6 drops betulla essential oil

Bring water and witch hazel to a boil. Add styrax benzoin gum and cinchona glycolic extract and stir. Remove from heat until lukewarm. Add betulla essential oil. Pour into a clean glass jar. Cover and shake to mix. Keep in a cool place or refrigerate.

Pure Copper Astringent (*all year*)

Copper water: Clean copper pieces or pennies by soaking in a natural lime solution for a few hours. Then rinse the pieces of lime residue. Put 1 ounce of copper pieces in 20 ounces of natural spring water and boil until 10 ounces of water remains. Remove the copper piece from solution and use the remaining copper solution for all formulas requiring copper water.

> 10 oz copper water
> 10 oz water
> 6 oz glycerine
> 2 Tbsp goldenseal powder
> 2 tsp jojoba oil

Bring water, glycerine, and goldenseal powder to a boil. Add copper water and remove from heat until lukewarm. Add jojoba oil to mixture. Pour into a clean glass jar. Cover and shake to mix. Keep in a cool place or refrigerate.

Kapha Tonics

Skin Tonic for Fatigue: See p. 243 for recipe. Replace corn oil instead of sunflower oil.

Occasional Day Skin Tonic

> 6 ripe strawberries
> $\frac{1}{4}$ tsp orris powder
> 1 tsp witch hazel
> 4 drops wheat germ oil

Pulp the strawberries in a suribachi or blender. Add the orris powder and witch hazel. Mix in thoroughly the wheat germ oil. Apply to a clean face for 15 minutes. Wash off with warm water before moisturizing or applying makeup.

Tonic for Excessive Oily Skin

> 1 tsp witch hazel
> 2 tsp glycolic extract of rhatany
> 2 drops sage oil

Warm the witch hazel and glycolic extract of rhatany together. Put in drops of sage oil. Mix thoroughly and apply to clean face. Leave on for 1 hour or longer if necessary.

Radiant Skin Tonic

> 4 Tbsp elderflower water (p. 213)

2 Tbsp honey
1 tsp lemon grass oil

Warm elderflower water and dissolve the honey. Add lemon grass oil. Use this paste to massage into face. Leave on for 15 minutes. Rinse off with warm water. Towel to semi dry and moisturize.

Tonic for Nervous Skin

1 tsp water
½ tsp white pine bark extract
¼ tsp orris powder
2 drops hops essential oil

Heat water with pine bark extract and orris powder. Apply to a clean face and leave on for 15 minutes. Wash off with warm water. Semi dry the face with towel. Massage the hops essential oil into face and leave on overnight.

Kapha Masks ─────────────

Kaolin Mask (*spring and summer*)

0.5 oz kaolin clay
0.2 oz witch hazel
0.5 oz aloe vera gel

Warm the witch hazel and aloe vera gel together and mix in the clay. Apply mask to a clean face. Leave on for 20 minutes. Rub off the dry, flaky clay. Then wash face with warm water.

Fuller's Earth Mask (*all year*)

0.5 oz fuller's earth
0.5 oz sweet birch astringent (p. 259)

Combine ingredients. Apply mask to a clean face. Leave on for 20 minutes. Rub off the dry, flaky clay. Then wash face with warm water.

Clay Mask I (*winter*):   See p. 245 for recipe.

Clay Mask II (*all year*)

0.5 oz kaolin clay or fuller's earth
0.1 oz brown algae extract
0.5 oz natural spring water

Dilute brown algae extract in warm spring water. Add clay to mixture. Apply to face. Algae extract will cause a film to form a mask. Leave on for 20 minutes. Peel mask off face. Wash face with warm water.

Clay and Gel Mask (*all year*): See p. 245 for recipe.

Clay-Lemon Mask (*summer*)

> 0.5 oz fuller's earth
> 0.1 oz fresh lemon juice
> 0.2 oz natural spring water
> 0.2 oz glycerine

Heat the water, glycerine, and lemon juice together. Add clay to mixture. Apply to a clean face. Leave on for 20 minutes. Wash face off with warm water.

Cucumber Mask (*summer*)

> 12 unpeeled cucumber slices
> 2 oz witch hazel
> 1 oz rice bran

Warm witch hazel and cucumber slices together. Strain and squeeze mixture through a clean musline bag into a clean bowl. Add the rice bran to mixture and make a paste. Apply paste to a clean face. Leave on for 20 minutes. Wash off face with lukewarm water.

Gentle Milk Mask (*all year*): See p. 218 for recipe. Apply to a clean face. Leave on for 20 minutes. Wash off face with warm water.

Clear Peel-off Mask (*all year*): See p. 219 for recipe. In the summer add a few drops of lemon juice to the rinse water for face.

Strawberry Mask (*summer*)

> 8 fresh ripe strawberries
> 1 oz natural spring water
> 0.5 oz glycerine
> 2 drops lemon oil

Heat water and glycerine together. Add strawberries and purée to a pulp with a fork. Add drops of lemon oil to mask. Allow to cool to lukewarm. Apply to face for 25 minutes. Rinse off with lukewarm water.

Slippery Elm Gel Mask (*all year*): See p. 219 for recipe. Apply to clean face for 25 minutes. Wash off with warm water.

Lime Mask (*summer*)

> 2 drops essential oil of lime
> 0.5 oz almond milk
> 0.5 oz witch hazel
> 0.2 oz fuller's earth
> 0.5 oz gram (chick-pea) flour

Heat almond milk and witch hazel together. Blend clay and gram flour into mixture. Add drops of essential oil of lime. Allow to cool to lukewarm. Apply to a clean face. Leave on for 25 minutes. Rub mask off face with clean fingers. Wash off with lukewarm water.

Apricot and Peach Mask (*spring and fall*)

0.2 oz ripe, unpeeled apricot pieces
0.2 oz ripe, unpeeled peach pieces
0.1 oz fruit pectin extract
0.3 oz natural spring water
0.3 oz witch hazel

Dissolve the fruit pectin extract in water. Pour witch hazel into water and heat. Put unpeeled apricot and peach pieces into water mixture and bring to a boil. Purée fruits with a fork. Mixture will thicken as a result of pulp and fruit pectin extract. Allow to cool to lukewarm. Apply to a clean face for 25 minutes. Wash off with lukewarm water. This mask like a jam can be kept for several applications. (The recipe lists the ingredients for one application.)

Kapha Emollient Creams

Sweet Birch Cream (*all year*)

10 oz sweet birch astringent (p. 259)
2 oz jojoba wax
1 oz sunflower oil
0.2 oz squalene extract (from olive oil)
1 oz almond oil
0.1 oz vitamin E oil
0.5 oz witch hazel
0.1 oz borax

Melt jojoba wax in sunflower oil on slow heat (jojoba wax melts at approximately 125°F). Dissolve squalene extract in oil-wax mixture and add almond and vitamin E oils. Heat mixture to 165°F. Simultaneously combine the sweet birch astringent, witch hazel, and borax in a separate container and heat to 165°F. Pour water mixture into oil mixture, while stirring briskly. Remove from heat and stir until mixture cools and thickens. Pour into a clean glass jar. Keep in a cool place.

Camellia and Licorice Cream

1.5 oz camellia oil
0.3 oz licorice extract
1 oz Japan wax
1 oz carrot oil
2 oz elderflower water (p. 213)
1 oz witch hazel
0.1 oz glycyrrhizic acid (from licorice root)

Melt Japan wax in camellia and carrot oils (Japan wax melts at 118°F) and slowly heat to approximately 155°F. Simultaneously combine elderflower water, witch hazel, licorice extract, and glycyrrhizic acid in a separate container and heat to 155°F. Pour in oil-wax mixture into the water-acid mixture. Remove from heat and stir briskly until moisture is cool and creamy. Pour in a clean glass jar. Keep in a cool place.

Aloe Vera Gel Cream (*summer*)

- 1 oz aloe vera gel
- 0.5 oz glycolic extract of butcher's broom
- 0.5 oz glycolic extract of horse chestnuts
- 0.5 oz glycolic extract of horsetails
- 0.2 oz orange peel oil
- 2 oz witch hazel
- 0.5 oz locust bean gum

Warm the aloe vera gel with glycolic extracts and orange peel oil. Heat witch hazel and dissolve locust bean gum in it. Add the warm gel mixture to witch hazel-gum mixture. Stir until an even gel consistency is reached. Pour into a clean glass jar. Keep in a cool place.

Jojoba Cream (*winter*)

- 1 oz jojoba butter
- 0.5 oz jojoba oil
- 1 oz cilantro water (Steep fresh cilantro leaves into boiling water. Allow to cool. Remove leaves and use water.)
- 1 oz vegetable glycerine
- 0.2 oz lecithin (natural lecithin from soybeans or avocado)
- 0.1 oz ascorbyl palmitate (natural fat-soluble vitamin C)
- 6 drops cetyl alcohol
- 6 drops honeysuckle essential oil

Heat jojoba butter and oil to 155°F. Simultaneously heat cilantro water, glycerine, lecithin, and ascorbyl palmitate in a separate container to 155°F. Remove from heat and pour astringent mixture into oil-butter mixture. Add drops of cetyl alcohol. Stir briskly until lotion emulsifies. Blend in the honeysuckle essential oil. Pour into a clean glass jar. Keep in a cool place.

Jasmine Herbal Cream (*summer*)

- 4 drops essential oil of jasmine
- 1 oz camomile
- 1 oz marigold
- 1 oz sage
- 6 oz natural spring water
- 1 oz vegetable glycerine
- 1 oz kuzu starch
- 1 oz almond oil

0.5 oz lemon peel oil

Combine camomile, marigold, and sage into 6 ounces of boiling water. Allow to steep until water cools. Remove herbs and use 4 ounces of herbal water. Heat the herbal water and glycerine together to 155°F. Dilute kuzu in a few tablespoons of water. Add kuzu mixture to hot water mixture and stir until it becomes a clear gel. Combine almond and lemon peel oils in a separate container and heat to 155°F. Combine hot oil with gel mixture. Stir to achieve a clear even consistency. Blend in the essential oil of jasmine. Pour into a clean glass jar. Keep in a cool place.

Rose Cream

> 6 oz rose water (p. 249)
> 2 oz rose oil
> 1 oz jojoba wax
> 2 oz almond oil
> 0.5 oz ascorbyl palmitate (a natural vegetable fat-soluble vitamin C)
> 0.2 oz borax

Melt jojoba wax in almond oil on slow heat, then raise to 155°F. Combine rose water, ascorbyl palmitate, and borax and heat to 155°F. Pour oil-wax mixture into water mixture. Add rose oil and stir briskly until cream stiffens and cools. Pour into a clean glass jar. Keep in a cool place.

Marigold Cream (*summer*)

> ½ lb fresh dried marigold flowers
> 2 oz natural vinegar
> 4 oz natural spring water
> 1 oz vegetable glycerine
> 0.5 oz glycolic extract of rhatany
> 1 oz jojoba wax
> 4 oz sunflower oil
> 1 oz sweet almond oil
> 6 drops grapefruit peel oil

Allow the marigold flowers to marinate in vinegar and water in a sealed glass jar for 1 week in the sun. Shake the mixture daily. Remove the flowers from jar and use 4 ounces of the marigold water. Mix with glycerine and glycolic extract of rhatany and heat to approximately 145°F. Melt the jojoba wax slowly in the mixture of sunflower and almond oils in a separate container and heat to approximately 145°F. Add the heated oil mixture to the marigold water mixture and add drops of grapefruit peel oil. Stir briskly until cream cools and thickens. Pour into a clean glass jar. Keep in a cool place.

Oil Blend Cream (*for occasional use when skin is unnaturally dry*)

> 0.5 oz jojoba oil
> 0.2 oz evening primrose oil

0.5 oz karite butter
0.5 oz elderflower water (p. 213)
1.5 oz vegetable glycerine
0.2 oz benzoin gum
6 drops cetyl alcohol
6 drops lily of the vally essential oil

Heat the jojoba and evening primrose oils and karite butter to 145°F. Combine the elderflower water, glycerine, and benzoin gum in a separate container and heat to 145°F. Add the cetyl alcohol to this mixture and stir actively as mixture thickens. Pour in the oil-butter mixture. Add the lily of the valley essential oil and stir mixture briskly until it cools. Pour into a clean glass jar. Keep in a cool place.

Copper Cream (*for healing and soothing Kapha skin; late fall and winter*)

8 oz pure copper water (p. 262)
2.5 oz sorbitol
0.1 oz borax
0.5 oz natural amino acid gel
0.5 oz gum arabic
1 oz rice oil
1 oz almond oil
0.1 oz vitamin E oil

Heat the copper water, sorbitol, borax, natural amino acid gel, and the gum arabic until mixture begins to thicken. Combine the rice oil, almond oil, and vitamin E oil in a separate container and heat. Pour oil mixture into copper water solution. Stir briskly until cream cools. Pour into a clean glass jar. Keep in a cool place.

Kapha Oils

Recommendation of oils from plants, seeds, roots, herbs, fruits, and barks for body and facial use.

The following are some of the oils and essential oils most suitable to the fullness of predominantly Kapha skin types. Kapha skin is generally very moist and oily. Depending on the varying degree of moisture inhibition or requirement of skin, the following oils may be used for facial or body massage. Very rarely does a predominantly Kapha type skin require both a facial massage with oil and a cream application to the face. One or the other will suffice. The following oils are listed in order of their least emolliency and heating factors.

More Common Oils	*More Expensive Oils*
Corn oil	Lemon grass oil (2 percent mix with water)
Sunflower oil	Sage oil (5 percent mix with water)
Almond oil	Sweet birch oil (5 percent mix with water)
Safflower oil	Ginger oil (3 to 5 percent mix with water)

More Common Oils	More Expensive Oils
Rapeseed oil	Citrus oils (peel or seed oils of grapefruit, lime, lemon, orange; use 2 percent mix with water)
Cottonseed oil	Wintergreen oil (use 2 percent mix with water)
Chaulmoogra oil	Pine needle oil (use 2 percent mix with water)
Carrot oil	St. John's wort oil (5 to 10 percent mix with water)
	Jojoba oil
	Balm of lavender oil
	Evening primrose oil
	Borage oil
	Black current seed oil

Essential Oils (In no specific order, use only a few drops.)

Hibiscus	Cardamom	Neroli
Lavender	Magnolia	Hops
Rose	Camellia	Echinacea
Lily of the valley	Ambrette musk	Elecampane
Jasmine	Elderflower	Arnica
Allspice	Sweet basil (tulsi)	Ivy
Almond	Sandalwood	Bedulla
Camomile	Ylang-ylang	Hyssop

Kapha Moisturizing Lotions

Sweet Birch Lotion

>   8 oz sweet birch astringent (p. 259)
>   0.5 oz witch hazel
>   2 oz almond milk
>   0.1 oz squalene extract (from olive oil)
>   1 oz almond oil
>   2 drops essential oil of lemon grass
>   4 drops lemon peel oil

Heat the sweet birch astringent, witch hazel, and almond milk together and dissolve the squalene extract in it. Heat the oils together in a separate container and add to the water mixture. Stir briskly until a creamy lotion is reached. Allow to cool. Pour into a clean glass jar. Keep in a cool place.

Camomile Lotion: See p. 224 for recipe.

Camellia and Licorice Lotion

>   1 oz camellia oil
>   0.5 oz licorice extract

6 oz elderflower water (p. 213)
2 oz witch hazel
0.5 oz willow bark extract
0.1 oz cetyl alcohol

Heat the elderflower water and witch hazel together. Dilute the licorice and willow bark extracts in water mixture. In a separate container heat the camellia oil. Pour oil and cetyl alcohol into the warm water mixture. Stir until mixture turns into a creamy consistency. Allow to cool. Pour into a clean glass jar. Cover and shake to mix. Keep in a cool place.

Aloe Vera Gel Lotion: See p. 252 for recipe.

Jojoba Lotion

1 oz jojoba oil
4 oz cilantro water (p. 266)
2 oz witch hazel
0.2 oz lecithin
6 drops essential oil of honeysuckle
4 drops vitamin E oil
6 drops cetyl alcohol

Heat the cilantro water and witch hazel together. Dissolve lecithin in mixture. In a separate container, heat the essential oil of honeysuckle, vitamin E oil, and jojoba oil together. Pour the oil mixture into water mixture and add the drops of cetyl alcohol. Stir briskly until a clear cool lotion is aquired. Pour into a clean glass jar. Keep in a cool place.

Jasmine Herbal Lotion

4 drops essential oil of jasmine
8 oz herbal water (p. 267)
2 oz glycerine
1 oz almond oil
0.5 oz grapefruit peel oil
0.5 oz cetyl alcohol

Heat herbal water and glycerine together. In a separate container, heat the essential oil of jasmine and almond and grapefruit peel oils together. Pour oil mixture into water mixture and add cetyl alcohol. Allow to cool. Pour into a clean glass jar. Cover and shake to mix. Keep in a cool place.

Rose Lotion

8 oz rose water (p. 249)
0.1 oz essential oil of rose
1 oz almond milk
0.1 oz corn acid
2 oz almond oil
4 drops storax oil

Heat rose water, almond milk, and corn acid together. In a separate container heat the essential oil of rose and almond oil. Pour water mixture into the oil mixture. Add drops of storax oil to preserve lotion. Stir briskly until lotion is cool and creamy. Pour into a clean glass jar. Keep in a cool place.

Marigold Lotion

8 oz marigold water (p. 267)
2 oz vegetable glycerine
0.5 oz gum arabic
0.5 oz glycolic extract of rhatany
1 oz sunflower oil
1 oz jojoba oil
6 drops evening primrose oil
6 drops grapefruit peel oil

Heat marigold water and glycerine together. Dissolve gum arabic and glycolic extract of rhatany into mixture. In a separate container, heat the oils. Pour water mixture into oil mixture and stir briskly until lotion is cool. Pour into a clean glass jar. Cover and shake to mix. Keep in a cool place.

Lily of the Valley Oil Blend Lotion

6 drops lily of the valley essential oil
0.5 oz jojoba oil
0.2 oz evening primrose oil
8 oz elderflower water (p. 213)
0.2 oz lecithin
0.2 oz benzoin gum
6 drops cetyl alcohol

Heat the jojoba and evening primrose oils together. In a separate container, heat the elderflower water, lecithin, and benzoin gum together. Pour oil mixture into water mixture and add the drops of cetyl alcohol. Stir briskly until mixture cools. Add the drops of lily of the valley essential oil to lotion. Pour into a clean glass jar. Cover and shake to mix. Keep in a cool place.

Pure Copper Lotion

8 oz copper water (p. 262)
2.5 oz sorbitol
0.1 oz borax
0.5 oz natural amino acid gel
1 oz rice oil
1 oz almond oil
0.1 oz vitamin E oil

Heat the copper water, sorbitol, borax, and natural amino acid gel until mixture begins to gel. Combine rice oil, almond oil, and vitamin E oil in a separate container and heat. Pour oil mixture into copper water solution. Stir briskly until lotion cools. Pour into a clean glass jar. Cover and shake to mix. Keep in a cool place.

Kapha Cleansing Creams

Azuki Cleanser (*perishable, for very oily skin; summer*)

> 1 oz azuki beans
> 1 oz sweet birch astringent (p. 259)
> 2 drops wheat germ oil

Ground azuki beans in a blender and keep in a clean glass jar. Adjust fineness of powder to suit oiliness of skin. The more oily the skin, the less fine the grain of powder. Warm astringent and add azuki powder and drops of wheat germ oil. Scrub the face thoroughly. Leave on for a few minutes. Wash off with warm water. Prepare only as much as you need for 1 use.

Cinchona Cleanser (*perishable, for very oily skin; summer*)

> 1 oz cinchona bark astringent (p. 261)
> 1 oz rice bran
> 2 drops rice bran oil

Warm cinchona bark astringent and add rice bran and rice bran oil. Scrub the face thoroughly, leave on for a few minutes, and wash off with warm water.

Aloe Vera Cleanser (*perishable, for semi-dry skin, dead cells remover*): See p. 255 for recipe. Use the azuki remnants in bag to scrub the face. Wash off with water. Mix the aloe vera gel with starch-azuki fluid, rub into face, and leave on for 15 minutes. Wash off with warm water.

Gentle Cleanser I (*for unnaturally dry skin; fall and winter*): See p. 228 for recipe.

Gentle Cleanser II (*for unnaturally dry skin; fall and winter*)

> 0.5 oz elderflower water (p. 213)
> 0.5 oz glycolic extract of bladder wrack (seaweed)
> 0.5 oz wheat germ
> 4 drops sandalwood oil
> 4 drops wheat germ oil

Heat elderflower water and glycolic extract of bladder wrack to approximately 135°F. Add drops of sandalwood and wheat germ oils into mixture. Blend in thoroughly and scrub face with cleanser. Leave on for 15 minutes and wash off with warm water.

Almond Meal Cleanser (*all year*)

> 3 oz almond meal
> 8 oz honey-citrus astringent (p. 261)
> 2 oz almond oil
> 2 drops storax oil

Heat the honey-citrus astringent to 145°F. Blend in the almond meal in astringent. Add warm almond oil and drops of storax oil. Blend in mixture thoroughly and put in a clean glass jar. Keep in a cool place.

Clay Cleanser (*perishable; all year*)

0.5 oz kaolin clay
1 oz elderflower water (p. 213)
0.4 oz rice flour
0.1 oz goldenseal powder

Warm the elderflower water. Blend in clay, rice flour, and goldenseal powder. Scrub face thoroughly and leave on for 5 minutes. Wash off with warm water.

Kapha Cold Creams

Almond Cold Cream (*all year*)

4 oz almond oil
1 oz jojoba wax
0.5 oz wheat germ oil
5 oz sweet birch astringent (p. 259)
0.05 oz borax
2 drops tincture of benzoin

Heat the jojoba wax over very low heat (jojoba wax melts at 132°F). Remove from heat and stir in the almond and wheat germ oils. In a separate container, heat the sweet birch astringent and borax. Pour the water mixture into the oil-wax mixture and stir briskly, adding drops of benzoin to preserve the cream. Stir until mixture cools and pour into a clean glass jar. Keep in a cool place.

Eucalyptus Cold Cream (*all year*)

0.5 oz eucalyptus water (p. 229)
6 drops eucalyptus oil
2 oz corn oil
2 oz cocoa butter
0.5 oz witch hazel
6 drops cetyl alcohol

Heat corn oil and cocoa butter to 155°F. In a separate container heat eucalyptus water and witch hazel to 155°F. Pour water mixture into oil-butter mixture. Add cetyl alcohol and eucalyptus oil to mixture. As it begins to thicken, stir briskly and pour into a clean glass jar. Keep in a cool place.

All Year Cleanser

1 oz elderflower water (p. 213)
0.2 oz vegetable glycerine
0.5 oz rice bran
0.5 oz grounded azuki

0.5 oz almond oil
2 drops camphor oil

Heat elderflower water and glycerine to approximately 135°F. Add rice bran and azuki powder and stir in warm almond oil to mixture. Add drops of camphor oil and apply to face for 5 minutes. Scrub and wash off with warm water.

Apricot Cleanser (*all year*)

0.5 oz finely grounded apricot kernels
2 drops essential oil of apricot
0.5 oz almond oil
0.5 oz elderflower water (p. 213)
0.5 oz vegetable glycerine
4 drops grapefruit peel oil

Warm the almond oil, elderflower water, and glycerine together. Mix in finely grounded apricot kernels. Blend in the essential oil of apricot and grapefruit peel oil. Scrub face, leave on for 5 minutes and wash off with warm water.

Jojoba Cold Cream (*all year*)

2 oz jojoba oil
1 oz jojoba butter
1 oz jojoba wax
4 oz sweet birch astringent (p. 259)
0.5 oz witch hazel

Combine jojoba oil, butter, and wax and slowly melt together to 145°F. Heat the sweet birch astringent and witch hazel together to 145°F. Add the oil mixture to the astringent mixture, stirring briskly until cream cools and thickens. Pour into a clean glass jar. Keep in a cool place.

Rose Cold Cream (*winter*): See p. 229 for recipe.

Apricot Cold Cream: See p. 229 for recipe.

Kapha Sun and Wind Protection Lotions

Note: The recommended sun and wind protection lotions are also applicable for men's and children's use.

Ultimate Sunscreen (*for maximum protection*): See p. 230 for recipe.

Comfrey-Aloe Sunscreen: See p. 230 for recipe.

Walnut-Yarrow Sunscreen: See p. 231 for recipe.

Mild Sunburn Cream: See p. 232 for recipe.

The following is a list of effective oils for the prevention of sun- and windburns.

Jojoba oil	Lavender oil	Marigold (calendula) oil
Walnut oil	Sandalwood oil	Chaulmoogra
Horse chestnut oil	Sunflower oil	(glynocardia) oil
Butcher's broom oil	Calamus root oil	Neroli oil
Balsam oil	Elderflower oil	(Aloe vera gel)

Kapha Shampoos

Rosemary and Sage Shampoo (*for dark brown and black hair*):   See p. 232 for recipe.

Camellia Shampoo (*for dry hair*):   See p. 232 for recipe.

Seaweed Shampoo: See p. 233 for recipe.

Kombu and Ivy Shampoo: See p. 233 for recipe.

Lavender and Evening Primrose Shampoo (*for all hair colors*):   See p. 234 for recipe.

Shampoo of the Sea: See p. 234 for recipe.

Kapha Hair Conditioners

Sage and Walnut Conditioner (*for black hair*):   See p. 235 for recipe.

Birch Conditioner (*for oily hair*)

> **0.5 oz birch glycolic extract (from betulla bark or leaves)**
> **0.3 oz witch hazel**
> **6 drops lemon juice**
> **3 drops essential oil of betulla**

Heat the witch hazel and lemon juice together. Add the birch glycolic extract and essential oil of betulla. Mix well and massage into wet hair. Leave on for 15 minutes. Rinse with warm water.

Seaweed Conditioner (*for normal hair of all colors*):   See p. 236 for recipe.

Ginseng and Walnut Conditioner (*for normal hair of all colors*):   See p. 236 for recipe.

Kapha Hair Rinses and Colors

Henna Rinse II (*for dark brown hair*):   See p. 236 for recipe.

Henna Rinse III (*for black hair*):   See p. 237 for recipe.

Camomile and Rosemary Rinse (*for blonde hair*):   See p. 237 for recipe.

Goldenrod and Vervain Rinse (*for light blonde hair*):   See p. 237 for recipe.

Mullein and Saffron Rinse (*for golden blonde hair*):   See p. 237 for recipe.

Sage, Birch, and Walnut Rinse (*for black hair*):   See p. 238 for recipe.

Twig and Musk Rinse (*for auburn hair*):   See p. 238 for recipe.

Thyme, Sage, and Rosemary Rinse (*for auburn and black hair; spring and summer*): See p. 238 for recipe.

Kapha Hair Oils ────────────────────────

Camellia Oil

Apply the pure camellia oil to hair for additional sheen occasionally. Use with a touch of water in the palm of hands.

Ylang-Ylang Oil (*for all hair colors*)

The pure oil of ylang-ylang is also excellent for additional hair sheen. Use with a touch of water in the palm of the hands.

Evening Primrose Oil (*for all hair colors; fall and winter*):   See p. 239 for recipe.

Golden Jojoba Oil (*for all hair colors; all year*):   See p. 239 for recipe.

Thyme-Sage Oil (*for dark hair; all year*):   See p. 239 for recipe.

Lavender Oil (*for all hair colors; spring and summer*):   See p. 239 for recipe.

Black Oil (*for black hair; spring and summer*):   See p. 240 for recipe.

Neroli-Orange Oil (*for light color hair; spring and summer*):   See p. 240 for recipe.

Gold Oil (*for blonde and black hair; all year*):   See p. 240 for recipe.

Transient-sensitive Skin and Hair

There is one other skin activity which is classified as the *transient-sensitive skin and hair type*. This can be any one of the seven types listed on page 157. It is called *transient* since it is generally a condition of the skin that is affected by change of diet, exercise, climate, and so on, and is not necessarily true to the symptoms of any of the seven categories of skin types. After a severe change of diet or living circumstances, one's skin type tends to indicate erratic symptoms such as spots, rashes, or extreme sensitivity to sunlight and cold. The body takes three to five years to adjust to new eating habits or new climate, even when the changes are for the better. In cleaning out fatty deposits, hard calcium deposits, and toxicity the body is generally adjusting to a new life form. Often times these rashes and sensitivities take months to disappear and reoccur during the summer months year after year. Sometimes pigmentation is affected and the area becomes lighter. The recommendations in the following category will assist in decreasing the symptoms of these erratic occurrences. Since the cleansing process is a continuous one, patience is necessary in the eventual achievement of exquisite skin.

The following formulas are for dry, damaged, excessively oily hair and for dandruff control. The transient-sensitive skin category of this section addresses dry, damaged, and wrinkled skin. There is an additional section for anti-aging formulas that addresses tired, wrinkled, aging, chapped, and nervous skins. A listing of healing oils for skin ailments is also included.

Transient-sensitive Skin

Ultimate Sunscreen (*for severe burns*):   See p. 230 for recipe.

Comfrey-Aloe Sunscreen (*for mild burns*):   See p. 230 for recipe.

Walnut-Yarrow Sunscreen (*for red, irritated skin*):   See p. 231 for recipe.

Karite Cream (*for dry skin patches*)

>   2 oz karite butter
>   0.5 oz carrot oil
>   0.1 oz vitamin E oil
>   0.5 oz hydroglycolic extract of marigold
>   0.5 oz hydroglycolic extract of camomile
>   2.5 oz PABA powder
>   0.1 oz ascorbyl palmitate

Heat karite butter, carrot oil, and vitamin E oil to 135°F. Blend in the hydroglycolic extracts of marigold and camomile to mixture and dissolve PABA powder and ascorbyl palmitate in mixture. Stir until mixture is buttery. Pour into a clean glass jar and refrigerate.

Allantoin Sun Protector (*for severe burns*): See p. 231 for recipe.

Cilantro Cream (*for red, irritated skin*): See p. 256 for recipe.

Transient-sensitive Hair

Jojaba Shampoo (*for damaged, dry hair*): See p. 234 for recipe.

Selenium and Honeysuckle Shampoo (*for dandruff*)

> 0.5 oz selenium
> 6 drops essential oil of honeysuckle
> 4 oz natural spring water
> 0.2 oz allantoin crystal
> 0.1 oz natural amino acid powder
> 0.2 oz vitamin B complex powder
> 2 oz coconut oil
> 0.5 oz aloe vera gel

Heat water and dissolve selenium, allantoin crystal, amino acid powder, and vitamin B complex powder in it. In a separate container, heat the coconut oil and blend in the water solution. Add the aloe vera gel and the essential oil of honeysuckle. Stir briskly until shampoo cools. Pour into a clean glass jar. Cover and shake to mix before each use. Keep in a cool place.

Rosemary and Camomile Shampoo (*for oil control of light color hair*)

Combine 1 ounce each of camomile, ivy, rhatany, and rosemary in 10 ounces of boiling spring water. Allow to steep until water cools. Remove herbs from water and use 8 ounces of herbal water for the following formula.

> 0.5 oz rosemary glycolic extract
> 8 oz herbal water
> 1 oz glycerine
> 1 oz yucca leaves extract
> 0.2 oz benzyl alcohol
> 1 oz palm kernel oil
> 1 oz essential oil of hyssop

Heat the herbal water and glycerine and add the rosemary glycolic extract, yucca leaves extract, and benzyl alcohol. Heat palm kernel oil in a separate container and add to water solution. Add the essential oil of hyssop. Allow to cool. Pour into a clean glass jar. Cover and shake to mix before use. Keep in a cool place.

Sage and Birch Shampoo

Combine 1 ounce each of birch, rhatany, red cinchona, and marigold flowers in 10 ounces of boiling spring water. Allow to steep until water cools. Remove herbs and use 8 ounces of the herbal water for the following formula.

0.5 oz sage oil
8 oz herbal water
1 oz witch hazel
1 oz quillai bark extract
0.2 oz benzyl alcohol
1 oz palm kernel oil
0.1 oz essential oil of betulla

Heat herbal water and witch hazel together. Add the quillai bark extract and benzyl alcohol. Heat the palm kernel oil and sage oil in a separate container. Add oils to water solution. Stir briskly and add essential oil of betulla. Allow to cool. Pour into a clean glass jar. Cover and shake to mix before use. Keep in a cool place.

Selenium Menthol Shampoo (*for dandruff*)

0.5 oz selenium
4 oz natural spring water
0.5 oz glycerine
0.2 oz allantoin
0.1 oz sulfur amino acid
0.2 oz glycolic extract of horsetail
0.2 oz glycolic extract of mallow
0.5 oz extract of quillai bark
0.2 oz aloe vera gel
0.5 oz palm kernel oil
0.2 oz wintergreen oil
0.5 oz jojoba oil

Heat the spring water and glycerine together. Dissolve the selenium, allantoin, sulfur amino acid, glycolic extracts of horsetail and mallow, extract of quillai bark, and aloe vera gel in water solution. In a separate container heat the palm kernel oil, wintergreen oil, and jojoba oil. Add oils to water solution. Stir briskly until shampoo cools. Pour into a clean glass jar. Cover and shake to mix before each use. Keep in a cool place.

Land and Sea Shampoo (*for damaged, sunburnt hair*)

Combine 1 ounce each of arnica, birch, horsetail, and coneflower in 10 ounces of boiling spring water. Allow herbs to steep until water cools. Remove herbs and use 4 ounces of herbal water for the following formula.

4 oz herbal water
1 oz sea kelp extract
0.5 oz blue green algae powder
0.5 oz extract of soybeans
0.1 oz natural amino acid powder
0.2 oz indigo fera
0.2 oz vitamin B powder
2 oz coconut oil

0.5 oz rosa masqueta oil (rose-hip seed oil)
0.5 oz vitamin E oil
0.2 oz benzyl alcohol

Heat the herbal water. Add the sea kelp extract, blue green algae powder, extract of soybeans, amino acid powder, indigo fera, and vitamin B powder to water and blend in thoroughly. In a separate container, heat the coconut and rosa mosqueta oils. Pour oils into water solution and then add the vitamin E oil and benzyl alcohol to mixture. Stir briskly until mixture cools. Pour into a clean glass jar. Cover and shake to mix before use. Keep in a cool place.

Hops Oil (*for dry, damaged hair of all hair colors; winter*)

0.5 oz hops
6 drops essential oil of hops
0.5 oz marigold
4 oz water
6 drops glycerine

Steep the hops and marigold in boiling water. Remove the herbs from water and add the essential oil of hops and glycerine. Pour hops-oil mixture into a clean glass jar. Use a few drops in the palm of hands and massage into the strands of hair.

Anti-aging Formulas

The term *anti-aging* is used advisedly. These formulas will improve tired, wrinkled, chapped, and nervous skins over a period of time. The degree to which your commitment is in caring for your personal health and nutritional program is the degree to which all the recommendations in this book will work for you. There are no miracles to gaining a healthy, clean, and beautiful body. It takes a commitment to and understanding of the body as one with the entire creation. It takes an understanding of what is beautiful. The *you* inside of the projected *you*. The idea of a miracle appeals to almost everyone, to live carelessly, and yet to be beautiful. The young years provide the concessions and time for this approach, but the price is named as we get older. Maturity is the gift we are given for getting older. A gift we often do not recognize because it is packaged with wrinkled cover. It is, however, the *Rasa*—the earned beauty where every wrinkle consciously gained is a mark of our true excellence. To undo this and to support the idea of holding back the natural process of time, is to deny this *Rasa*. However to make the marks of time more subtle is to be kind to the ravishments of aging. These formulas and recommendations provide you with such a guide. All constitutional skin types will benefit from these formulas, however, the predominantly Vata skin type will benefit the most since it is the skin type that usually wrinkles the most.

Rosa Mosqueta, Borage, Sage, and Fennel Cream

Combine 0.5 ounce each of horsetails, St. John's wort, fennel, echinacea, and marigold in 15 ounces of boiling natural spring water. Allow herbs to steep until water cools. Remove herbs from water and use 10 ounces of herbal water for the following formula.

- 0.5 oz rosa mosqueta oil (rose-hip seed oil)
- 0.2 oz borage oil
- 0.5 oz sage oil
- 0.2 oz fennel oil
- 10 oz herbal water
- 2 oz sorbitol
- 0.5 oz natural vitamin A powder (from vegetable or dairy sources)
- 3 oz guar gum (powder extract)
- 1 oz squalene extract (from olive, wheat germ, or rice germ)
- 2 oz olive oil
- 0.5 oz wheat germ oil
- 0.05 oz benzyl alcohol
- 0.1 oz essential oil of echinacea

Heat the herbal water and sorbitol together. Dissolve the powdered extracts of vitamin A, guar gum, and squalene. In a separate container, heat the olive, borage, rosa mosqueta, fennel, sage, and wheat germ oils. Pour the oils into the water mixture. Add the benzyl alcohol to mixture and stir until cream cools and thickens. Add the essential oil of echinacea to cream. Pour into a clean glass jar. Keep in a cool place.

Camellia, Ylang-Ylang, Ginseng, and Licorice Cream

- 1 oz camellia oil
- 0.5 oz ylang-ylang oil
- 0.5 oz glycolic extract of ginseng
- 0.5 oz extract of licorice
- 1 oz beeswax
- 0.5 oz black currant oil
- 0.2 oz borax
- 0.5 oz extract of yarrow
- 0.2 oz cetyl alcohol
- 0.5 oz vitamin E oil

Slowly melt the beeswax in a combination of camellia, ylang-ylang, and black currant oils. Add the borax to oil-wax mixture. In a separate container combine the glycolic extract of ginseng and extracts of licorice and yarrow and add to warm oil mixture. Add the cetyl alcohol and vitamin E oil. Stir briskly until a firm cream is achieved. Pour into a clean glass jar. Keep in a cool place.

Anti-aging Bark Gel

- 0.5 oz extract of China bark
- 2 oz vegetable glycerine
- 0.5 oz extract of arnica
- 0.5 oz extract of cinchona
- 0.5 oz extract of rosemary
- 1 oz Siam benzoin gum

0.2 oz benzyl alcohol
0.1 oz tincture of benzoin
2 oz cocoa butter
0.5 oz essential oil of *Laminaria digitata* (seaweed)

Heat the glycerine. Combine the extracts and benzoin gum and dissolve in glycerine. Add the benzyl alcohol and tincture of benzoin to mixture. In a separate container, heat the cocoa butter and essential oil of *Laminaria digitata*. Pour oil-butter mixture into the glycerine-extract combination. Mix the gel briskly until an even, firm consistency is achieved. Pour into a clean glass jar. Store in a cool place.

Jojoba-Shea Butter

1 oz jojoba oil
1 oz jojoba butter
0.3 oz jojoba wax
1 oz shea butter
0.01 oz borax
1 oz sorbitol
0.1 oz essential oil of fennel

Slowly melt the jojoba wax in jojoba oil, jojoba butter, and shea butter. Dissolve the borax in the mixture. Heat the sorbitol in a separate container and add to the oil-wax mixture. Stir cream briskly and add the essential oil of fennel to cream. Pour into a clean glass jar. Keep in a cool place.

Milk Cream

1 oz fresh cow's milk*
0.2 oz aloe vera gel
2 drops tincture of benzoin
0.5 oz rice flour

Heat the milk and stir in aloe vera gel and benzoin. Add the rice flour to milk and make a thin paste. Apply to face and leave on overnight.

Rose Lotion

0.5 oz rose water (p. 249)
3 drops essential oil of rose
0.5 oz glycerine
1 oz guar gum
1 oz olive oil
0.1 oz rice germ oil

Heat the rose water and glycerine together and dissolve the guar gum. In a separate container, heat the olive and rice germ oils together. Add the oils to the water mixture. Stir lotion briskly and pour into a clean glass jar. Store in a cool place.

---

*The milk of the cow, after she has given birth, is best for the anti-aging process.

Oils of Youth (*for extreme dryness only*)

> 0.5 oz evening primrose oil
> 0.5 oz borage oil
> 0.5 oz black currant seed oil
> 0.5 oz rosa mosqueta oil (rose-hip seed oil)

Mix the oils and pour into a clean glass jar. Use a few drops on a clean face before bed.

Avocado, Carrot, Sesame, and Ghee Cream

> 0.5 oz avocado oil
> 0.2 oz carrot oil
> 0.2 oz dark sesame oil
> 0.5 oz ghee (unsalted clarified butter)
> 0.5 oz cocoa butter
> 2 oz vegetable glycerine
> 0.1 oz natural amino acid powder
> 0.1 oz lecithin powder
> 0.1 oz cetyl alcohol
> 0.1 oz tincutre of benzoin
> 0.5 oz wheat germ oil

Heat the avocado oil, carrot oil, dark sesame oil, ghee, and cocoa butter together. In a separate container, heat the glycerine and dissolve the amino acid and lecithin powders. Add the cetyl alcohol and tincture of benzoin to glycerine mixture. Pour in the oil mixture. Stir briskly until mixture is cool and creamy. Add the wheat germ oil to mixture. Pour into a clean glass jar. Keep in a cool place.

Eye Care

Sweet Fennel Eye Cream

> 4 oz fennel water (p. 215)
> 1 oz jojoba wax
> 4 oz cocoa butter
> 4 drops grapefruit peel oil

Heat the fennel water to approximately 155°F. Melt jojoba wax slowly in cocoa butter in a separate container and heat to approximately 155°F. Pour water mixture into wax-butter mixture and stir briskly. Remove from heat, add the grapefruit peel oil to preserve it, and continue stirring until cream cools. Pour into a clean glass jar. Keep in a cool place.

Rich Oil Blend Eye Cream: See recipe of rich oil blend cream on p. 222.

Rose Eye Cream

> 6 oz rose water (p. 249)
> 0.5 oz rose oil

1 oz beeswax
1 oz camellia oil
1 oz almond oil
0.5 oz ascorbyl palmitate (a natural vegetable source fat-soluble vitamin C)
0.2 oz borax

Melt the beeswax in the camellia and almond oils on slow heat. Raise heat to approximately 155°F. Combine rose water, ascorbyl palmitate, and borax in a separate container and heat to approximately 155°F. Pour oil-wax mixture into water mixture. Add rose oil and stir briskly until cream stiffens and cools. Pour in a clean glass jar.

Healing Oils for Ailments

Marigold (Calendula) Herb and Oil

The marigold or calendula blossoms which grace the cover of this book have been used for ages for every possible damage done to the skin tissues as well as for beautification of the skin. Apart from the beauty of this field of blossoms, its healing capacity is extensive. The blossoms are used as poultice for burns, sunburn, slow-healing wounds, eczemas, chapped skin, and inflamed mucous membranes, amongst other skin ailments. The marigold blossoms accelerate the healing process of serious wounds. The extract of the marigold flowers, leaves, and herb are used as a skin freshner, softener, and stimulant. When purchasing this oil, be sure that it is pure. Pure, unadulterated marigold oil is extracted in soybean oil without synthetic solvents.

Carrot Oil

Both the carrot seed oil and the carrot root oil are used for medicinal as well as cosmetic purposes. The carrot oil is naturally high in vitamin A and beta-carotene. Both factors contribute to maintain the body's metabolic processes. Carrot oil compensates the skin's deficiency of vitamin A. External application of carrot oil accelerates the formation of new cells. It produces and moisturizes skin that produces insufficient sebum, such as dried and chapped skin.

Avocado Oil

The avocado tree grows in South and Central America, Florida, southern California, and Mexico. The pulp of its fruit yields an oil that is considered superior to all other vegetable oils. It is an active ingredient in cosmetic formulas. The oil itself is rich in vitamin A, vitamin D, vitamin E, carbohydrates, protein, sugars, amino acids, glycerides of oleic, linoleic, and palmoleic acids. It is highly unsaponifiable in that it does not decompose into an acid, alcohol or salt, as do the coconut and palm kernel oils. Both the fresh pulp of the fruit and its oil can be used for creams, massage oils, and numerous healing cosmetic formulas. It accelerates the crusting of the skin over wounds and is thus effective for skin diseases such as eczema.

Tea-tree Oil

Tea-tree oil is from the northern coast of South Wales, Australia, and is used for topical skin problems. The leaves were used originally by the aboriginal people to make tea. The oil from a specific species known as the *malalenca alternifolia* is used for antiseptic and fungicidal actions. It is used for vaginal infection, burns, infections, cuts and scrapes, pimples, stings, toothache, gum infections, and sore throats. (For sore throat oil is put into steaming hot water and is inhaled through the nose and mouth.) Dilute with 8 parts almond, coconut, sesame or olive oil when used as a topical application on skin. Use a drop with a cotton swab (undiluted) when applying to burns, pimples, cuts, stings, tooth or gums, cuts and scrapes. Should a reaction develop from using this potent oil, desist the use of it.

Neem Oil

The neem tree is grown profusely in India, Pakistan, Ceylon, Southeast Asia, Japan, and Africa, among other countries. A very tall tree, approximately 50 feet, this evergreen with its fragrant white flowers purifies the air abundantly.

The neem tree is one of the most sacred of trees for Hindus. Five branches and a coconut are traditionally offered in ceremonies. The five branches represent the five elements of nature, and the coconut represents the human body, or the *jagat*, which is the entity of creation. The bark, leaves, and fruit of the neem tree are used in Ayurvedic medicine. Neem oil is excellent for skin afflictions of a stubborn nature, such as psoriasis and eczema. It is used in India on leprosy victims.

Borage Oil

Borage oil was used in the Middle Ages for many medicinal purposes. Originally from Syria, it was used also for alleviating depression. Borage oil is higher in gamma linolenic acid (GLA), a unique fatty acid found in mother's milk, than is either evening primrose oil or black currant seed oil, according to natural cosmetic chemist and herbalist Aubrey Hampton.

Borage oil is also high in calcium, potassium, and mineral acids. It is used externally for extremely stubborn dry skins such as psoriasis and eczema. The borage herbs can be used as a poultice for inflammatory swellings. It is used also internally as a supplement to diet.

Jojoba Oil

Jojoba oil is extracted and cold-pressed from the jojoba bean. This desert plant's endurance is truly miraculous. It survives the arid deserts of Arizona, California, and Mexico. During the hot days of summer and cold desert nights the pores of the plant are covered by a wax. This prevents the evaporation process that would normally kill any plant. Its life span exceeds that of the human being.

The oil which is often called "liquid gold" has a diverse and long list of excellent contributions to the cosmetic and pharmaceutical industries. It is one of the best emollients for hair and skin, and is considered superior even to sperm whale oil which was recently outlawed for use in the United States. It is also used as a stabilizer for penicillin. The American Indians were the first known consumer of this oil. They used it for cooling and anointing their bodies and hair. The oil is considered calorie-free in foods, as the digestive enzymes of the human body cannot hydrolyze this polyunsaturated oil. It is considered to be more a liquid wax than a plant oil.

About the Ingredients of Natural Beauty Formulas

The following is a list of the lesser known derivatives used in the formulas in this chapter. Most of these derivatives are from the plant kingdoms. and a few are from the animal kingdom. It is highly recommended that the derivatives you use in your formulas come from the plant kingdom.

As these formulas were created with the natural harmony of the body and the universe in mind, the plant kingdom offers a clear, and brilliant energy. It is also a much more superior product to any that hails from the animal and chemical kingdom.

The most reliable sources of purchasing your ingredients is through your local health food store's proprietors. You may also inquire as to the names of national mail order companies that offer natural ingredients from the plant kingdom.

Allantoin: Crystalline derived from the urine of animals and humans as well as from herbs such as comfrey and usa ursi. Recommendation of allantoin in formulas is from herbal source only. Allantoin is a healing agent for dry, damaged hair and skin.

Ascorbyl palmitate: Fat-soluble form of vitamin C.

Balsam: Healing agent. Resins that contain benzoil acid or its ester (balsam peru, styrax, benzoin gum).

Beeswax: Produced by the honeybee to build the honeycomb. Color varies from deep brown to a light amber shade. Test on skin for allergy before using in formulas.

Benzyl alcohol: A fragrant alcohol made up of many herbs—balsam peru, cananga oil, cassie absolute, castoreum, cherry laurel leaves, jasmine, and storax.

Borage oil, black currant seed oil, and evening primrose oil: Apart from mother's milk, these three oils are the only known sources of a less common fatty acid called *gamma-linolenic acid (GLA)*. GLA is formed in the body as part of the process of manufacturing postaglandin which is a hormone-like substance that contributes to the control of every organ of the body.

Carrageen (carrageenen or Irish moss: A seaweed which is dried and made into a powdered extract. It is a very good natural emulsifier and binding agent in cosmetics.

Cetyl: Wax-like powder. Powder produced from spermaceti and coconut oil.

Fruit pectin: Natural thickener from fruits, also from vegetables. Used as a preservative in jams and recommended in this chapter as a preservative for cosmetics or as a natural emulsifier and thickener.

Glycerine: Also known as glycerol it is a syrupy alcohol that can be produced from synthetic alcohol or from vegetable oils. Only the natural source glycerine is recommended for use in the formulas.

Glycolic extract: A semi-thick or light olefinic extract of a plant.

Glycyrrhizic acid: Organic acid derived from licorice root.

Japan wax: An ivory color vegetable wax from the coating on the berry kernels of the Japanese hazel (sumac) trees.

Jojoba wax: A hard wax made by hydrogenating the liquid wax of the jojoba shrub.

Karite (African or shea) butter: The African butter trees grown on the Ivory Coast produce a dark gum berry. The pits are dried and cold pressed. This butter is used as a nondairy substitute in Africa and Japan. It is also an excellent emollient.

Kuzu: A starch from the kuzu plant root. It is used for medicinal purposes in Japan and is recommended in this chapter as a softener, thickener, and emulsifier in cosmetics.

Lecithin: A naturally occurring mixture of stearic, palmitic, and oleic acid compounds found in plants, egg yolks, soybeans, avocado, and also from the animal kingdom. Only the lecithin from plants and beans is recommended for use in formulas.

Musk: This is obtained from skin of the abdomen of the male musk deer, as well as from musk-ox, the civet cat and muskrat. The herbal sources are the musk seed (ambrette seed), musk clover, and musk mallow. Only herbal sources are recommended for use in the formulas.

Naringen extract: Extracted from the peel and seed of the grapefruit. The grapefruit peel and seed is also used as a preservative in cosmetics.

PABA (para amino benzoic acid): Water-soluble B vitamin found in molasses, brewers yeast, eggs, liver, milk, bran, rice, organ of animals, wheat germ, and whole wheat. It is used as a protective screen from harmful ultraviolet rays. Only the vegetable and grain derivatives are recommended for use in formulas.

Panthenol: This is converted in the body to panthothenic acid, a member of B vitamins. It prevents hair loss and is absorbent through the scalp and into the hair keratin.

Rice bran wax: This comes from the bran of the rice. It is light beige to caramel in color.

Rosa mosqueta oil (rose-hip seed oil): This oil is recommended for reducing wrinkles, scars, and marks on face and body. It also helps sunburns and damaged hair. The oil comes from the tiny amber seeds of the fruit known as rose hips. The oil is high in essential fatty acids and is used therapeutically for severe burns. This rosa mosqueta oil grows in the Andes of South America. (Do not use on oily skin.)

Sorbitol: Slightly sweet alcohol in crystalline form, occurring naturally in mountain ash. It is produced industrially by a reaction process of D-glucose. It is used, like glycerine or mannitol, as a moisturizer and binder in cosmetics.

Squalene: Saturated hydrocarbon from oil of shark, olive oil, wheat germ oil, rice bran oil, and lanolin which is derived from sheep's wool. The use of shark's oil and lanolin are not recommended.

Stearyl: Similar to cetyl but is derived from both animal and vegetable sources.

Storax oil: Oil from the balsam of the bark. It is used as a preservative in cosmetics and also as an ingredient to make benzoic tincture.

■ *Avoid All Chemicals and Animal Extracts and Especially the Following:*

• Propylene glycol, fatty acid esters of ethylene glycol, diethylene glycol, polyethylene glycol (PEG), polyoxyethylene, sorbitol, and sorbitan; all mineral oils, petroleum, paraffin, ceresin, ozokerite, silicone waxes, silicone oils; all petrochemical by-products (paraben family of petrochemicals, i.e., methyl paraben, propyl paraben); spermaceti (sperm whale oil, it is outlawed in the United States); all commercial bubble baths, nail polish and nail polish removers; all cellular extracts; and animal collagen.

• All ingredients beginning with "coca" and followed by a chemical name, for example cocamide, DEA, MEA, or MIPA, cocamidopropyl, cocoa betaine, MEA (monoethanolamine), DEA (diethanolamine), TEA (triethanolamine), NDELA (nitrosodiethanolamine). The chemicals are suspect of nitrosamine contamination which can enter the bloodstream from external use.

• Two-bromo, 2-nitroprophane, 1- and 3-diol (aka bronopol, onyxide 500 and BNPD) and sodium lauryl sulfate, alkyl sulfate. These chemicals are suspect of contamination with nitrosamines, a carcinogenic agent and are often used in so-called "natural beauty products" as well as commercial beauty products.

• Cellulose gum (it is synthetic).

Note: The following ingredients are also available from vegetable sources and are recommended as the superior alternative to the animal derived substances which are more readily available: animal collagen elastin (amino by-product, wool wax), lanolin, squalene (from shark liver oil), spermaceti (sperm whale oil), cetyl and stearyle, alcohols (derived from animal fats), animal musk oil, and glycerine (from animal fats and synthetic derivatives).

■ *Some Noteworthy Cosmetic Terminology*

Collagen: Collagen is the elastic fibrous protein that holds the skin together. It is a white substance which when boiled converts to gelatin. It constitutes a third of the total body's protein. The term *soluble collagen* refers to connective skin tissues that have good moisture absorbing capacity as in youthful skin. Insoluble collagen is connective tissue that are cross-linked and have lost the ability to absorb moisture. Be careful of using products which list collagen as an ingredient. Most collagen in cosmetics are from animal sources such as the beef industry and many are insoluble to the skin.
  Vegetarian collagen: More positive effects can be obtained on the skin by using the herbs that encourage the formulation of collagen fibrils. Herbs high in organic silica such as coltsfoot, horsetails, St. John's wort, coneflower, and marigold are all collagen effective. Also the rosa mosqueta oil (rose-hip seed oil) is excellent for increasing the elasticity of the skin, to compensate for collagen loss, and to stimulate the formation of new collagen fibrils.

EFAs (essential fatty acids—vitamin F):   EFAs are part of the membranes in all tissues of the body. They are a vital part of the structure of all cells. EFAs are not synthesized by the human body. They can only be obtained in the blood through the skin or through the diet. Vitamin F is known as the cosmetic vitamin for it plays a primary role in the maintenance of healthy skin, hair, and nails. EFAs control the secretions of body oils and guard against disease causing organisms entry through the skin. They are responsible for respiration of vital organs, lubrication of cells, and assist in regulating normal glandular activity. EFAs' most appealing ability for the skin is that it attracts moisture retaining properties. It maintains a healthy level of water to the skin and keeps supple and soft. It is an excellent base for cosmetics, for it helps penetrate the skin. A good source of EFAs is lecithin found in egg yolks, avocados, and black soybeans. Although EFAs are easily available through unrefined oils such as sesame oil, corn oil, flax seed oil, sunflower oil, soybean oil, and evening primrose oil, their conversion to usable essential fatty acids to the body is a complex process. According to scientists, only the cislinoleic acid form of EFAs found in the above listed unrefined oils, converts biologically in the body.

Emollient: An emollient is a lubricant to soften the skin tissue and protect the skin from dryness. The skin's natural water content is its primary emollient. Oil is a secondary emollient to the skin as it depends on the water content of the skin in order to be effective. In essence, the skin absorbs through its oil glands, but it moisturizes with its water content.

Emollient oils are most good vegetable oils, olive oil, cod liver oil, avocado oil, castor oil, and so on. Lanolin is also considered an emollient oil but it comes from the animal kingdom. It is present in sheep's wool and is removed by ether or by scrubbing with a soap solution. Musk oil is also derived from animals. (There is a natural "musk" scent available from the ambrette seed.)

Since there is such a wide variety of good vegetable oils to be used, it is not necessary to use the natural oils of animals and animal skins. Recommended emollient oils are those obtained through steam distillation process of plants. There are a few essential oils or *absolutes* of therapeutic value to the skin and hair derived from flowers and herbs such as the jasmine, rose, camomile, lavender, and camellia flowers. Emollient oils are excellent for absorption by the skin and hair. A recommended list of oils is included in this chapter expressively for each different skin types.

Emulsifiers: A emulsifier is a catalytic element that binds water to oil. A good example is the wax that holds the oil and water together in a cold cream.

Essential oils: They are the mixtue of organic compounds such as sulfur compounds, acids, oxides, ethers, and so on. Essential oils aid absorption through the skin.

PH: The pH factor is the measure of acidity or alkalinity of the skin.

Macrobiotic Resources

● **Macrobiotic Way of Life Seminar**

The *Macrobiotic Way of Life Seminar* is an introductory program offered by the Kushi Institute in Boston. It includes classes in macrobiotic cooking, home care, and kitchen setup, lectures on the philosophy of macrobiotics and the standard diet, and individual way of life guidance. It is presented monthly and includes introductory and intermediate level programs. Information on the *Macrobiotic Way of Life Seminar* is available from:

The Kushi Institute
17 Station Street
Brookline, Massachusetts 02147
(617) 738–0045

● **Macrobiotic Residential Seminar**

The *Macrobiotic Residential Seminar* is an introductory program offered at the Kushi Foundation Berkshires Center in Becket, Massachusetts. It is a one week live-in program that includes hands-on training in macrobiotic cooking and home care, lectures on the philosophy and practice of macrobiotics, and meals prepared by a specially trained cooking staff. It is presented monthly and includes introductory and intermediate levels. Information on the *Macrobiotic Residential Seminar* is available from:

Kushi Foundation Berkshires Center
Box 7
Becket, Massachusetts 01223
(413) 623–5742

● **Kushi Institute Leadership Studies**

For those who wish to study further, the Kushi Institute in Boston offers instruction for individuals who wish to become trained and certified macrobiotic teachers. Similar leadership training programs are offered at Kushi Institute affiliates in London, Amsterdam, Antwerp, Florence, as well as in Portugal and Switzerland. Information on *Leadership Studies* is available from the Kushi Institute in Boston.

● **Other Programs**

The Kushi Institute offers a variety of public programs including an annual Summer Conference in western Massachusetts, special weight loss and natural beauty seminars, and intensive cooking and spiritual development training at the Berkshires Center. Information on these programs is available at either of the above addresses. Moreover, macrobiotic educational centers throughout the United States, Canada, and the world offer a variety of introductory and special programs. The Kushi Foundation publishes a *Worldwide Macrobiotic Directory* every year listing these centers and individuals. Please consult the *Directory* for the nearest macrobiotic center or qualified instructor.

● **Publications**

Books and publications with information on macrobiotics are available from the Kushi

Foundation, or at other macrobiotic centers, natural food stores, and bookstores. Ongoing developments are reported in the Kushi Foundation's periodicals, including the *East West Journal*, a monthly magazine begun in 1971 and now with an international readership of 200,000. The *EWJ* features regular articles on the macrobiotic approach to health and nutrition, as well as related subjects. Moreover, Michio and Aveline Kushi have authored numerous books on macrobiotic philosophy, cooking, diet, and way of life. The following titles are especially recommended for further study:

● **Books by Michio Kushi**

Health and Diet

1. *The Cancer-Prevention Diet* (with Alex Jack, St. Martin's Press, 1983)
2. *Diet for a Strong Heart* (with Alex Jack, St. Martin's Press, 1985)
3. *Natural Healing through Macrobiotics* (edited by Edward Esko and Marc Van Cauwenberghe, M.D., Japan Publications, Inc., 1979)
4. *Macrobiotic Home Remedies* (edited by Marc Van Cauwenberghe, M.D., Japan Publications, Inc., 1985)
5. *Macrobiotic Diet* (coauthored with Aveline Kushi; edited by Alex Jack, Japan Publications, Inc., 1985)
6. *Cancer and Heart Disease: The Macrobiotic Approach to Degenerative Disorders* (with various contributors; edited by Edward Esko, Japan Publications, Inc., 1982)
7. *Crime and Diet: The Macrobiotic Approach* (with various contributors; edited by Edward Esko, Japan Publication, Inc., 1987)
8. *Macrobiotic Health Education Series—Diabetes and Hypoglycemia; Allergies; Obesity, Weight Loss and Eating Disorder; Infertility and Reproductive Disorders; Arthritis; Stress and Hypertension* (with various editors, Japan Publications, Inc., 1985–91)
9. *How to See Your Health: The Book of Oriental Diagnosis* (Japan Publications, Inc., 1980)
10. *Your Face Never Lies* (Avery Publishing Group, 1983)
11. *AIDS, Macrobiotics, and Natural Immunity* (with Martha C. Cottrell, M.D. and Mark N. Mead, Japan Publications, Inc., 1990)

Phylosophy and Way of Life

1. *One Peaceful World* (with Alex Jack, St. Martin's Press, 1986)
2. *The Book of Macrobiotics: The Universal Way of Health, Happiness and Peace* (with Alex Jack, Japan Publications, Inc., revised edition, 1986)
3. *The Macrobiotic Way* (with Stephen Blauer, Avery Publishing Group, 1985)
4. *The Book of Dō-In: Exercises for Physical and Spiritual Development* (Japan Publications, Inc., 1979)
5. *Macrobiotic Palm Healing: Energy at Your Finger-Tips* (with Olivia Oredson, Japan Publications, Inc., 1989)
6. *On the Greater View* (Avery Publishing Group, 1986)

● **Books by Aveline Kushi**

Cooking

1. *Aveline Kushi's Complete Guide to Macrobiotic Cooking for Health, Harmony, and Peace* (with Alex Jack, Warner Books, 1985)

2.   *Aveline Kushi's Introducing Macrobiotic Cooking* (with Wendy Esko, Japan Publications, Inc., 1987)

3.   *Aveline Kushi's Wonderful World of Salads* (with Wendy Esko, Japan Publications, Inc., 1989)

4.   *The Changing Seasons Macrobiotic Cookbook* (with Wendy Esko, Avery Publishing Group, 1985)

5.   *How to Cook with Miso* (Japan Publications, Inc., 1979)

6.   *Macrobiotic Family Favorites* (with Wendy Esko, Japan Publications, Inc., 1987)

7.   *The Macrobiotic Cancer Prevention Cookbook* (with Wendy Esko, Avery Publishing Group, 1988)

8.   *Macrobiotic Food and Cooking Series—Diabetes and Hypoglycemia; Allergies; Obesity, Weight Loss and Eating Disorder; Arthritis; Stress and Hypertension* (with various editors, Japan Publications, Inc., 1985–88)

Family Health

1.   *Macrobiotic Pregnancy and Care of the Newborn* (with Michio Kushi; edited by Edward and Wendy Esko, Japan Publications, Inc., 1984)

2.   *Macrobiotic Child Care and Family Health* (with Michio Kushi; edited by Edward and Wendy Esko, Japan Publications, Inc., 1986)

3.   *Lessons of Night and Day* (Avery Publishing Group, 1985)

Philosophy and Way of Life

1.   *Aveline: The Life and Dream of the Woman Behind Macrobiotics Today* (with Alex Jack, Japan Publications, Inc., 1988)

Recommended Reading

Aihara, Cornellia: *The Dō of Cooking*. Chico, Calif.: George Ohsawa Macrobiotic Foundation, 1972.

——. *Macrobiotic Childcare*. Oroville, Calif: George Ohsawa Macrobiotic Foundation, 1971.

——. *Macrobiotic Kitchen: Key to Good Health*. Tokyo & New York: Japan Publications, Inc., 1982.

Aihara, Herman. *Basic Macrobiotics*. Tokyo & New York: Japan Publications, Inc., 1985.

Benedict, Dirk. *Confessions of a Kamikaze Cowboy*. Van Nuys, Calif.: Newcastle, 1987.

Brown, Virginia, with Susan Stayman. *Macrobiotic Miracle: How a Vermont Family Overcame Cancer*. Tokyo & New York: Japan Publications, Inc., 1985.

Dietary Goals for the United States. Washington, D. C.: Select Committee on Nutrition and Human Needs, U.S. Senate, 1977.

Diet, Nutrition, and Cancer. Washington, D. C.: National Academy of Sciences, 1982.

Dufty, William. *Sugar Blues*. New York: Warner Books, 1975.

Esko, Wendy. *Aveline Kushi's Introducing Macrobiotic Cooking*. Tokyo & New York: Japan Publications, Inc., 1987.

Esko, Edward and Wendy. *Macrobiotic Cooking for Everyone*. Tokyo & New York: Japan Publications, Inc., 1980.

Fukuoka, Masanobu. *The Natural Way of Farming: The Theory and Practice of Green Philosophy*. Tokyo & New York: Japan Publications, Inc., 1985.

——. *The Road Back to Nature: Regaining the Paradise Lost*. Tokyo & New York: Japan Publications, Inc., 1987.

——. *The One-Straw Revolution*. Emmaus, Pa.: Rodale Press, 1978.

Hampton, Aubrey. *Natural Organic Hair and Skin Care*. Tampa, Fla.: Organic Press, 1987.

Healthy People: The Surgeon General's Report on Health Promotion and Disease Prevention. Washington, D. C.: Government Printing Office, 1979.

Heidenry, Carolyn. *Making the Transition to a Macrobiotic Diet*. Wayne, N. J.: Avery Publishing Group, 1987.

Hippocrates. *Hippocratic Writings*. Edited by G. E. R. Lloyd. Translated by J. Chadwick and W. N. Mann. New York: Penguin Books, 1978.

I Ching or *Book of Changes*. Translated by Richard Wilhelm and Cary F. Baynes. Princeton: Bollingen Foundation, 1950.

Ineson, John. *The Way of Life: Macrobiotics and the Spirit of Christianity*. Tokyo & New York: Japan Publications, Inc., 1986.

Ishida, Eiwan. *Genmai: Brown Rice for Better Health*. Tokyo & New York: Japan Publications, Inc., 1988.

Jack, Alex, ed. *The New Age Dictionary*. Tokyo & New York: Japan Publications, Inc., 1990.

Jack, Gale, with Alex Jack. *Promenade Home: Macrobiotics and Women's Health*. Tokyo & New York: Japan Publications, Inc., 1988.

Jacobs, Barbara and Leonard. *Cooking with Seitan: The Delicious Natural Food from Whole Grain*. Tokyo & New York: Japan Publications, Inc., 1986.

Jacobson, Michael. *The Changing American Diet*. Washington, D. C.: Center for Science in the Public Interest, 1978.

Kaibara, Ekiken. *Yojokun: Japanese Secrets of Good Health*. Tokyo: Tokuma Shoten, 1974.

Kohler, Jean, and Mary Alice. *Healing Miracles from Macrobiotics*. West Nyack, N. Y.: Parker, 1979.

Kotzsch, Ronald. *Macrobiotics: Yesterday and Today*. Tokyo & New York: Japan Publications, Inc., 1985.

——. *Macrobiotics Beyond Food*. Tokyo & New York: Japan Publications, Inc., 1988.

Kushi, Aveline. *How to Cook with Miso*. Tokyo & New York: Japan Publications, Inc., 1978.

——. *Lessons of Night and Day*. Wayne, N. J.: Avery Publishing Group, 1985.

——. *Macrobiotic Food and Cooking Series: Arthritis; Stress and Hypertension*. Tokyo & New York: Japan Publications, Inc., 1988.

——. *Macrobiotic Food and Cooking Series: Diabetes and Hypoglycemia; Allergies*. Tokyo & New York: Japan Publications, Inc., 1985.

——. *Macrobiotic Food and Cooking Series: Obesity, Weight Loss and Eating Disorder; Infertility and Reproductive Disorders*. Tokyo & New York: Japan Publications, Inc., 1987.

Kushi, Aveline, with Alex Jack. *Aveline Kushi's Complete Guide to Macrobiotic Cooking*. New York: Warner Books, 1985.

——. *Aveline: The Life and Dream of the Woman Behind Macrobiotics Today*. Tokyo & New York: Japan Publications, Inc., 1988.

Kushi, Aveline and Michio. *Macrobiotic Pregnancy and Care of the Newborn*. Edited by Edward and Wendy Esko. Tokyo & New York: Japan Publications, Inc., 1984.

——. *Macrobiotic Child Care and Family Health*. Tokyo & New York: Japan Publications, Inc., 1986.

Kushi, Aveline, and Tom Monte. *Thirty Days: A Program to Lower Cholesterol, Achieve Optimal Weight, and Prevent Serious Disease*. Tokyo & New York: Japan Publications, Inc., 1991.

Kushi, Aveline, and Wendy Esko. *Macrobiotic Family Favorites*. Tokyo & New York: Japan Publications, Inc., 1987.

——. *The Changing Seasons Macrobiotic Cookbook*. Wayne, N. J.: Avery Publishing Group, 1983.

——. *The Macrobiotic Cancer Prevention Cookbook*. Wayne, N. J.: Avery Publishing Group, 1986.

——. *The Quick and Natural Macrobiotic Cookbook*. New York & Chicago: Contemporary Books, 1989.

Kushi Aveline, with Wendy Esko. *The Macrobiotic Cancer Prevention Cookbook*. Garden City Park, N.Y.: Avery Publishing Group, 1988.

Kushi, Michio. *The Book of Dō-In: Exercise for Physical and Spiritual Development*. Tokyo & New York: Japan Publications, Inc., 1979.

——. *The Book of Macrobiotics: The Universal Way of Health, Happiness and Peace*. Tokyo & New York: Japan Publications, Inc., 1986 (Rev. ed.).

——. *Cancer and Heart Disease: The Macrobiotic Approach to Degenerative Disorders*. Tokyo & New York: Japan Publications, Inc., 1986 (Rev. ed.).

——. *Crime and Diet: The Macrobiotic Approach*. Tokyo & New York: Japan Publications, Inc., 1987.

——. *The Era of Humanity*. Brookline, Mass.: East West Journal, 1980.

——. *How to See Your Health: The Book of Oriental Diagnosis*. Tokyo & New York:

Japan Publications, Inc., 1980.

——. *Macrobiotic Health Education Series: Arthritis.* Tokyo & New York: Japan Publications, Inc., 1988.

——. *Macrobiotic Health Education Series: Diabetes and Hypoglycemia; Allergies.* Tokyo & New York: Japan Publications, Inc., 1985.

——. *Macrobiotic Health Education Series: Obesity, Weight Loss and Eating Disorder; Infertility and Reproductive Disorders.* Tokyo & New York: Japan Publications, Inc., 1987.

——. *Natural Healing through Macrobiotics.* Tokyo & New York: Japan Publications, Inc., 1978.

——. *On the Greater View: Collected Thoughts on Macrobiotics and Humanity.* Wayne, N. J.: Avery Publishing Group, 1985.

——. *Your Face Never Lies.* Wayne, N. J.: Avery Publishing Group, 1983.

Kushi, Michio, and Alex Jack. *The Cancer-Prevention Diet.* New York: St. Martin's Press, 1983.

——. *Diet for a Strong Heart.* New York: St. Martin's Press, 1984.

Kushi, Michio, and Phillip Jannetta. *Macrobiotics and Oriental Medicine: An Introduction to Holistic Health.* Tokyo & New York: Japan Publications, Inc., 1991.

Kushi, Michio, with Alex Jack. *One Peaceful World.* New York: St. Martin's Press, 1987.

Kushi, Michio, and Associates. *Doctors Look at Macrotiotics.* Edited by Edward Esko. Tokyo & New York: Japan Publications, Inc., 1988.

Kushi, Michio and Aveline, with Alex Jack. *Food Governs Your Destiny: The Teachings of Namboku Mizuno.* Tokyo & New York: Japan Publications, Inc., 1991.

——. *Macrobiotic Diet.* Tokyo & New York: Japan Publications, Inc.; 1985.

Kushi, Michio, and Martha C. Cottrell with Mark N. Mead. *AIDS, Macrobiotics, and Natural Immunity.* Tokyo & New York: Japan Publications, Inc., 1990.

Kushi, Michio, and the East West Foundation. *The Macrobiotic Approach to Cancer.* Wayne, N. J.: Avery Publishing Group, 1982.

Kushi, Michio, with Olivia Oredson. *Macrobiotic Palm Healing: Energy at Your Finger-Tips.* Tokyo & New York: Japan Publications, Inc., 1988.

Kushi, Michio, with Stephen Blauer. *The Macrobiotic Way.* Wayne, N.J.: Avery Publishing Group, 1985.

Lad, Vasant. *Ayurveda: The Science of Self-healing.* Santa Fe, N. Mex.: Lotus Press, 1984.

Levin, Cecile Tovah. *Cooking for Regeneration: Macrobiotic Relief from Cancer, AIDS, and Degenerative Disease.* Tokyo & New York: Japan Publications, Inc., 1988.

Mendelsohn, Robert S., M.D. *Confessions of a Medical Heretic.* Chicago: Contemporary Books, 1979.

——. *Male Practice.* Chicago: Contemporary Books, 1980.

Mishra, Satyenda P. *Yoga and Ayurveda.* (Sanskrit edition) Varanasi, India: Chaukhambha Orientalia, 1989.

Nussbaum, Elaine. *Recovery: From Cancer to Health through Macrobiotics.* Tokyo & New York: Japan Publications, Inc., 1986.

Nutrition and Mental Health. Washington, D. C.: Select Committee on Nutrition and Human Needs, U.S. Senate, 1977, 1980.

Ohsawa, George, *Cancer and the Philosophy of the Far East.* Oroville, Calif.: George Ohsawa Macrobiotic Foundation, 1971 edition.

——. *You Are All Sanpaku.* Edited by William Dufty, New York: University Books, 1965.

——. *Zen Macrobiotics.* Los Angeles: Ohsawa Foundation, 1965.

Ohsawa, Lima. *Macrobiotic Cuisine.* Tokyo & New York: Japan Publications, Inc., 1984.

Polatin, Betsy. *Macrobiotics in Motion: Yin and Yang in Moving Spirals*. Tokyo & New York: Japan Publications, Inc., 1987.

Price, Western, A., D.D.S. *Nutrition and Physical Degeneration*. Santa Monica, Calif.: Price-Pottenger Nutritional Foundation, 1945.

Sattilaro, Anthony, M.D., with Tom Monte. *Recalled by Life: The Story of My Recovery from Cancer*. Boston: Houghton-Mifflin, 1982.

Sawami Saraswati, Dayananda. *Japa Meditation*. Saylorsburg, Pa.: Aresha Vidya Pitham, 1989.

Schauss, Alexander. *Diet, Crime, and Delinquency*. Berkeley, Calif.: Parker House, 1980.

Scott, Neil E., with Jean Farmer. *Eating with Angels*. Tokyo & New York: Japan Publications, Inc., 1986.

Sergel, David. *The Macrobiotic Way of Zen Shiatsu*. Tokyo & New York: Japan Publications, Inc., 1989.

Tara, William. *Macrobiotics and Human Behavior*. Tokyo & New York: Japan Publications, Inc., 1985.

Vagabhata. *Astanga Hrdaya Samhita*. (Sanskrit edition) Vol. 1. Varanasi, India: Chauhambha Orientalia, 1948.

Wood, Rebecca. *Quinoa the Supergrain: Ancient Food for Today*. Tokyo & New York: Japan Publications, Inc., 1988.

Yamamoto, Shizuko. *Barefoot Shiatsu*. Tokyo & New York: Japan Publications, Inc., 1979.

The Yellow Emperor's Classic of Internal Medicine. Translated by Ilza Veith, Berkeley: University of California Press, 1949.

Index